D1527112

Borna Disease Virus
and Its Role in Neurobehavioral Disease

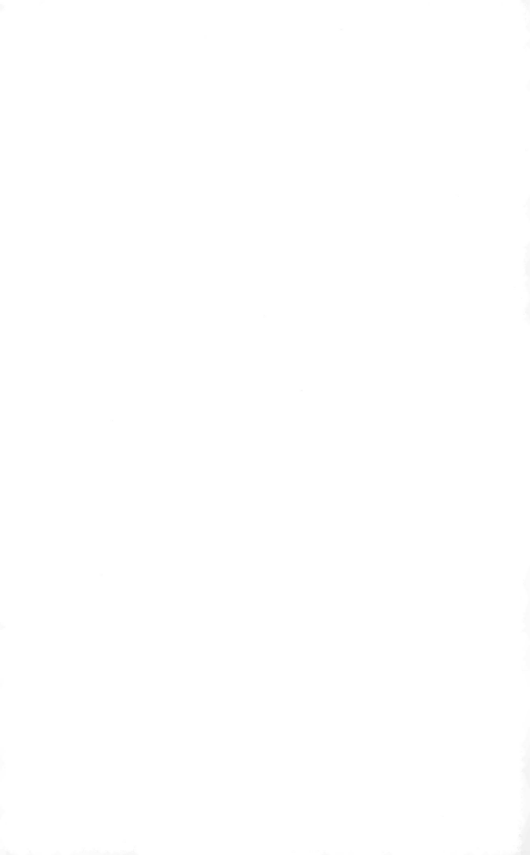

Borna Disease Virus
and Its Role in Neurobehavioral Disease

EDITED BY Kathryn M. Carbone

Office of the Director
Center for Biologics Evaluation and Research
Food and Drug Administration
Bethesda, Maryland

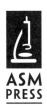

WITHDRAWN

WASHINGTON, D.C.

Address editorial correspondence to ASM Press, 1752 N St. NW, Washington, DC 20036-2904, USA

Send orders to ASM Press, P.O. Box 605, Herndon, VA 20172, USA
Phone: (800) 546-2416 or (703) 661-1593
Fax: (703) 661-1501
E-mail: books@asmusa.org
Online: www.asmpress.org

Library of Congress Cataloging-in-Publication Data

Borna disease virus and its role in neurobehavioral disease / edited by
Kathryn M. Carbone.
      p. ; cm.
Includes bibliographical references and index.
    ISBN 1-55581-235-X (hardcover)
    1. Borna disease. 2. Borna disease virus. 3. Neurobehavioral
disorders—Etiology. 4. Central nervous system—Infections.
    [DNLM: 1. Borna Disease—virology. 2. Borna disease
virus—pathogenicity. 3. Central Nervous System Viral
Diseases—physiopathology. SF 959.E5 B736 2002] I. Carbone, Kathryn M.

QR201.B66 B67 2002
616.89'0194—dc21

                                                              2002009541

10 9 8 7 6 5 4 3 2 1

Cover photos: (Top) A representative autoradiogram of specific binding of serotonin reuptake sites to [^{125}I]RTI-55 in a Borna disease virus-infected rat. Reprinted from M. V. Pletnikov, S. A. Rubin, M. W. Vogel, T. H. Moran, and K. M. Carbone, *Brain Res.* **944**:108–123, 2002, with permission of Elsevier Science. (Bottom) A sagittal section of the dentate gyrus of the hippocampus in a Borna disease virus-infected rat. Double staining with anti-glial fibrillary acidic protein (GFAP) antibody (green) and anti-serotonin 1a receptor antibody (red) was done. Courtesy of Mikhail V. Pletnikov.

To Rudolf Rott, on behalf of all BDV scientists, in appreciation of his foresight, devotion, and many contributions to modern BDV research, and
to my greatest mentor and supporter, my father, Paul P. Carbone (1931–2002), Lasker Award recipient, clinical researcher, and talented clinical oncologist, who provided the foundation for scientific careers for myself and many young researchers; from him I learned always to take the most interesting path, not the path of least resistance

Contents

Contributors

Karl A. Bechter • Department of Psychosomatics/Psychotherapy and Department of Psychiatry II, University of Ulm, Ludwig-Heilmeyer-Strasse 2, 89312 Günzburg, Germany

Kathryn M. Carbone • Office of the Director, Center for Biologics Evaluation and Research, U.S. Food and Drug Administration, HFM 20, 8800 Wisconsin Ave., Bethesda, MD 20892

Juan Carlos de la Torre • Department of Neuropharmacology, Division of Virology, IMM-6, The Scripps Research Institute, 10550 N. Torrey Pines Rd., La Jolla, CA 92037

Daniel Gonzalez-Dunia • Unité des virus lents, CNRS URA 1930, Institut Pasteur, 28 rue du Dr Roux, 75724 Paris Cedex, France

Katsuro Hagiwara • Department of Veterinary Microbiology, Faculty of Veterinary Medicine, Rakuno Gakuen University, Ebetsu, Hokkaido 069-8501, Japan

Kazuyoshi Ikuta • Department of Virology, Research Institute for Microbial Diseases, Osaka University, 3-1 Yamadaoka, Suita, Osaka 565-0871, Japan

Masahiko Kishi • Tsukuba Central Laboratories, Kyoritsu Seiyaku Corporation, Inashiki-gun, Ibaraki, Japan

Patrick Lai • Bioscience, Carlson Hall, Salem International University, Salem, WV 26426-0500

Tetsuya Mizutani • Laboratory of Public Health, Department of Environmental Veterinary Sciences, Graduate School of Veterinary Medicine, Hokkaido University, Kita-ku, Kita-18, Nishi-9, Sapporo 060-0818, Japan

Norbert Nowotny • Clinical Virology Group, Institute of Virology, University of Veterinary Sciences, Vienna, A-1210 Vienna, Austria, and Department of Medical Microbiology, Faculty of Medicine and Health Sciences, United Arab Emirates University, P.O. Box 17666, Al Ain, United Arab Emirates

Oliver Planz • Institute for Immunology, Federal Research Center for Virus Diseases of Animals, Paul-Ehrlich-Strasse 28, 72076 Tübingen, Germany

Mikhail V. Pletnikov • Department of Psychiatry and Behavioral Sciences, The Johns Hopkins University School of Medicine, Ross 618, 720 Rutland Ave., Baltimore, MD 21205

Christian Sauder • Department of Virology, Institute for Medical Microbiology and Hygiene, University of Freiburg, Hermann-Herder-Strasse 11, 79104 Freiburg, Germany

Martin Schwemmle • Institute of Medical Virology, University of Zürich, Gloriastrasse 30, 8028 Zürich, Switzerland

Lothar Stitz • Institut für Immunologie, Bundesforschungsanstalt für Viruskrankheiten der Tiere, Paul-Ehrlich-Strasse 28, 72076 Tübingen, Germany

Hiroyuki Taniyama • Department of Pathology, Faculty of Veterinary Medicine, Rakuno Gakuen University, Ebetsu, Hokkaido 069-8501, Japan

Keizo Tomonaga • Department of Virology, Research Institute for Microbial Diseases, Osaka University, 3-1 Yamadaoka, Suita, Osaka 565-0871, Japan

Kazunari Yamaguchi • Blood Transfusion Service and Internal Medicine, Kumamoto University School of Medicine, Honjo 1-1-1, Kumamoto 860-8556, Japan

Foreword

This book represents a singular event for all virologists, especially those interested in neuropathogenesis and virus-related neuropsychiatric disorders. The virus du jour is Borna disease virus (BDV), which is the etiological agent of Borna disease (BD). BD is a fatal neurological disease of horses that has been known for over 100 years and is now emerging as a disease in cats, dogs, certain birds, and possibly all warm-blooded animals, including humans. However, due to the difficulty of isolation and detection of BDV, there remains controversy about possible links between BDV and human neuropsychiatric disorders.

Kathryn Carbone and her colleagues have put together a definitive tome that examines real criteria for establishing a BDV infection and the pitfalls of overinterpreting highly sensitive assays. Twenty-five years ago, I was intently researching the assembly of murine and avian retroviruses, focusing on retroviral proteases. At the time, there was suggestive evidence that a human retrovirus might also exist; after several false starts, human T-cell leukemia virus type 1 was isolated and characterized as the etiological agent of adult T-cell leukemia and, later, tropical spastic paraparesis. About 10 years later, these findings and culture methods laid the groundwork for the classical isolation of human immunodeficiency virus type 1 as the etiological agent of AIDS. In some ways, links between BDV in horses and rats are awaiting a similar fate for a direct link to neuropsychiatric diseases in humans. As of now, there is a smoking gun but no definitive association. However, as with the retroviruses, it may only be a matter of time before an association is firmly established.

In closing, I thank Kathryn Carbone, as well as Jeff Holtmeier of ASM Press, for asking me to write a foreword for this important text in a new and emerging area of virology. I hope that the authors, by bringing BDV into the limelight, will spur greater activity in the field of viral neuropathogenesis.

Ronald Luftig

Preface

In the field of Borna disease virus (BDV) research, where each experiment reveals a new mystery more often than an answer, where the subject repeatedly refuses to play by the rules of traditional virology, where revelations of scientific interest in BDV often lead to responses of "What virus?" and where grant funding opportunities are difficult to realize, it is amazing and gratifying to see that worldwide interest in BDV has increased exponentially over the past 20 years. Despite the unique challenges of BDV research, or perhaps because of them, those in the field have always seen tremendous potential benefits from studying this agent. I acknowledge, first and foremost in the BDV field, Rudolf Rott of the Institute for Virology, University of Giessen, Giessen, Germany, who is considered the founder of modern BDV research. Virtually all BDV investigators trace the beginning of their experiences in BDV research to Rudolf Rott or to someone trained by him (see chapter 1).

Despite the increasing international interest in BDV research, the field is still young and controversial. I have tried to bring together BDV scientists whose stars are rising or have already risen to craft an encyclopedia of modern BDV research. Each chapter author was asked to present an overview of the data in the assigned area, to provide a critique of these data with a discussion of the controversies therein (and there are many), and, perhaps most importantly, to suggest the direction in which the future of BDV research should go. In a field where conflicting, unresolved issues tend to polarize, these accomplished BDV researchers have worked hard to provide a balanced view of up-to-date BDV knowledge for other scientists, clinicians, and the public, and I thank them for their selfless efforts and quality performance. It is also important to emphasize that the support and guidance of leaders in the American Society of Microbiology, such as Ronald Luftig, and the ASM Press staff, especially the director, Jeff Holtmeier, were the final common denominators in realizing the efforts of all the BDV scientists who worked diligently on this book.

From 1985 and my baptism in BDV research in Opendra Narayan's laboratory at Johns Hopkins University, the first laboratory in the United States to take up BDV study, to my role in 2002 as editor of an exciting and up-to-date summary of modern BDV research, I remain enthusiastic about past discoveries and those we have yet to make in the BDV field. Working in an area considered obscure by some and groundbreaking by others, I am constantly reminded of a delightful letter to the editor of *The Lancet* by

J. Morris ("Originality: who is to judge?" [*Lancet* **342**:930, 1993]): "If the work receives acclaim then it means that it is part of the conventional wisdom, and is not original. If rejected it might be original; if dismissed out of hand, it probably is." Having worked in the field for almost 2 decades, I have seen all three outcomes in response to BDV discoveries, yet, by these criteria, I hope never to see new BDV research accepted without controversy. I am sure that BDV research will continue to surprise, frustrate, and delight scientists for decades to come.

Kathryn M. Carbone

Borna Disease Virus and Its Role in Neurobehavioral Disease
Edited by K. M. Carbone
© 2002 ASM Press, Washington, D.C.

Chapter 1

Borna Disease Virus: Spanning a Century of Science

Keizo Tomonaga and Kathryn M. Carbone

In 1885, a large number of horses of a German cavalry regiment died of a fatal neurological disease in the town of Borna in Saxony, southeastern Germany. The diseased horses exhibited abnormal behaviors, e.g., running about excitedly, walking into walls, being unable to chew food, and standing with heads and necks strained forward and down. Many of the afflicted animals died. This disease had been noted, but rarely, in horses and sheep for over a hundred years in the areas of endemicity, southern Germany and Switzerland. Veterinary handbooks published in Germany at the end of the 18th century described this disease, believed due to "sexual frustration and overeating," calling this disease *hitzige Kopfkrankheit* (acute head disease) or *Kopfkrankheit der Pferde* (head disease of horses). Later, this disease was called *Bornasche Krankheit* (Borna disease [BD]), for the small town where the 1885 outbreak took place.

BD in horses and sheep is the result of a progressive, mononuclear cell encephalomyelitis. Horses and sheep are believed to be the major natural hosts of BD, and those with BD show neurologic signs such as ataxia, depression, circular movement, standing in awkward positions, collapse, running into obstacles, and paralysis. Clinical illness usually lasts 1 to 3 weeks, and death rates for horses are 80 to 100% (Becht and Richt, 1996; Rott and Becht, 1995).

In the early 20th century, German scientists developed a great base of scientific literature regarding BD and demonstrated that the brain from dis-

Keizo Tomonaga • Department of Virology, Research Institute for Microbial Diseases, Osaka University, 3-1 Yamadaoka, Suita, Osaka 565-0871, Japan. **Kathryn M. Carbone** • Office of the Director, Center for Biologics Evaluation and Research, U.S. Food and Drug Administration, HFM 20, 8800 Wisconsin Ave., Bethesda, MD 20892.

1

eased horses contained the transmissible etiological agent of BD (Zwick, 1939; Zwick and Seifried, 1925). The BD virus (BDV) could experimentally infect many vertebrates from rabbits to monkeys to chickens and caused neurological symptoms (Zwick, 1939; Zwick and Seifried, 1925; Zwick et al., 1927). Furthermore, more-recent epidemiological data demonstrate that natural infection with BDV also exists in cats, cattle, dogs, donkeys, goats, and ostriches, indicating that host range of this virus is likely to include all warm-blooded animals (Ludwig and Bode, 2000; Rott and Becht, 1995; Staeheli et al., 2000). Asymptomatic natural infection in various animal species has also been reported worldwide, but neither a reservoir nor clear mode of transmission of natural infection has been confirmed.

Recent molecular biological analysis demonstrated that BDV is a non-segmented, negative-sense, single-strand (NNS) RNA virus that belongs to the *Mononegavirales* (Briese et al., 1994; Cubitt et al., 1994). BDV is highly neurotropic and typically has a noncytolytic strategy for replication in cells. Despite the similarity in genome organization to other members of this order such as *Rhabdoviridae*, *Paramyxoviridae*, and *Filoviridae*, BDV replicates and transcribes in the nucleus of infected cells, while other animal viruses of this order undergo their life cycle in the cell cytoplasm (de la Torre et al., 1990; Carbone et al., 1991). Based on its unique features, BDV has been classified into a new family: *Bornaviridae*.

Although the number of animals diagnosed with BD has decreased in the areas of endemicity in recent years (Caplazi et al., 1999; Herzog et al., 1994; Staeheli et al., 2000), since the late 1970s, research interest in BDV has rapidly increased. It was proposed that expression of BD, which in animals is identified by specific neurological and emotional disturbances, might be expressed as various forms of psychiatric disease in humans. Thus, researchers became interested in the possible existence of a specific psychiatric disorder-related virus in human brain, and a new cadre of researchers began studying BDV. The broad host range of BDV, originally identified as a virus of animal origin, also enhanced the interest of the possibility of a zoonotic infection in humans.

In 1985, a hundred years after the equine epidemic in Borna, Germany, the first reports were published of BDV-specific antibodies detected in patients with psychiatric disorders from Germany and the United States (Amsterdam et al., 1985; Rott et al., 1985). Subsequently, a higher prevalence of evidence of BDV infection has been reported in neuropsychiatric patients than in controls in several countries outside the areas of endemicity (as reviewed elsewhere [Jordan and Lipkin, 2001; Richt and Rott, 2001]). Isolation of human BDV from the peripheral blood or brain of neuropsychiatric patients from Germany (Bode et al., 1996; Planz et al., 1999), the United States (de la Torre et al., 1996), and Japan (Nakamura et al.,

2000) has also been described. These and other recent studies strongly suggested that BDV is a human pathogen and raised the question of a possible link between BDV and certain human mental disorders. However, other scientists believe there is a substantial risk of artifactual results (e.g., contamination of human samples by laboratory BDV strains), making the establishment of any relationship between human BDV and psychiatric disorders highly controversial (Schwemmle et al., 1999).

The study of BD and BDV has broad impact on diverse areas of biology and medicine, notably on molecular genetics of RNA virus, neurobiology, biological psychiatry, and public health. Although our knowledge regarding BD and BDV has progressed remarkably in the past 2 decades, we still have some fundamental questions that need to be resolved in the future. In this chapter, we briefly summarize the history of BD and BDV research in the past century and showcase the direction of BDV science as we enter a new century.

BRIEF HISTORY OF BORNA DISEASE RESEARCH IN THE EARLY 20TH CENTURY

Around the turn of the 20th century, studies concerning the neuropathology and etiology of BD became a primary interest for veterinary public health in Germany, because of the severe outbreaks that occurred in an area around the city of Borna. The disease was diagnosed not only in farm animals but also in military horses. The histopathological picture of spontaneous BD in horses was described in detail by Joest and Degen (1911), who discovered small acidophilic inclusion bodies in the nuclei of neurons of the diseased horses, named Joest-Degen bodies. Schmidt's (1912) investigations of more than 500 cases presenting the classical clinical symptomatology and progression of the disease in horses demonstrated that the nature of BD is a mononuclear cell encephalomyelitis with a predilection for gray matter of the cerebral hemispheres and brain stem and that the inflammatory response is commonly found in the form of perivascular cuffs around venules. In the 1920s and 1930s, the virus etiology of BD was proven by Zwick and coworkers by successful transmission to laboratory animals using brain homogenates from infected horses. The clinical course, histopathology, and virological aspects of the agent were studied in rabbits, chickens, rhesus monkeys, and guinea pigs (Zwick, 1939; Zwick and Seifried, 1925; Zwick et al., 1927). Some biochemical data on the BD agent were reported by Nicolau and Galloway (1928). In addition, the size of the agent was also estimated by filtration experiments (Elford and Galloway, 1933). Another milestone in BD research in the early 20th century was the detection in 1955 of virus-specific antigens and antibodies by immunological techniques by von Sprockhoff and Nitzschke, who demonstrated that BDV produces a soluble antigen (s-antigen) now known as the BDV nucleoprotein (N) (40 or 38 kDa) and phosphoprotein (P) (24 kDa) (von Sprockhoff and Nitzschke, 1955). von Sprockhoff also identified anti-BDV antibodies in sera from diseased and asymptomatic BDV-infected guinea pigs. These primary studies have provided a substantial foundation for subsequent BDV research, taking advantage of the cell culture, immunological, and molecular biological techniques that were developed in the late 20th century.

BDV RESEARCH: SPREAD FROM CENTRAL EUROPE TO THE REST OF THE WORLD

To date, more than 500 papers have been published in the field of BDV research. Until 1980, almost all papers in the field were from scientists in countries where BD is endemic, including Germany and Switzerland. Publications from regions of nonendemicity, including Europe, North America, and Asia, however, represented about 75% of BDV-related papers published in 1999 and 2000 (Fig. 1). Here we outline the spread of BDV research from central Europe throughout the world over the past 2 decades.

Europe

Without a doubt, German scientists initiated the first European BDV research. In the 1980s, BDV research was concentrated in independent groups in Giessen and Berlin, Germany. These scientists extended the primary knowledge of the biological and pathogenic aspects of BDV using persistently BDV-infected cell cultures and experimental animal models such as rats and rabbits. During this period, German scientists were also able to demonstrate antibodies specific for BDV antigens in humans and vigorously surveyed the seroprevalence in humans, not in the areas of endemicity and in other areas of Germany (Bode, 1995). In addition, a Zurich group in Switzerland demonstrated BDV infection in sheep during the same period (Waelchi et al., 1985).

With the exception of Nicolau and Galloway (1928), working in France and England in the 1930s, who reported on the viral nature and the etiology of BD and provided valuable information on BD pathogenesis through experimental infection of small animals, the publications from the original countries without endemic BD have been limited until very re-

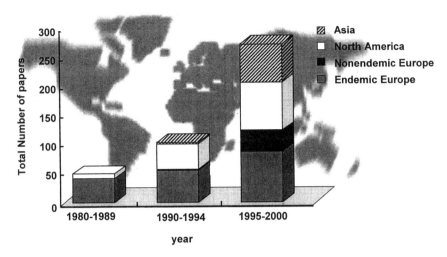

Figure 1. Spread of BDV research throughout the world. Total numbers of publications concerning BDV from European regions of endemicity (Germany and Switzerland), European regions of nonendemicity, North America, and Asia between 1980 and 2000 as indicated by the PubMed search program at the National Library of Medicine website are shown. Papers containing authors in different areas were counted in each area.

cently. BD research in the European countries of nonendemicity began in the early 1990s with surveillance of BDV infection in domestic animals, with the first report from Sweden in 1993 demonstrating that cats with neurological signs of staggering disease and typical neuropathology had a high prevalence of BDV-specific antibodies (Lundgren and Ludwig, 1993). Subsequently, antibodies to BDV were demonstrated in cats from Austria, Switzerland, and the United Kingdom (Bornand et al., 1998; Nowothy and Weissenböck, 1995; Reeves et al., 1998). Swedish scientists suggested that BDV infection in cats might lead to various disease patterns depending on differences in viral pathogenicity (Berg and Berg, 1998). In addition to feline BDV, BDV infection was reported in dogs with neurological symptoms in Austria, Sweden, and south Germany (Ludwig and Bode, 2000; Weissenböck et al., 1998a). BDV infection in horses has been also demonstrated in the European countries where the virus is not endemic, including Austria, Sweden, France, The Netherlands, Poland, Russia, Luxembourg, and Liechtenstein (Caplazi et al., 1999; Herzog et al., 1994; Rott and Becht, 1995) (see also chapter 4).

    Since the original report in 1985, evidence of BDV infection in patients with various neurological disorders has been reported in many European countries (see chapter 6). In 1999, the seroprevalence of BDV in Swiss patients with neurological disorders with or without human immunodeficiency virus infection was reported. Two groups have demonstrated negative and positive evidence of BDV infection in chronic fatigue syndrome (CFS) patients from Sweden and Austria, respectively. Furthermore, the Dutch and Danish groups have investigated BDV infection in schizophrenic patients in Surinamese immigrants and fibromyalgia patients, respectively, claiming no relationship between BDV infection and these disorders in those countries.

Reports concerning molecular and cellular biology of BDV have also gradually increased in European countries. The groups in Sweden and France have published data on the interaction between BDV-specific antigens and mitogen-activated kinase activation in persistently BDV-infected neuronal cells (see chapter 2).

North America

In the early 1980s a U.S.-German collaboration between Rudolf Rott of the University of Giessen and Jay Amsterdam and Hilary Koprowski at the University of Pennsylvania demonstrated evidence of BDV seropositivity (by indirect immunofluorescence assay [IFA]) in humans with neurological disease, a finding that has sparked the worldwide search for evidence of BDV human infection for the past 2 decades (Amsterdam et al., 1985; Rott et al., 1985; reviewed in Carbone, 2001). More modern tests for BDV infection were subsequently developed in the United States, including Western blotting (Fu et al., 1993; Waltrip et al., 1995; Waltrip et al., 1997), enzyme-linked immunosorbent assay (ELISA) (Briese et al., 1995), and reverse transcription (RT)-PCR (Sierra-Honigmann et al., 1993; de la Torre et al., 1996) and used to test human samples for evidence of BDV.

Also in the early 1980s, Rott collaborated with Opendra Narayan of Johns Hopkins University to establish the rat model of BDV infection (Narayan et al., 1983a, 1983b). The second generation of U.S. scientists who took up the study of BDV pathogenesis continued to advance the understanding of important host responses to BDV using animal models (Carbone et al., 1987; Carbone et al., 1991a, 1991b; reviewed by Pletnikov et al., 2001), leading to exciting discoveries of BDV immunology and neurobehavioral, neuroanatomical, and neurochemical abnormalities associated with BDV-induced damage to the mature and developing nervous system (see chapter 5).

The BDV research effort worldwide has been substantially supported by the initial technical advancements that occurred in BDV research in the United States during the 1980s and 1990s. For example, molecular biological research initiated in the United States led to the discovery of the first

BDV-specific cDNA clones (Lipkin et al., 1990; VandeWoude et al., 1990). Until this discovery, researchers working in the field were uncertain as to whether BDV was a DNA or an RNA virus or, even, possibly a novel non-virus agent. The availability of BDV-specific cDNA clones permitted the surprising discovery that BDV was the only negative-sense, single-strand RNA animal virus to replicate in the cell nucleus, first discovered by in situ hybridization using single-strand RNA probes (Carbone et al., 1991a) and confirmed by further molecular biology characterization (Briese et al., 1992; Cubitt et al., 1994). The first BDV-specific nested RT-PCR permitted the detection of BDV RNA from peripheral blood mononuclear cells (PBMCs) in persistently infected rats, clearly documenting the previously unsuspected infection of cells of the hematogenous system (Sierra-Honigmann et al., 1993). This animal model work provided the basis for future efforts at BDV recovery from humans, since, for the first time, autopsy specimens (e.g., brain) were not required for BDV isolation attempts. Rather, samples easily obtained from patients (e.g., blood) were realized to be viable sources for BDV isolation.

The molecular biology talents of two independent groups in the United States resulted in elucidation of the first full-length genomic sequence of BDV (Briese et al., 1994; Cubitt et al., 1994). These and other groups have gone on to contribute substantially to the understanding of the molecular biology of this unique agent (see chapter 2).

Asia

The research interest in BDV moved to include Asia in the middle of the 1980s, with specific interests in virus infection and human neuropsychiatric diseases. In 1988, the first cases of Borna-like disease in Asia Minor were reported to have occurred in young ostriches in Israel that died of a BD-like syndrome between 1989 and 1992 on farms (Malkinson et al., 1993). Natural infection with BDV has not been proven in any other species of bird in Asia. BDV epidemiology research in domestic animals in Asia has also been initiated. Until recently, BDV infection in animals had been found only in a few countries in Asia, including Japan, Israel, Iran, China, and Bangladesh (see chapter 4). In the early 1990s, a group in Japan began to investigate BDV infection in domestic animals in Hokkaido, the land most prominently used for livestock in Japan. Kazuyoshi Ikuta demonstrated a high prevalence of subclinical BDV infection in several healthy-appearing animals, including horses, cattle, and sheep (Ikuta, 1997). Nakamura et al. (1996) also reported evidence of BDV infection in domestic cats in Japan and detected BDV RNAs in the brains of cats with neurological disorders. BDV infection in wild horses was also demonstrated in Kyushu Island, Japan, in 1999 (Yamaguchi et al., 1999). Very recently, Hiroyuki Taniyama at Rakuno Gakuen University in Hokkaido clearly identified horses in Japan with the classical signs of BD (Taniyama et al., 2001). The group surveyed a great number of horses, which showed movement disorders (previously diagnosed as wobbler's syndrome) at farms in Hokkaido and diagnosed BD in the horses by serological, histological, and molecular techniques. They also detected the presence of BD-like syndromes in cattle and dogs in Japan (Okamoto et al., 2002a; Okamoto et al., 2002b). These studies suggested that BDV is more widely spread in Japan than previously thought.

A relationship between BDV and human psychiatric or neurological disorders in Asia was suggested first in a publication in 1991 of a collaborative study between Rudolf Rott in Germany and Kazuhiro Ikeda in Japan (Rott et al., 1991). To date, epidemiological studies of BDV infection in humans have been reported in several Asian countries, including Japan, South Korea, Thailand, Taiwan, and Bangladesh (see chapter 6). In 1995, Kishi et al. reported finding a high prevalence of BDV RNA in the PBMCs from Japanese psychiatric patients (Kishi et al., 1995). Later, BDV RNA and antibodies were also demonstrated in CFS patients as well as in healthy blood donors. Due to the controversy surrounding the validity of evidence of BDV infection in humans from the early studies in the 1990s, BDV research groups in Japan started a multicenter study of diagnostic techniques to detect BDV infection in humans in 1997 using PBMCs from blood donors. Six different laboratories independently tested the same samples with different methods that were developed in each laboratory, such as Western blotting, reverse-type sandwich ELISA, or electrochemiluminescence immunoassay. Although each group could detect BDV RNAs or antibodies in blood donors, positive samples did not necessarily correspond among the groups. Furthermore, positive results were also not necessarily reproduced in the same laboratory. This study suggested that, for technical reasons, acquisition of solid evidence for BDV infection is quite difficult, at least in samples from blood donors. On the other hand, some Japanese groups have apparently successfully demonstrated BDV RNAs in the PBMCs or brain samples from psychiatric patients (Haga et al., 1997; Iwata et al., 1998). Very recently, an isolation of BDV from an autopsy brain from a psychiatric patient has been demonstrated in a collaboration between groups in Japan and the United States (Nakamura et al., 2000).

Besides the epidemiological study of BDV infection in animals and humans in Asia, biological analysis of the virus has also originated from Japan, and the number of such publications has gradually increased since 1997. Japanese groups have contributed to the research field of BDV biology, such as information on transcription and nucleocytoplasmic export mechanisms of the virus, and also have developed a novel animal model of the infection using Mongolian gerbils (see chapters 2 and 5). Very recently, a Japanese group reported that the BDV phosphoprotein (P) binds a neurite outgrowth factor in host cells, demonstrating a possible mechanism for the BDV-induced damage to developing central nervous systems (CNSs) (Kamitani et al., 2001).

MAJOR CONTRIBUTIONS TO UNDERSTANDING THE NEUROPATHOGENICITY OF BDV BETWEEN 1980 AND 2001

Virology

Successful cultivation and titration of BDV in cell culture at the end of 1970s was a watershed event for scientists' ability to analyze the biological properties of the virus. The unique biological features of BDV such as noncytopathic replication, low-level production of infectious virus, and viral persistence in infected cells were demonstrated by the early experiments in this period. Herzog and Rott (1980) and Pauli and Ludwig (1985) were able to show specific biochemical properties, as well as the virion size and replication cycle, of the agent of BD. The persistently BDV-infected cell lines generated by cocultivation of infected animal brains with cultured cells greatly aided further characterization of BDV biology in the 1980s and 1990s. The establishment of sensitive immunoassays using infected culture cells also contributed to the characterization of virus-specific antibodies. These assays were relevant for the diagnostic investigations and the characterization of viral antigens (Pauli et al., 1984; Rott et al., 1985; Schädler et al., 1985). An animal model using rats was also widely applied for understanding BDV biology. Using the rat model, Narayan et al. (1983a, 1983b), Hirano et al. (1983), Herzog et al. (1984), and Carbone et al. (1987) demonstrated that the agent is highly neurotropic, causes immunopathogenic disease, and spreads intra-axonally (see chapter 5).

Along with the remarkable progress in understanding the biological nature of BDV in the 1980s, application of molecular genetic approaches laid significant new groundwork in the field (see chapter 2). The isolation and characterization of BDV cDNA clones were first demonstrated in 1990 (Lipkin et al., 1990; VandeWoude et al., 1990). The BDV-specific cDNA clones clearly identified viral transcripts in infected animal brains and cultured cells by hybridization techniques, demonstrating that the BDV genome is NNS RNA. About that time, the nucleus-dependent replication and RNA splicing of the viral transcripts were also determined (Briese et al., 1992; Carbone et al., 1991a; de la Torre et al., 1990; Schneider et al., 1994). In 1993, the first identification of BDV sequences by RT-PCR techniques occurred (Sierra-Honigmann et al., 1993). In 1994, two independent groups, Briese et al. and Cubitt et al. were the first to determine the full-length sequences and the genome organization of two different strains of BDV derived from horses (Briese et al., 1994; Cubitt et al., 1994). Another contribution in BDV virology in the past decade was the identification and characterization of the virus-encoded proteins. At present, at least six different proteins have been identified in BDV-infected cells. The studies concerning translation, processing, interaction, intercellular localization, and nucleocytoplasmic transport of these proteins strongly advanced our understanding not only of the biological nature of this unique NNS RNA virus but also of the neuropathogenesis of BDV. BDV virology is described in more detail in chapter 2.

Epidemiology: Diagnosis and BDV Infection in Animals

Diagnosis of BDV infection in animals is now evaluated by several alternative methods using serological and molecular techniques. The demonstration of BDV-specific antibodies in serum and/or cerebrospinal fluid has been widely used by researchers in this field since the first attempts in the late 1970s. IFA using persistently BDV-infected cell lines is still a valuable method. ELISA and Western blotting developed in the early 1990s, using natural purified or recombinant viral proteins, are frequently employed (see chapter 3). To detect virus-specific antigens in infected samples, antigen capture ELISA or fluorescence-activated cell sorting techniques have been reported. Nucleic acid amplification using the nested RT-PCR method has become another powerful tool made possible by the information on BDV genome published in the early 1990s.

Until very recently the evidence of endemic BDV infection in horses and sheep had been described only in Central Europe. The reason why BDV infection had heretofore not been identified outside these areas may be that BD is rare and outbreaks are usually sporadic, and therefore, diseased horses and other animals might have been misdiagnosed. The development of an array of diagnostic tools used in epidemiological studies in the 1990s and beyond has clearly revealed the presence of BDV infection in horses and sheep outside Europe. The first evidence of BDV infection in horses in the countries where the virus is not endemic was published from the United States in 1993 by Kao et al. (1993). Natural BDV infection in horses has now been reported in Austria, France, Sweden, The Netherlands, Japan, Israel, Iran, the People's Republic of China, and Australia

(Hagiwara et al., 2001; Herzog et al., 1994; Ikuta, 1997; Ludwig and Bode, 2000; Richt and Rott, 2001; Rott and Becht, 1995; Weissenböck et al., 1998b). Although only asymptomatic BDV-infected horses were initially identified in the areas of nonendemicity, Nowotny et al. (2000) and Taniyama et al. (2001) recently found classical BD in horses in Austria and Japan, respectively (see chapter 4).

Natural BDV infection has been observed in other animal species, including rabbits, cattle, goats, donkeys, and deer, in Central Europe since the early 20th century. Detailed investigations in the 1990s also revealed that natural BDV infection occurs in other species such as cats (Lundgren and Ludwig, 1993), dogs (Weissenböck et al., 1998a), lynxes (Degiorgis et al., 2000), foxes (Dauphin et al., 2001), and ostriches (Malkinson et al., 1993) and can occur worldwide. These epidemiological studies have clearly suggested that almost all warm-blooded animals are likely to be susceptible to BDV and BD is not likely to be limited to Central Europe. The details of epidemiology and BDV infection in natural hosts are described in chapter 4.

Animal Models

In vivo studies of experimentally BDV-infected animals such as rabbits, chickens, guinea pigs, and rhesus monkeys have been undertaken since the early 20th century. In addition, infection in the rat system was also first reported by Nitzschke (1963) and further developed by Narayan et al. (1983) and Hirano et al. (1983). In the past 2 decades, rats have taken a principal position in the experimental infection of BDV and have become the best-characterized animal model for BD.

The results of BDV infection in animals depend on strains within a species, immune status of the host and route of inoculation. In 1983, based on background information such as enhanced virulence of brain-passaged virus and immune tolerance in young animals, two independent laboratories, those of Narayan et al. and Hirano et al., were the first to develop an animal model of immunopathogenicity of BDV in Lewis and Wistar rats, respectively (Hirano et al., 1983; Narayan et al., 1983b). Those investigators demonstrated that newborn rats show a persistent, tolerant infection without signs of BD or encephalitis. In 1989, Dittrich et al. published an evaluation of intriguing behavioral abnormalities in infected neonatal rats presenting abnormal learning and hyperactivity (Dittrich et al., 1989). Carbone et al. (1991b) showed that the neonatal infection causes significant alternations in the development of the CNS, including site-specific lysis of neurons and developmental injury in the cerebellum and hippocampus due to BDV infection. This work has been further developed in this laboratory (Bautista et al., 1995; Pletnikov et al., 1999; Rubin et al., 1999), providing evidence of direct viral effects on cell and organism function in the absence of traditional immunopathological responses, and leading to the use of neonatal rats as a valuable animal model of developmental neurobehavioral diseases such as autism (Pletnikov et al., 1999). The mechanism of neuronal disturbances found in the infected newborn rats has not been conclusively determined. Recent experiments, however, produced some intriguing findings, such as abnormal expression of cytokines, neurotransmitters, and neurotropic factors (Hornig et al., 1999; Plata-Salaman et al., 1999; Sauder and de la Torre, 1999), as well as loss of neuroplasticity in the infected brains (Gonzalez-Dunia et al., 2000).

The immune-mediated neurological disorder in adult rats following BDV infection was demonstrated first by Narayan et al. (1983a). The experiments conducted in the 1980s demonstrated that adult rats show signs of disease such as hyperactivity and aggressiveness in the acute phase of infection and the clinical onset of disease is directly correlated with the appearance of inflammatory cells in the brain (Carbone et al., 1987; Narayan et al., 1983a), leaving the adult-infected rat as the most utilized animal model of classical BD. Studies using immunosuppressed rats revealed that BD is likely to be due to a virus-induced immunopathological reaction of the T cells (Stitz et al., 1989). In the 1990s, Planz et al. (1993) demonstrated that both neurons and astrocytes in BDV-infected rats express major histocompatibility complex class I and that lymphocytes from these rats lyse infected cells in a major histocompatibility complex class I-restricted manner. Furthermore, the role of $CD8^+$ T cells in the induction of atrophy in BDV-infected rat brain has been also determined (Bilzer and Stitz, 1994). The association of cytokines with the neuropathogenesis of BDV in adult rats has been also published (Shankar et al., 1992). The distinct changes in neurotransmitters such as dopamine or serotonin in the CNS of BD-infected rats have been discussed in association with behavioral disorders (Solbrig et al., 1995, 1996).

In addition to rats, mice and Mongolian gerbils have been also used as experimental models of BDV infection. As in rats, the mouse model indicated that the incidence and severity of BDV-induced neurological disease varied dramatically among the strains tested and that severe clinical disease in susceptible mice was mediated by $CD8^+$ cytotoxic T cells (Hallensleben et al., 1998). BDV-infected newborn gerbils showed severe neurological disease without any neuroanatomical abnormalities or neuronal cell loss (Watanabe et al., 2001). Furthermore, animal models using monkeys, cats, and ponies have also appeared in the 1980s and 1990s. These animal models have provided new insights into the neuropathogenicity of BDV. See chapter 5 for details on animal models of BDV infection.

BDV Infection in Humans

BDV infection in humans is the most controversial issue in the research field of BDV. In the late 1970s, the broad experimental host range of BDV and the observation of the behavioral abnormalities in experimentally infected animals provided some clues that BDV might be implicated in the pathogenesis of human neuropsychiatric disease. The first reports of evidence of BDV infection in humans appeared in 1985. Amsterdam et al. (1985) and Rott et al. (1985) detected BDV-specific antibodies in human sera by IFA using persistently BDV-infected cells as the antigen. In these investigations, BDV-specific antibodies were found in some psychiatric patients, whereas such antibodies were not detected in healthy controls. In the 1990s, using various serological techniques, many studies were published that supported the original finding, suggesting that BDV infection in humans occurs worldwide and seems to be associated with certain mental diseases. In contrast, a number of studies have been published that do not support these findings and associations (see chapter 6). BDV-specific antibodies have also been detected in some neurological disorders, including CFS, multiple sclerosis, motor neuron disease, and panic disorders (reviewed by Jordan and Lipkin, 2001). However, the seroprevalence differed widely among the various laboratories, and the titers of reactive antibodies were usually very low. Recently, it has also been suggested that reactive human sera exhibit low avidity for BDV antigens, a finding that suggests a cross-reactive rather than specific antibody-antigen interaction (Allmang et al., 2001).

Following the finding of BDV RNA in infected rat PBMCs by a highly sensitive nested RT-PCR technique (Sierra-Honigmann et al., 1993), BDV researchers used a similar technique to detect BDV-specific RNA in PBMCs of several psychiatric patients and CFS patients (2 to 50%), as well as in control blood donors (0 to 5%). However, several groups have failed to confirm these results (Kim et al., 1999; K. Lieb et al., letter, Lancet **350**:1002, 1997), suggesting the possibility of contamination artifact, not uncommon in the exquisitely sensitive nested RT-PCR method.

BDV antigen and/or RNA have been also detected in human autopsy brain samples from patients with a history of mental disorders (de la Torre et al., 1996; Nakamura et al., 2000; Salvatore et al., 1997) and also from healthy controls (Haga et al., 1997). de la Torre et al. (1996) demonstrated BDV-specific antigen and RNA in three psychiatric patients by using immunohistochemistry, nested RT-PCR, and in situ hybridization. The presence of BDV-specific RNA in three of those autopsy brains was confirmed by an independent laboratory (Czygan et al., 1999). To date, there are several reports of isolation of an infectious BDV from human blood samples

(Bode et al., 1996, de la Torre et al., 1996; Planz et al., 1999) or brain tissue (Nakamura et al., 2000) of psychiatric patients. The validity of these findings was confirmed by isolation of infectious BDV from human tissues in two independent laboratories in Japan and the United States using two different techniques (Nakamura et al., 2000). However, some researchers have questioned the origin of "human" BDV isolates reported so far, because the genomes of these BDV isolates are virtually identical to those of strains of BDV frequently used in the various laboratories (Schwemmle et al., 1999). Although there is a consensus that humans are likely to be susceptible to BDV infection, the epidemiology and clinical consequences of human infection remain controversial. This issue will be thoroughly discussed in chapter 6.

BDV RESEARCH AS WE ENTER A NEW CENTURY

BDV research in its early and middle stages of development was a rather regional interest. The geographical restriction of known BDV infections made access to the field difficult for the scientists in countries where the virus is not endemic. This geographical isolation of BDV research was opened when Narayan, who first decided to import the virus for study into the United States, began the original BDV laboratory at Johns Hopkins University. During much of its 200-year history, BDV research was clearly of interest to veterinarians but had only a tenuous claim to relevance for human disease. This isolation from human medicine began to disappear with the novel work by Rott and Amsterdam, who demonstrated evidence of antibodies to BDV in psychiatric patients. Thus, the known neurological and emotional disturbances documented in BDV-infected animals began to stimulate hypotheses of virus-associated psychiatric disease in humans. In the past 2 decades, BDV research has had increasing impact on various research fields, not only the fields of biology of neurotropic RNA viruses and developmental neurobiology but also the field of neuropsychiatry.

Although we have achieved many BDV research milestones during the past century, some major issues with broad consequences for biology and medicine remain to be resolved. Despite numerous reports of BDV infection in humans, problems such as the lack of a universal, validated diagnostic test, the variability of the seroprevalence among different laboratories, and low levels of apparently low affinity of human anti-BDV antibody continue to stimulate controversy about the validity of claims of isolation of human BDV, raising fundamental questions of whether BDV infects humans and truly contributes to neuropsychiatric disorders. In order to begin to resolve these controversies, first, we need a valid and validated test for BDV diagnosis in humans and animals. Although the broad potential host range of BDV suggests that humans are targets for infection, the sources and routes of human infection are not clear, and transmission from domestic animals to humans has not been demonstrated. Furthermore, it is not known yet how much neurological disease is caused by BDV in animals outside the classical areas of endemicity. Once a test for BDV is developed, then detailed epidemiology and surveillance need to be done in domestic and wild animals in classical areas of endemicity and around the world.

Less controversial are the recent data of multiple mechanisms possibly linked to the neurological signs of BDV infection. The immune-mediated disruption of neuronal cells produces severe neurological disorders in horse, sheep, and adult-infected rat BD. The unique characteristics of this virus, such as persistent and noncytolytic infections, however, suggest that classical immune-mediated BD might be only one outcome of natural BDV infection. Experimental infections have clearly shown that BDV can cause behavioral and neuroanatomical disturbances without immune-mediated brain destruction. Moreover, BDV-infected animals with neurological symptoms but without encephalitis or brain inflammation have now been demonstrated in the field (Berg and Berg, 1998; Taniyama, 2001).

The direct effects and mechanisms of BDV infection on brain dysfunction, in the absence of immunopathological brain injury, need to be determined for a better understanding of BD pathogenesis but also for a better understanding of the links between BDV, human infection, and noninflammatory neuropsychiatric disease. Further studies using immunoincompetent models such as neonatal or prenatal infection, including vertical transmission of this virus, are needed. These models can be used to search for host brain factors, such as cytokines, chemokines, neurotrophins, and neurotransmitters, that are altered by BDV infection and would help provide us with molecular mechanisms of the neuropathological damage in infected animals.

A more thorough understanding of the biological properties of BDV is also needed to explain the neuropathogenesis of this virus. The functions of each viral protein, as well as the mechanism of persistent infection of the virus in the nuclei of infected cells, have not been fully determined. The long-awaited generation of an infectious molecular clone of BDV would be a significant breakthrough to further this aspect of BDV research. The mystery of the extremely high degree of genetic conservation of BDV in different species needs to be solved on the molecular level, and the virus genome-specific contribution to differences in disease outcome needs to be determined as well. Key issues for understanding the neu-

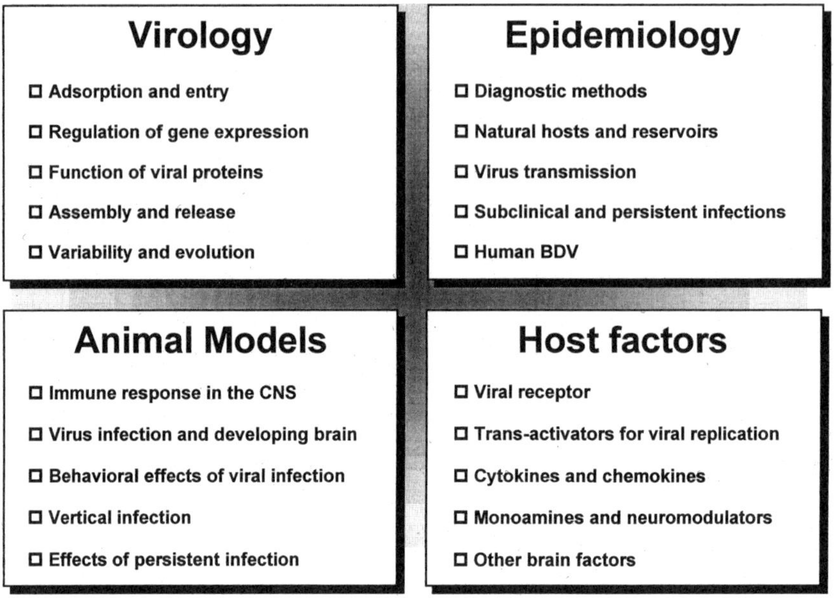

Figure 2. Key issues in understanding the neuropathogenesis of BDV.

ropathogenesis of BDV are summarized in Fig. 2 and are discussed elsewhere in this book.

BDV research is an old but rapidly advancing area of virology that encompasses broad interests in several different research fields. The intellectual foundations established in the past century will give rise to paradigm changes in the related-research fields of BDV science as we enter a new century.

REFERENCES

Allmang, U., M. Hofer, S. Herzog, K. Bechter, and P. Staeheli. 2001. Low avidity of human serum antibodies for Borna disease virus antigens questions their diagnostic value. *Mol. Psychiatry* **6:**329–333.

Amsterdam, J. D., A. Winokur, W. Dyson, S. Herzog, F. Gonzalez, R. Rott, and H. Koprowski. 1985. Borna disease virus. A possible etiologic factor in human affective disorders? *Arch. Gen. Psychiatry* **42:**1093–1096.

Bautista, J. R., S. A. Rubin, T. H. Moran, G. J. Schwartz, and K. M. Carbone. 1995. Developmental injury to the cerebellum following perinatal Borna disease virus infection. *Dev. Brain Res.* **90:**45–53.

Becht, H., and J. Richt. 1996. Borna disease, p. 235–244. *In* M. J. Studdert (ed.), *Virus Diseases of Equines.* Elsevier Science Publishers BV, Amsterdam, The Netherlands.

Berg, A. L., and M. Berg. 1998. A variant form of feline Borna disease. *J. Comp. Pathol.* **119:**323–331.

Bilzer, T., and L. Stitz. 1994. Immune-mediated brain atrophy. CD8+ T cells contribute to tissue destruction during Borna disease. *J. Immunol.* **153:**818–823.

Bode, L. 1995. Human infections with Borna disease virus and potential pathogenic implications. *Curr. Top. Microbiol. Immunol.* **190:**103–130.

Bode, L., R. Dürrwald, F. A. Rantam, R. Ferszt, and H. Ludwig. 1996. First isolates of infectious human Borna disease virus from patients with mood disorders. *Mol. Psychiatry* **1:**200–212.

Bornand, J. V., R. Fatzer, K. Melzer, D. G. Jmaa, P. Caplazi, and F. Ehrensperger. 1998. A case of Borna disease in a cat. *Eur. J. Vet. Pathol.* **4:**33–35.

Briese, T., J. C. de la Torre, A. Lewis, H. Ludwig, and W. I. Lipkin. 1992. Borna disease virus, a negative-strand RNA virus, transcribes in the nucleus of infected cells. *Proc. Natl. Acad. Sci. USA* **89:**11486–11489.

Briese, T., C. G. Hatalski, S. Kliche, Y. S. Park, and W. I. Lipkin. 1995. Enzyme-linked immunosorbent assay for detecting antibodies to Borna disease virus-specific proteins. *J. Clin. Microbiol.* **33:**348–351.

Briese, T., A. Schneemann, A. J. Lewis, Y. S. Park, S. Kim, H. Ludwig, and W. I. Lipkin. 1994. Genomic organization of Borna disease virus. *Proc. Natl. Acad. Sci. USA* **91:**4362–4366.

Caplazi, P., K. Meizer, R. Goetzmann, A. Rohner-Cotti, V. Bracher, K. Zlinszky, and F. Ehrensperger. 1999. Borna disease in Switzerland and in the principality of Liechtenstein. *Schweiz. Arch. Tierheilkd.* **141:**521–527.

Carbone, K. M. 2001. Borna disease virus and human disease. *Clin. Microbiol. Rev.* **14:**513–527.

Carbone, K. M., C. S. Duchala, J. W. Griffin, A. L. Kincaid, and O. Narayan. 1987. Pathogenesis of Borna disease in rats: evidence that intra-axonal spread is the major route for virus dissemination and the determinant for disease incubation. *J. Virol.* **61:**3431–3440.

Carbone, K. M., T. R. Moench, and W. I. Lipkin. 1991a. Borna disease virus replicates in astrocytes, Schwann cells and ependymal cells in persistently infected rats: location of viral genomic and messenger RNAs by in situ hybridization. *J. Neuropathol. Exp. Neurol.* **50:**205–214.

Carbone, K. M., S. W. Park, S. A. Rubin, R. W. Waltrip II, and G. B. Vogelsang. 1991b. Borna disease: association with a maturation defect in the cellular immune response. *J. Virol.* **65:**6154–6164.

Cubitt, B., C. Oldstone, and J. C. de la Torre. 1994. Sequence and genome organization of Borna disease virus. *J. Virol.* **68:**1382–1396.

Czygan, M., W. Hallensleben, M. Hofer, S. Pollak, C. Sauder, T. Bilzer, I. Blümcke, P. Riederer, B. Bogerts, P. Falkai, M. J. Schwarz, E. Masliah, P. Staeheli, F. T. Hufert, and K. Lieb. 1999. Borna disease virus in human brains with a rare form of hippocampal degeneration but not in brains of patients with common neuropsychiatric disorders. *J. Infect. Dis.* **180:**1695–1699.

Dauphin, G., V. Legay, C. Sailleau, S. Smondack, S. Hammoumi, and S. Zientara. 2001. Evidence of Borna disease virus genome detection in French domestic animals and in foxes (Vulpes vulpes). *J. Gen. Virol.* **82:**2199–2204.

Degiorgis, M.-P., A.-L. Berg, C. Hård Af Segerstad, T. Mörner, M. Johansson, and M. Berg. 2000. Borna disease in a free-ranging lynx (*Lynx lynx*). *J. Clin. Microbiol.* **38:**3087–3091.

de la Torre, J. C., L. Bode, R. Dürrwald, B. Cubitt, and H. Ludwig. 1996. Sequence characterization of human Borna disease virus. *Virus Res.* **44:**33–44.

de la Torre, J. C., K. M. Carbone, and W. I. Lipkin. 1990. Molecular characterization of the Borna disease agent. *Virology* **179:**853–856.

Dittrich, W., L. Bode, H. Ludwig, M. Kao, and K. Schneider. 1989. Learning deficiencies in Borna disease virus-infected but clinically healthy rats. *Biol. Psychiatry* 26:818–828.

Elford, W. J., and I. A. Galloway. 1933. Filtration of the virus of Borna disease through graded collodion membranes. *Br. J. Exp. Pathol.* 14:196–205.

Fu, Z. F., J. D. Amsterdam, M. Kao, V. Shankar, H. Koprowski, and B. Dietzschold. 1993. Detection of Borna disease virus-reactive antibodies from patients with affective disorders by western immunoblot technique. *J. Affect. Disord.* 27:61–68.

Gonzalez-Dunia, D., M. Watanabe, S. Syan, M. Mallory, E. Masliah, and J. C. de la Torre. 2000. Synaptic pathology in Borna disease virus persistent infection. *J. Virol.* 74:3441–3448.

Haga, S., M. Yoshimura, Y. Motoi, K. Arima, T. Aizawa, K. Ikuta, M. Tashiro, and K. Ikeda. 1997. Detection of Borna disease virus genome in normal human brain tissue. *Brain Res.* 770:307–309.

Hagiwara, K., M. Asakawa, L. Liao, W. Jiang, S. Yan, J. Chai, Y. Oku, K. Ikuta, and M. Ito. 2001. Seroprevalence of Borna disease virus in domestic animals in Xinjiang, China. *Vet. Microbiol.* 80:383–389.

Hallensleben, W., M. Schwemmle, J. Hausmann, L. Stitz, B. Volk, A. Pagenstecher, and P. Staeheli. 1998. Borna disease virus-induced neurological disorder in mice: infection of neonates results in immunopathology. *J. Virol.* 72:4379–4386.

Herzog, S., K. Frese, J. A. Richt, and R. Rott. 1994. Ein Beitrag zur Epizootiologie der Bornaschen Krankheit beim Pferd. *Wien. Tierarzti. Monatsschr.* 81:374–379.

Herzog, S., C. Kompter, K. Frese, and R. Rott. 1984. Replication of Borna disease virus in rats: age-dependent differences in tissue distribution. *Med. Microbiol. Immunol.* 173:171–177.

Herzog, S., and R. Rott. 1980. Replication of Borna disease virus in cell cultures. *Med. Microbiol. Immunol.* 168:153–158.

Hirano, N., M. Kao, and H. Ludwig. 1983. Persistent, tolerant or subacute infection in Borna disease virus-infected rats. *J. Gen. Virol.* 64:1521–1530.

Hornig, M., H. Weissenböck, N. Horscroft, and W. I. Lipkin. 1999. An infection-based model of neurodevelopmental damage. *Proc. Natl. Acad. Sci. USA* 96:12102–12107.

Ikuta, K. 1997. Possible association of Borna disease virus with human diseases. *Uirusu* 47:37–47.

Iwata, Y., K. Takahashi, X. Peng, K. Fukuda, K. Ohno, T. Ogawa, K. Gonda, N. Mori, S. Niwa, and S. Shigeta. 1998. Detection and sequence analysis of Borna disease virus p24 RNA from peripheral blood mononuclear cells of patients with mood disorders or schizophrenia and of blood donors. *J. Virol.* 72:10044–10049.

Joest, E., and K. Degen. 1911. Untersuchngen über die pathologische Histologie, Pathogenese und postmortale Diagnose der seuchenhaften Gehirn-Rückenmarksentzündung (Bornasche Krankheit) des Pferdes. *Z. Infekt. Krankh. Haustiere* 9:1–98.

Jordan, I., and W. I. Lipkin. 2001. Borna disease virus. *Rev. Med. Virol.* 11:37–57.

Kamitani, W., Y. Shoya, T. Kobayashi, M. Watanabe, B. J. Lee, G. Zhang, K. Tomonaga, and K. Ikuta. 2001. Borna disease virus phosphoprotein binds a neurite outgrowth factor, amphoterin/HMG-1. *J. Virol.* 75:8742–8751.

Kao, M., A. N. Hamir, C. E. Rupprecht, Z. F. Fu, V. Shankar, H. Koprowski, and B. Dietzschold. 1993. Detection of antibodies against Borna disease virus in sera and cerebrospinal fluid of horses in the USA. *Vet. Rec.* 132:241–244.

Kim, Y. K., S. H. Kim, S. H. Choi, Y. H. Ko, L. Kim, M. S. Lee, K. Y. Suh, D. I. Kwak, K. J. Song, Y. J. Lee, R. Yanagihara, and J. W. Song. 1999. Failure to demonstrate Borna disease virus genome in peripheral blood mononuclear cells from psychiatric patients in Korea. *J. Neurovirol.* 5:196–199.

Kishi, M., T. Nakaya, Y. Nakamura, Q. Zhong, K. Ikeda, M. Senjo, M. Kakinuma, S. Kato, and K. Ikuta. 1995. Demonstration of human Borna disease virus RNA in human peripheral blood mononuclear cells. *FEBS Lett.* 364:293–297.

Lieb, K., W. Hallensleben, M. Czygan, L. Stitz, P. Staeheli, and the Bornavirus Study Group. 1997. No Borna disease virus-specific RNA detected in blood from psychiatric patients in different regions of Germany. *Lancet* **350**:1002.

Lipkin, W. I., G. H. Travis, K. M. Carbone, and M. C. Wilson. 1990. Isolation and characterization of Borna disease agent cDNA clones. *Proc. Natl. Acad. Sci. USA* **87**:4184–4188.

Ludwig, H., and L. Bode. 2000. Borna disease virus: new aspects on infection, disease, diagnosis and epidemiology. *Rev. Sci. Tech.* **19**:259–288.

Lundgren, A. L., and H. Ludwig. 1993. Clinically diseased cats with non-suppurative meningoencephalomyelitis have Borna disease virus-specific antibodies. *Acta Vet. Scand.* **34**:101–103.

Malkinson, M., Y. Weisman, E. Ashash, L. Bode, and H. Ludwig. 1993. Borna disease in ostriches. *Vet. Rec.* **133**:304.

Nakamura, Y., S. Asahi, T. Nakaya, M. K. Bahmani, S. Saitoh, K. Yasui, H. Mayama, K. Hagiwara, C. Ishihara, and K. Ikuta. 1996. Demonstration of Borna disease virus RNA in peripheral blood mononuclear cells derived from domestic cats in Japan. *J. Clin. Microbiol.* **34**:188–191.

Nakamura, Y., H. Takahashi, Y. Shoya, T. Nakaya, M. Watanabe, K. Tomonaga, K. Iwahashi, K. Ameno, N. Momiyama, H. Taniyama, T. Sata, T. Kurata, J. C. de la Torre, and K. Ikuta. 2000. Isolation of Borna disease virus from human brain tissue. *J. Virol.* **74**:4601–4611.

Narayan, O., S. Herzog, K. Frese, H. Scheefers, and R. Rott. 1983a. Behavioral disease in rats caused by immunopathological responses to persistent Borna virus in the brain. *Science* **220**:1401–1403.

Narayan, O., S. Herzog, K. Frese, H. Scheefers, and R. Rott. 1983b. Pathogenesis of Borna disease in rats: immune-mediated viral ophthalmoencephalopathy causing blindness and behavioral abnormalities. *J. Infect. Dis.* **148**:305–315.

Nicolau, S., and I. A. Galloway. 1928. Borna disease and enzootic encephalomyelitis of sheep and cattle. *Rep. Ser. Med. Res. Counc.* **121**:7–90.

Nitzschke, E. 1963. Untersuchungen über die experimentelle Bornavirus-Infektion bei der Ratte. *Zentbl. Vetmed. Reihe B* **10**:470–527.

Nowotny, N., J. Kolodziejek, C. O. Jehle, A. Suchy, P. Staeheli, and M. Schwemmle. 2000. Isolation and characterization of a new subtype of Borna disease virus. *J. Virol.* **74**:5655–5658.

Nowotny, N., and H. Weissenböck. 1995. Description of feline nonsuppurative meningoencephalomyelitis ("staggering disease") and studies of its etiology. *J. Clin. Microbiol.* **33**:1668–1669.

Okamoto, M., H. Furuoka, K. Hagiwara, W. Kamitani, R. Kirisawa, K. Ikuta, and H. Taniyama. 2002a. Borna disease in a heifer in Japan. *Vet. Rec.* **150**:16–18.

Okamoto, M., Y. Kagawa, W. Kamitani, K. Hagiwara, R. Kirisawa, H. Iwai, K. Ikuta, and H. Taniyama. 2002b. Borna disease in a dog in Japan. *J. Comp. Pathol.* **126**:312–317.

Pauli, G., J. Grunmach, and H. Ludwig. 1984. Focus-immunoassay for Borna disease virus-specific antigens. *Zentbl. Vetmed. (B)* **31**:552–557.

Pauli, G., and H. Ludwig. 1985. Increase of virus yields and releases of Borna disease virus from persistently infected cells. *Virus Res.* **2**:29–33.

Planz, O., T. Bilzer, M. Sobbe, and L. Stitz. 1993. Lysis of major histocompatibility complex class I-bearing cells in Borna disease virus-induced degenerative encephalopathy. *J. Exp. Med.* **178**:163–174.

Planz, O., C. Rentzsch, A. Batra, A. Batra, T. Winkler, M. Büttner, H.-J. Rziha, and L. Stitz. 1999. Pathogenesis of Borna disease virus: granulocyte fractions of psychiatric patients harbor infectious virus in the absence of antiviral antibodies. *J. Virol.* **73**:6251–6256.

Plata-Salaman, C. R., S. E. Ilyin, D. Gayle, A. Romanovitch, and K. M. Carbone. 1999. Persistent Borna disease virus infection of neonatal rats causes brain regional changes of mRNAs for cytokines, cytokine receptor components and neuropeptides. *Brain Res. Bull.* **49**:441–451.

Pletnikov, M. V., M. L. Jones, S. A. Rubin, T. H. Moran, and K. M. Carbone. 2001. Rat model of autism spectrum disorders. Genetic background effects on Borna disease virus-induced developmental brain damage. *Ann. N. Y. Acad. Sci.* **939**:318–319.

Pletnikov, M. V., S. A. Rubin, K. Vasudevan, T. H. Moran, and K. M. Carbone. 1999. Developmental brain injury associated with abnormal play behavior in neonatally Borna disease virus-infected Lewis rats: a model of autism. *Behav. Brain Res.* **100**:43–50.

Reeves, N. A., C. R. Helps, D. A. Gunn-Moore, C. Blundell, P. L. Finnemore, G. R. Pearson, and D. A. Harbour. 1998. Natural Borna disease virus infection in cats in the United Kingdom. *Vet. Rec.* **143**:523–526.

Richt, J. A., and R. Rott. 2001. Borna disease virus: a mystery as an emerging zoonotic pathogen. *Vet. J.* **161**:24–40.

Rott, R., and H. Becht. 1995. Natural and experimental Borna disease in animals. *Curr. Top. Microbiol. Immunol.* **190**:17–30.

Rott, R., S. Herzog, K. Bechter, and K. Frese. 1991. Borna disease, a possible hazard for man? *Arch. Virol.* **118**:143–149.

Rott, R., S. Herzog, B. Fleischer, A. Winokur, J. Amsterdam, W. Dyson, and H. Koprowski. 1985. Detection of serum antibodies to Borna disease virus in patients with psychiatric disorders. *Science* **228**:755–756.

Rubin, S. A., P. Sylves, M. Vogel, M. Pletnikov, T. H. Moran, G. J. Schwartz, and K. M. Carbone. 1999. Borna disease virus-induced hippocampal dentate gyrus damage is associated with spatial learning and memory deficits. *Brain Res. Bull.* **48**:23–30.

Salvatore, M., S. Morzunov, M. Schwemmle, W. I. Lipkin, and the Bornavirus Study Group. 1997. Borna disease virus in brains of North American and European people with schizophrenia and bipolar disorder. *Lancet* **349**:1813–1814.

Sauder, C., and J. C. de la Torre. 1999. Cytokine expression in the rat central nervous system following perinatal Borna disease virus infection. *J. Neuroimmunol.* **96**:29–45.

Schädler, R., H. Diringer, and H. Ludwig. 1985. Isolation and characterization of a 14500 molecular weight protein from brains and tissue cultures persistently infected with Borna disease virus. *J. Gen. Virol.* **66**:2479–2484.

Schmidt, J. 1912. Untersuchungen über das klinische Verhalten der seuchenhaften Gehirn-Rückenmarksentzündung (Bornasche Krankheit) des Pferdes nebst Angaben über diesbezügliche therapeutische Versuche. *Berl. Tierarztl. Wochenschr.* **28**:581–586, 597–603.

Schneider, P. A., A. Schneemann, and W. I. Lipkin. 1994. RNA splicing in Borna disease virus, a nonsegmented, negative-strand RNA virus. *J. Virol.* **68**:5007–5012.

Schwemmle, M., C. Jehle, S. Formella, and P. Staeheli. 1999. Sequence similarities between human Bornavirus isolates and laboratory strains question human origin. *Lancet* **354**:1973–1974.

Shankar, V., M. Kao, A. N. Hamir, H. Sheng, H. Koprowski, and B. Dietzschold. 1992. Kinetics of virus spread and changes in levels of several cytokine mRNAs in the brain after intranasal infection of rats with Borna disease virus. *J. Virol.* **66**:992–998.

Sierra-Honigmann, A. M., S. A. Rubin, M. G. Estafanous, R. H. Yolken, and K. M. Carbone. 1993. Borna disease virus in peripheral blood mononuclear and bone marrow cells of neonatally and chronically infected rats. *J. Neuroimmunol.* **45**:31–36.

Solbrig, M. V., J. H. Fallon, and W. I. Lipkin. 1995. Behavioral disturbances and pharmacology of Borna disease. *Curr. Top. Microbiol. Immunol.* **190**:93–99.

Solbrig, M. V., G. F. Koob, J. N. Joyce, and W. I. Lipkin. 1996. A neural substrate of hyperactivity in Borna disease: changes in brain dopamine receptors. *Virology* **222**:332–338.

Staeheli, P., C. Sauder, J. Hausmann, F. Ehrensperger, and M. Schwemmle. 2000. Epidemiology of Borna disease virus. *J. Gen. Virol.* **81:**2123–2135.

Stitz, L., D. Soeder, U. Deschl, K. Frese, and R. Rott. 1989. Inhibition of immune-mediated meningoencephalitis in persistently Borna disease virus-infected rats by cyclosporine A. *J. Immunol.* **143:**4250–4256.

Taniyama, H. 2001. Borna disease of animals in Japan. *J. Jpn. Vet. Med. Assoc.* **54:**1–6.

Taniyama, H., M. Okamoto, K. Hirayama, K. Hagiwara, R. Kirisawa, W. Kamitani, N. Tsunoda, and K. Ikuta. 2001. Equine Borna disease in Japan. *Vet. Rec.* **148:**480–482.

VandeWoude, S., J. A. Richt, M. C. Zink, R. Rott, O. Narayan, and J. E. Clements. 1990. A Borna virus cDNA encoding a protein recognized by antibodies in humans with behavioral diseases. *Science* **250:**1278–1281.

von Sprockhoff, H., and E. Nitzschke. 1955. Unterschungen über das komplementbindende Antigen in Gehirnen bornavirus-infizierter Kaninchen. 1. Mitteilung: Nachweis eines löslichen Antigens. *Zentbl. Vetmed.* **2:**185–192.

Waelchi, R. O., F. Ehrensperger, A. Metzler, and C. Winder. 1985. Borna disease in a sheep. *Vet. Rec.* **117:**499–500.

Waltrip, R. W., II, R. W. Buchanan, W. T. Carpenter, Jr., B. Kirkpatrick, A. Summerfelt, A. Breier, S. A. Rubin, and K. M. Carbone. 1997. Borna disease virus antibodies and the deficit syndrome of schizophrenia. *Schizophr. Res.* **23:**253–257.

Waltrip, R. W., II, R. W. Buchanan, A. Summerfelt, A. Breler, W. T. Carpenter, Jr., N. L. Bryant, S. A. Rubin, and K. M. Carbone. 1995. Borna disease virus and schizophrenia. *Psychiatry Res.* **56:**33–44.

Watanabe, M., B. J. Lee, W. Kamitani, T. Kobayashi, H. Taniyama, K. Tomonaga, and K. Ikuta. 2001. Neurological diseases and viral dynamics in the brains of neonatally Borna disease virus-infected gerbils. *Virology* **282:**65–76.

Weissenböck, H., N. Nowotny, P. Caplazi, J. Kolodziejek, and F. Ehrensperger. 1998a. Borna disease in a dog with lethal meningoencephalitis. *J. Clin. Microbiol.* **36:**2127–2130.

Weissenböck, H., A. Suchy, P. Caplazi, S. Herzog, and N. Nowotny. 1998b. Borna disease in Austrian horses. *Vet. Rec.* **143:**21–22.

Yamaguchi, K., T. Sawada, T. Naraki, R. Igata-Yi, H. Shiraki, Y. Horii, T. Ishii, K. Ikeda, N. Asou, H. Okabe, M. Mochizuki, K. Takahashi, S. Yamada, K. Kubo, S. Yashiki, R. W. Waltrip II, and K. M. Carbone. 1999. Detection of Borna disease virus-reactive antibodies from patients with psychiatric disorders and from horses by electrochemiluminescence immunoassay. *Clin. Diagn. Lab. Immunol.* **6:**696–700.

Zwick, W. 1939. Bornasche Krankheit und Encephalomyelitis der Tiere, p. 252–354. *In* E. Gildenmeister, E. Haagen, and O. Waldmann (ed.), *Handbuch der Viruserkrankungen,* vol. 2. Gustav Fischer Verlag, Jena, Germany.

Zwick, W., and O. Seifried. 1925. Ubertragbarkeit der seuchenhaften Gehirnrückenmarksentzündung des Pferdes (Bornasche Krankheit) auf kleine Versuchstiere (Kaninchen). *Berl. Tierarztl. Wochenschr.* **41:**129–132.

Zwick, W., O. Seifried, and J. Witte. 1927. Experimentelle Untersuchungen über die suchenhafte Gehirn- und Rückenmarksentzündung der Pferde (Bornasche Krankheit). *Z. Infekt. Krankh. Haustiere* **30:**42–136.

Chapter 2

Borna Disease Virus Molecular Virology

Masahiko Kishi, Keizo Tomonaga, Patrick Lai,
and Juan Carlos de la Torre

BIOLOGICAL CHARACTERISTICS

Host Range

Horses and sheep have been regarded as the main natural hosts of Borna disease (BD) virus (BDV). In these species BDV can cause BD, a frequently fatal neurologic disease manifested by profound behavioral abnormalities. However, more-recent evidence indicates that the natural host range of BDV is wider than originally thought. Naturally occurring BDV infections have been documented in cattle and cats and also sporadically in a variety of other species, including dogs, donkeys, mules, ostriches, alpacas, and pygmy hippopotami (Hatalski et al., 1997; Richt et al., 1997; Rott and Becht, 1995; Staeheli et al., 2000). Experimentally, BDV has a remarkably wide host range, including phylogenetically distant species from birds to rodents and nonhuman primates (Hatalski et al., 1997; Richt et al., 1997; Rott and Becht, 1995). Moreover, serological data and recent molecular epidemiological studies indicate that BDV can infect humans and might be associated with certain neuropsychiatric disorders; however, BDV has not been implicated as a human pathogen yet (Gonzalez-Dunia et al., 1997b; Lipkin et al., 1997). Nevertheless, technical difficulties

Masahiko Kishi • Tsukuba Central Laboratories, Kyoritsu Seiyaku Corporation, Inashiki-gun, Ibaraki, Japan. **Keizo Tomonaga** • Department of Virology, Research Institute for Microbial Diseases, Osaka University, 3-1 Yamadaoka, Suita, Osaka 565-0871, Japan. **Patrick Lai** • Bioscience, Carlson Hall, Salem International University, Salem, WV 26426-0500. **Juan Carlos de la Torre** • Department of Neuropharmacology, Division of Virology, IMM-6, The Scripps Research Institute, 10550 North Torrey Pines Rd., La Jolla, CA 92037.

and limitations of the currently existing diagnostic tools for BDV have led some investigators to question the worldwide distribution of BDV and its relevance as a human virus (Staeheli et al., 2000). Improved knowledge of the immunobiology as well as the molecular and cellular biology of BDV may facilitate the development of more-sensitive and reliable assays for the investigation of the epidemiology of BDV.

BDV infectivity and RNA have been detected in bodily secretions and excretions, suggesting that BDV can be transmitted through salival, nasal, and conjunctival secretions and, particularly, urine and feces (Sierra-Honigmann et al., 1993). Although this theory is not yet firmly established, infection may result from direct contact with these body fluids or by exposure to contaminated water and food (Rott and Becht, 1995). BDV infection produces a significant range of phenotypic disease expression. However, despite a wide host range and phenotypic disease variability, molecular epidemiological data have shown a remarkable sequence conservation, not only among BDV isolates within the same host species but also among isolates from different animal species (Gonzalez-Dunia et al., 1997b; Hatalski et al., 1997; Richt et al., 1997).

Tissue and Cell Tropism

BDV is noncytolytic and highly neurotropic. Although BDV infects a wide range of species, within a specific host BDV replicates preferentially in the central and peripheral nervous systems. Neurons and astrocytes are the primary cell targets of BDV, but oligodendrocytes and ependymal and Schwann cells can be also infected (Rott and Becht, 1995). In addition, ectoderm-derived cells become infected in vivo as a consequence of the centrifugal axonal spread of BDV (Rott and Becht, 1995). The virus can be also present in peripheral blood mononuclear cells from naturally and experimentally infected animals (Hatalski et al., 1997; Richt et al., 1997; Sierra-Honigmann et al., 1993).

BDV can be grown in a variety of brain- and non-brain-derived established cell lines by cocultivation with infected brain cells or by inoculation with brain homogenates from infected animals (Rott and Becht, 1995). In all known cases infected culture cells do not produce significant levels of extracellular cell-free virus and have low cell-associated infectivity, ranging from less than 0.01 to 0.1 infectious unit per cell. Treatment of BDV-infected cells with a hypertonic buffer (250 mM $MgCl_2$) for 90 min at 37°C can release up to 50% of the total cell-associated infectivity (Briese et al., 1992), a technique which provided researchers with a source of cell-free virus. Cell survival does not appear to be significantly compromised by this treatment, indicating that the release of cell-free virus is unlikely to be due to cell death caused by the hypertonic treatment. Homogenates from BDV-infected cells and tissues, as well as cell-free virus, can be quantified by using an immunofocus assay.

VIRION MORPHOLOGY AND PHYSICAL CHARACTERISTICS

Electron microscopy studies of negatively stained cell-free BDV infectious particles have shown that virions have a spherical morphology, with a diameter ranging from 70 to 130 nm (Gonzalez-Dunia et al., 1997a; Kohno et al., 1999; Zimmermann et al., 1994). These particles contain an internal electron-dense core (diameter, 50 to 60 nm) and a limiting outer membrane envelope, which appears to be covered with spikes approximately 7.0 nm long (Kohno et al., 1999). Partially purified BDV infectious particles have a buoyant density in CsCl of 1.16 to 1.22 g/cm^3, and that in sucrose is 1.22 g/cm^3. Virus infectivity is rapidly lost by heat treatment at 56°C. Virions are relatively stable at 37°C, but after incubation for 24 h in the presence of serum, only minimal infectivity is recovered. Virions are inactivated below pH 5 and above pH 12 and by treatment with organic solvents, detergents, formaldehyde, and exposure to UV radiation.

GENOME ORGANIZATION AND ENCODED PROTEINS

BDV has a non-segmented, negative-stranded (NNS) RNA genome (ca. 8.9 kb in size; M_r, ca. 3×10^6) (de la Torre, 1994; Schneemann et al., 1995). The RNA genome is not polyadenylated. Extracistronic sequences are found at the 3' (leader) and 5' (trailer) ends of the BDV genome. As with other negative-strand RNA viruses, the ends of BDV genome RNA exhibit partial inverted complementarity. Full-length plus-strand (antigenomic) RNAs are present in infected cells and viral ribonucleoproteins.

Six major open reading frames (ORFs) are found in the BDV genome sequence (de la Torre, 1994; Schneemann et al., 1995) (Fig. 1). These ORFs code for polypeptides with predicted molecular masses of 40 kDa (p40), 24 kDa (p24), 10 kDa (X), 16 kDa (p16), 56 kDa (p56), and 180 kDa (p180), respectively. Based on their positions in the viral genome and abundance in infected cells and virion particles, together with their biochemical and sequence features, p40, p24 and p16 BDV polypeptides correspond to the viral nucleoprotein (N), the phosphoprotein (P) transcriptional activator, and the matrix (M) proteins, respectively, found in other NNS RNAs. Two isoforms of the BDV N (p40 and p38) are found in BDV-infected cells. These two forms of the viral N may be encoded by two different mRNA species (Pyper and Gartner, 1997), but differential usage of two inframe initiation codons present in the BDV N gene could also contribute to the production of BDV p40/38. BDV P is an acidic polypeptide (predicted pI, 4.8), that has a high Ser-Thr content (16%), with phosphorylation at serine residues that is mediated by both protein kinase C and casein kinase II (Schwemmle et al., 1997). In addition to P, a second polypeptide (16 kDa), termed P′ (p16), is also translated from the second in-frame AUG codon present within the P ORF. P′ has been detected in BDV-infected cultured cells and brain cells of experimentally infected animals (Kobayashi et al., 2000), but its role in the virus life cycle is currently unknown. An additional ORF, ORF X, encodes a polypeptide of 10 kDa present in BDV-infected cells and tissues (Wehner et al., 1997). BDV X starts within the same mRNA transcription unit, 49 nucleotides (nt) upstream from P, and overlaps, in a different frame, with the 71 N-terminal amino acids of P. In contrast to other NNS RNA viruses, the putative BDV M protein appears to be glycosylated and has a molecular mass of 18 kDa (gp18) (Kliche et al., 1994). M was originally characterized as a biantennary complex-type glycoprotein sensitive to endoglycosidase F (endo F), but not to endo H or O-glycosidase (Kliche et al., 1994). Intriguingly, M does not contain any typical consensus sequence for N glycosylation. In addition, M was proposed to be present in the virus envelope and to participate in viral attachment to the cell (Kliche et al., 1994). However, recent evidence has shown that BDV M is a nonglycosylated protein that lines the inner side of a lipid-containing viral envelope (Kraus et al., 2001). Therefore, BDV M has features similar to those found in the M proteins of other mononegaviruses. BDV ORF IV (p56), the putative virus surface glycoprotein (G), overlaps, in a different frame, with the C terminus of M and is capable of encoding a 503-amino-acid polypeptide with a predicted molecular mass of 56 kDa. The G gene directs the synthesis of two glycosylated polypeptides of about 84 to 94 kDa (gp84/94) and 43 kDa (gp43), corresponding to the full length and the C terminus, respectively, of G (Gonzalez-Dunia et al., 1997a). gp43 is produced via cleavage of gp84/94 by the cellular protease furin. BDV ORF V (p180) is capable of encoding a polypeptide whose deduced amino acid sequence displays strong homology to other NNS RNA virus polymerases, members of the L protein family (de la Torre, 1994; Schneemann et al., 1995). Several additional viral polypeptides can be translated from spliced forms of BDV mRNAs (see "Transcription and Replication"), which increases the proteomic complexity of BDV.

The genomic polarity of the RNA has a very limited coding capability, consisting only of very small ORFs that are not flanked by recognizable putative transcription initiation and termination or polyadenylation signals. Thus, presently there is no evidence that BDV might use an ambisense coding strategy.

CYCLE OF INFECTION

Virus Adsorption and Entry

There is evidence that a proteinaceous cellular receptor, of unknown identity, is required for BDV infection. Antibodies to both the virus G and M (gp18) proteins have neutralizing activity, suggesting that both are implicated in BDV adsorption and/or entry (Gonzalez-Dunia et al., 1997a; Kliche et al., 1994). Nevertheless, monoclonal antibodies directed to gp84/94, but not to M, exhibited neutralizing activity against BDV (Furrer et al., 2001). It is plausible that antibodies against M-associated carbohydrates, which might be present also in gp84/94, could explain the reported neutralizing activity of anti-M antibody. Whether the carbohydrate modifications found in G and M contribute to the adsorption process is unknown. Lysosomotropic drugs and chemical treatments that cause depletion of cellular energy block BDV infection, indicating that BDV entry occurs by receptor-mediated endocytosis and requires an acidic intracellular compartment to allow the fusion between viral and cellular membranes (Gonzalez-Dunia et al., 1998). Reduction in the pH of the endocytic compartment triggers this fusion event and releases the BDV ribonucleoprotein (RNP), which is then transported to the cell nucleus where viral transcription and replication occur.

Both gp84/94 and gp43 are associated with cell-free infectious BDV particles and appear to participate in virus entry. A plausible model for BDV cell entry is that the N-terminal part of the virion-associated gp84/94 is involved in BDV receptor binding and endocytosis, whereas gp43 would mediate the pH-dependent fusion event required for BDV infection. The role of gp43 in membrane fusion is supported by the observation that it is the only known BDV polypeptide that has been detected at the cell surface, and cells persistently infected with BDV form extensive syncytia upon exposure to low-pH medium (Gonzalez-Dunia et al., 1998). Interestingly, near the N terminus of gp43 there is a highly hydrophobic sequence that is reminiscent of the fusogenic domain described for the surface glycoproteins of other enveloped viruses. Nonetheless, we cannot rule out the possibility that other viral proteins not expressed at the cell surface could influence fusion, as has been described for the herpes simplex virus gK protein (Hutchinson et al., 1995). Results from pseudotype studies have provided evidence that the N-terminal part (amino acids 1 to 244) of BDV p56 is sufficient for receptor recognition and virus entry (Perez et al., 2001). This pseudotype approach was based on a recently developed recombinant vesicular stomatitis virus (VSV) in which the gene for green fluorescent protein (GFP) was substituted for the VSV G protein gene (VSV-G*). Complementation of VSV-G* with BDV p56 resulted in infectious VSV-G* pseudotypes that contained both BDV gp84 and gp43. A chimeric glycoprotein that contained the N-terminal 244 amino acids of BDV p56 fused to the transmembrane (TM) domain and cytoplasmic domain (CTD) of VSV G protein was efficiently incorporated into VSV-G* particles, resulting in pseudotype infectious virions that were neutralized by BDV-specific antiserum (Perez et al., 2001).

Transcription and Replication

BDV has the property, unique among known NNS RNA animal viruses, of a nuclear site for genome transcription and replication (de la Torre, 1994; Schneemann et al., 1995). The nucleolus has been proposed as the site where BDV RNA synthesis occurs (Pyper et al., 1998). The genomic and antigenomic RNA molecules are neither capped nor polyadenylated. These RNAs exist as infectious RNPs in the nuclei of infected cells (de la Torre, 1994).

Sequential and polar transcription results in decreasing molar quantity of BDV transcripts from the 3'- to the 5'-encoded cistrons. RNA species corresponding to the leader RNA have not been detected in BDV-infected cells. The viral mRNAs are polyadenylated and contain a 5' cap structure, but sequences at the 5' end of the BDV mRNAs are homogeneous and genome encoded (Schneemann et al., 1994). Thus, it is unlikely that transcription initiation of BDV mRNAs involves a cap-snatching mechanism similar to the one used by influenza viruses. Monocistronic viral mRNAs in BDV-infected cells are detected only for the N gene (Fig. 1). The BDV genome contains three transcription initiation sites (S signals) and four transcription termination or polyadenylation sites (E signals) (de la Torre, 1994; Schneemann et al., 1995) (Fig. 1). The S signals contain a semiconserved U-rich motif that is partially copied into the respective transcripts. A similar motif is not found within the S signals of previously described NNS RNA viruses. BDV E signals consist of six or seven U residues preceded by a single A residue, resembling the E signal motif found in other NNS RNA viruses. The BDV genome lacks the characteristic configuration of E signal-intergenic region-S signal, found at the gene boundaries of other NNS RNA viruses. Instead, BDV transcription units and transcriptive signals frequently overlap. Thus, for example, signal S2 of the P gene is located 18 nt upstream of signal E1 of the N gene. Likewise, the BDV E2

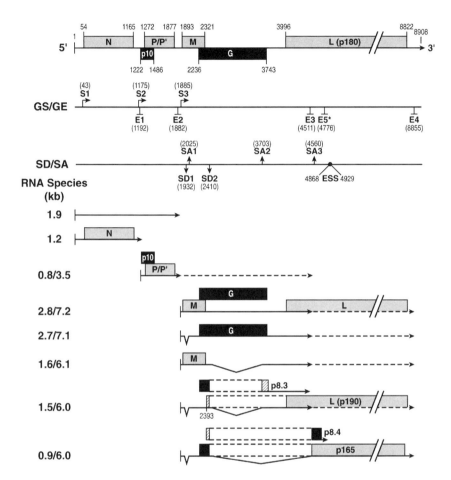

Figure 1. Genomic organization and transcriptional map of BDV. BDV ORFs are represented by boxes at the top. Nucleotide positions (antigenomic polarity) corresponding to the AUG and stop codons for each ORF are indicated. Different shades correspond to usage of different reading frames within the antigenomic polarity of the BDV genomic RNA. The locations of transcription initiation (GS) and transcription termination sites (GE) are indicated by S and E, respectively. Positions of splicing donor (SD) and splicing acceptor (SA) sites for BDV introns I, II, and III are indicated. The location of the ESS element is indicated. The sizes of subgenomic viral mRNAs detected in BDV-infected cells are indicated. Sizes on the left and right sides of the slash correspond to transcripts that initiate at the same GS but terminate at a different GE, respectively.

signal for the P gene is completely contained within the S3 signal of the third transcription unit. Overlapping genes have been documented for several NNS RNA viruses, and such arrangement is thought to contribute to gene expression regulation. In the case of respiratory syncytial virus (RSV), the E signal of the M2 gene lies downstream of the S signal of L polymerase, separated by 45 nucleotides (Fearns and Collins, 1999). This arrangement leads to termination at the M2 E signal of about 90% of the transcripts initiated at the L S signal, suggesting a down-regulatory mechanism for the expression of the RSV L gene. Work with RSV has shed some light about the mechanisms by which the virus polymerase can access an S signal located upstream of an overlapping E signal. These studies showed that the virus polymerase accesses the S signal only following arrival at the M2 E signal and that RSV L is capable of being efficiently recycled from the M2 E signal to the L S signal. The latter scenario provides an explanation for the unexpectedly high level of accumulation of L mRNA in RSV-infected cells. It is reasonable to expect that L polymerases of other mononegaviruses, including BDV, use similar mechanisms to access overlapping E and S signals. It is worth noting that RSV polymerase is capable of efficiently transcribing from an L S signal placed downstream of the M2 E signal (Fearns and Collins, 1999). This finding raises the possibility that the gene overlap exhibited by several mononegaviruses, including BDV, might not have a significant impact on the biology of these viruses.

Readthrough at transcriptional termination sites can be observed with several mononegaviruses. This phenomenon is usually considered to be aberrant and of low, or no, biological significance for the virus. However, for some viruses transcriptional readthrough may be critical for their viability. Thus, readthrough of BDV E3 signal is strictly required for the synthesis of the virus L polymerase, which may provide an additional regulatory mechanism for the control of BDV genome expression.

Two of the BDV primary transcripts are posttranscriptionally processed by the cellular RNA splicing machinery (de la Torre, 1994; Schneemann et al., 1995). Three introns (introns I, II, and III) have been identified in the BDV genome. BDV introns I and II span nt 1932 to 2025 and nt 2410 to 3703, respectively, in the BDV antigenomic sequence. Splicing of intron I results in mRNA species where the amino acid in position 13 of the M protein is followed by a stop codon, whereas splicing of intron II, and that of introns I and II, results in an mRNA containing an ORF that corresponds to the first 58 amino acids of G fused to a new C terminus of 20 amino acids, resulting in a polypeptide with a predicted molecular mass of 8.3 kDa (p8.3 kDa). RNA species resulting from splicing of intron II, and that of introns I and II, also predict an additional ORF that would consist of BDV ORF V (p180) extended by 153 amino acid residues at its N terminus, resulting in a putative BDV L protein with a predicted molecular mass of 190 kDa (p190). Whether all these new predicted BDV polypeptides are synthesized in infected cells and tissues is unknown. However, recent evidence suggests that p190, rather than p180, is likely to be the BDV L polymerase preset in infected cells (Walker et al., 2000). Intron III is generated by alternative choice of the 3′ splicing acceptor site (Cubitt et al., 2001; Tomonaga et al., 2000; Walker et al., 2000). Intron III spliced mRNAs were detected in cells from different types and species and have the capability to code for two new viral proteins with predicted molecular masses of 8.4 (p8.4) and 165 (p165) kDa. These findings underscore the proteomic complexity exhibited by BDV.

Assembly, Release, and Cell-to-Cell Propagation

Thin sections of BDV-infected cells revealed the presence of intracytoplasmic virus-like particles with morphological characteristics similar to those described for partially purified cell-free BDV infectious particles (Compans et al., 1994). These particles were observed below the plasma membrane of infected cells and were rarely seen in cytoplasmic vacuoles. They showed no association with cisternae of the endoplasmic reticulum (ER), the Golgi complex, or other intracytoplasmic membranes. The assembly process and site of BDV maturation have not been identified. BDV RNPs accumulate in the nuclei of infected cells. These RNPs are biologically active as determined by their ability to direct synthesis of BDV macromolecules and production of infectious virus upon transfection into susceptible cells (Cubitt and de la Torre, 1994). The nuclear envelope is continued by the ER, and BDV gp84/94 appears to accumulate at the ER and perinuclear space. This may facilitate the interaction of gp84/94 with viral RNPs during their nuclear egress. Budding of BDV particles has only been observed at the cell surface of BDV-infected MDCK cells after treatment with *n*-butyrate (Kohno et al., 1999). Whether this reflects a natural pathway for the exit of BDV remains to be determined.

An intriguing aspect of the biology of BDV is the mechanism by which BDV spreads within the central nervous system (CNS). BDV appears to propagate transsynaptically, but full virus particles have never been observed at the site of synaptic junctions (Carbone et al., 1987; Gosztonyi et al., 1993; Gosztonyi and Ludwig, 1995). A similar situation has been described for rabies virus (RV) (Gosztonyi et al., 1993). These observations led to the attractive hypothesis that bare RNP could be the infectious unit being transported transsynaptically within the CNS. However, recent findings have indicated that RV G is absolutely required for the propagation of RV in neuronal culture cells, as well as within the mouse CNS (Etessami et al., 2000). Whether this finding applies also to the propagation of BDV is unknown.

REGULATION OF GENE EXPRESSION

Mononegaviruses use a variety of mechanisms to direct and control expression of their genomes. These include (i) overlap of transcription units and transcriptive signals, (ii) readthrough of transcription termination signals, (iii) differential use of translational initiation codons, and (iv) efficient translation of ORFs placed downstream within polycistronic mRNAs. Remarkably, all these mechanisms, together with RNA splicing, are concurrently employed for the control of the expression of the BDV compact genome, representing a unique situation among known mononegaviruses. There is presently only very limited knowledge about the details of the molecular mechanisms responsible for the control of BDV genome expression. This section focuses only on a few selected processes to illustrate the complexity underlying the execution of the BDV gene expression program.

Expression of BDV dORF

In eukaryotes, the majority of mRNAs are monocistronic. However, examples of downstream ORF (dORF) expression have been described for several cell and viral polycistronic transcripts. BDV polypeptides, with the exception of N, are translated from polycistronic mRNAs, a unique situation among known mononegaviruses. Expression of dORF can be achieved by a leaky ribosome-scanning mechanism, resumption of scanning after termination of an upstream ORF, or cap-independent internal initiation. Experimental evidence indicates that a leaky ribosome-scanning mechanism contributes to the expression of the ORFs P' and G (Etessami et al., 2000; Kobayashi et al., 2000; Schneider et al., 1997), whereas at the present time there is no evidence that cap-independent internal initiation is used for translation of BDV mRNAs.

Regulation of BDV G Expression

The expression and functions of virus surface glycoproteins have been extensively studied for other NNS RNA viruses, comprising the families *Paramyxoviridae, Filoviridae,* and *Rhabdoviridae.* The *Paramyxoviridae* possess two integral membrane proteins, one of which (HN) is involved in cell attachment and the other of which (F) is involved in mediating pH-independent fusion of the viral envelope with cellular membranes (Lamb, 1996). The *Filoviridae* have a single surface G (Peters, 1996). Expression of this G results from a complex regulatory mechanism involving both transcriptional editing and translational frameshifting

(Sanchez et al., 1996). Finally, the *Rhabdoviridae* also have a single G present at the surface of the virus (Wagner, 1996). In all cases, synthesis of these glycoproteins involves maturation by trafficking through the Golgi complex. Eventually, these viral Gs are expressed at the cell surface and assembly of infectious virions occurs through budding on plasma membranes. In contrast, expression of full-length BDV G (gp84) appears to be mainly restricted to the ER and nuclear envelope, and only the C terminus (gp43), resulting from posttranslational cleavage by the cellular protease furin, is detected at the cell surface (Gonzalez-Dunia et al., 1998; Gonzalez-Dunia et al., 1997a; Perez et al., 2001). Both products are associated with infectious virions and are involved in the initiation of infection by BDV, resembling the situation seen in filoviruses. However, in the case of BDV the predicted N-terminal part of G (gp41), generated upon cleavage by furin, has not been detected in BDV-infected cells, suggesting a rapid degradation of this product upon cleavage of gp84/94. It is also intriguing that in BDV-infected cells, both gp84/94 and gp43 remained sensitive to both endo F and endo H (Gonzalez-Dunia et al., 1997a), suggesting that these polypeptides do not mature in the Golgi complex. Together, these features are indicative of a novel mechanism for the maturation of an NNS RNA virus surface glycoprotein and hence for the assembly of BDV particles. Also intriguing is the observation that G expression is usually detected only in a low percentage (1 to 10%) of BDV persistently infected cells. These features of BDV G expression might contribute to the paucity of infectious viral particles produced and the exquisite ability of BDV to establish persistence.

Regulation of BDV RNA Splicing

Alternative splicing of mRNA precursors is a versatile mechanism of gene expression regulation that accounts for a considerable proportion of proteomic complexity in higher eukaryotes. Its modulation is achieved through the combined interplay of positive and negative regulatory signals present in the RNA that are recognized by complexes composed of members of the hnRNP and SR protein families (Chabot, 1996; Lopez, 1998; Smith and Valcarcel, 2000). Alternative splicing has been shown to play an important role in the life cycle of several viruses, including influenza virus (Lamb and Horvath, 1991), adenovirus (Kanopka et al., 1998), human immunodeficiency virus (Berget, 1995), and bovine papillomavirus type 1 (Barksdale and Baker, 1995). Moreover, in the case of BDV, RNA splicing can modulate the efficiency of termination-reinitiation of translation and leaky scanning mechanisms that are also involved in the regulation of the expression of BDV gene products.

Virus-derived BDV mRNAs are spliced with significantly lower efficiency than the same plasmid-derived mRNAs (Cubitt et al., 2001; Jehle et al., 2000; Tomonaga et al., 2000). It has been also documented that splicing of plasmid-derived BDV 2.8-kb primary transcript is not influenced by co-expression of the BDV proteins N, P, and X in BDV-infected cells (Jehle et al., 2000). These findings indicate that BDV-encoded factors, or virally induced cellular factors, rather than cis-acting RNA elements, determine the low efficiency of RNA splicing in virus-infected cells. In addition, a similar splicing pattern has been observed in different cell types from different species, and such a pattern was not altered in response to osmotic shock-mediated stress (Cubitt et al., 2001). These findings suggest that BDV might have developed strategies to acquire a certain degree of insulation from cellular influences that could have unwanted effects on the regulation of virus RNA processing. These mechanisms could also prevent BDV-induced disturbances in the regulation of the cellular RNA processing machinery. This, in turn, could facilitate virus persistence without compromising cell viability.

Introns II and III share the 5' splicing donor (SD) site (Cubitt et al., 2001; Tomonaga et al., 2000). Interestingly, alternative splicing of introns II and III is regulated by the use of an alternative transcription termination or polyadenylation signal (GE6), and a cis-acting exon splicing suppressor (ESS) element located within the L gene (Tomonaga et al., 2000). This ESS resembles those found in other viral and cellular pre-mRNAs. BDV mRNAs that terminate at GE6 will not contain the ESS and can be spliced more efficiently than those pre-mRNAs terminating at GE5. The regulation of the use of alternative GE signals by the BDV polymerase is presently unknown.

NUCLEOCYTOPLASMIC TRANSPORT DURING THE LIFE CYCLE OF BDV

Completion of the BDV life cycle requires a variety of nuclear transport events involving viral macromolecules, namely, (i) import of RNP containing the incoming viral genome, (ii) export of transcribed BDV mRNA for translation in the cytosol, (iii) import of viral proteins required for control of virus RNA synthesis and formation of RNP, and (iv) export of assembled BDV RNP. Each of these processes is distinct, and the same viral components can be part of multiple transfer events in and out of the nucleus, each of which may utilize different mechanisms and different signals (Gorlich, 1998; Nakielny and Dreyfuss, 1999; Whittaker and Helenius, 1998). The mechanisms involved in the control of trafficking of viral RNP across the nuclear envelope and BDV mRNA nuclear export remain largely unknown. In contrast, several of the signals and interactions involved in nucleocytoplasmic transport of BDV proteins have been elucidated during the last few years, and these are the focus of this section. Whenever possible, we relate this information to the problem of BDV RNP trafficking.

Nucleocytoplasmic Transport of BDV N

The nucleoprotein (N) is the most abundant BDV protein present in virus-infected cells both in tissue culture systems and in BDV-infected animals. Immunofluorescence studies using specific antibodies showed that N was mainly found in the nucleus, although it was present also at lower levels in the cytoplasm of BDV-infected cells (Bause-Niedrig et al., 1991; Haas et al., 1986; Nakielny and Dreyfuss, 1999; Thiedemann et al., 1992; Whittaker and Helenius, 1998). Likewise, N predominantly localized in the nuclei of cells transfected with an N-expression plasmid (Kobayashi et al., 2001; Kobayashi et al., 1998; Pyper and Gartner, 1997). These results suggested that BDV N contained a nuclear localization signal (NLS). Based on computer predictions it was initially proposed that positively charged residues $K^{163}KRFK^{167}$ and $R^{338}YRRREISR^{346}$ within BDV N might serve as NLSs because of their similarity to short basic amino acid previously found to be bona fide NLSs that mediate nuclear localization of proteins in eukaryotes (Boulikas, 1993). However, BDV N mutants with amino acid substitutions within the $K^{163}KRFK^{167}$ and the $R^{338}YRRREISR^{346}$ motifs were found to accumulate in the nuclei of transiently transfected cells, indicating that these two motifs were dispensable for nuclear targeting activity of BDV N (Kobayashi et al., 1998; Pyper and Gartner, 1997). Cells transfected with plasmids independently encoding each of the two N isoforms, p40 and p38, revealed that Np38 and Np40 accumulate in the nucleus and cytoplasm, respectively (Kobayashi et al., 2001; Kobayashi et al., 1998; Pyper and Gartner, 1997). This finding suggested that the nuclear targeting activity of BDV N was associated with the 13 amino-terminal residues, containing the basic amino acid-rich sequence P^3KRR^6. Consistent with this finding, Np40 mutants containing deletions or amino acid substitutions that disrupted the putative P^3KRR^6 NLS showed a cytoplasmic localization instead of the nuclear one associated with the wild-type Np40 isoform (Kobayashi et al., 1998). In addition, β-galactosidase, which normally resides in the cytoplasm, exhibited a nuclear localization after its fusion to the nonapeptide $P^3KRRLVDDA^{11}$ from the N terminus of Np40 (Kobayashi et al., 1998). Together, these results demonstrated that $P^3KRRLVDDA^{11}$ represents a bona fide NLS of BDV N.

The isoform p38 of N lacks the NLS present in N, and as predicted Np38 accumulates in the cytoplasm of cells transfected with the corresponding expression plasmid. Interestingly, immunoprecipitation of lysates prepared after subcellular fractionation of BDV-infected cells showed that Np38 and Np40 were present in both nuclear and cytoplasmic fractions (Pyper and Gartner, 1997). Both Np38 and Np40 proteins were also found in the nucleus and cytoplasm of cells cotransfected with plasmids expressing Np38 and Np40, suggesting an interaction between the two N isoforms (Kobayashi et al., 2001; Kobayashi et al., 1998). This intracellular interaction between Np40 and Np38 had been suggested earlier by results of coimmunoprecipitation studies. These findings suggest that Np38 can be imported into the nucleus through interaction with Np40. Furthermore, the cytoplasmic retention of Np40 when interacting with Np38 raised the possibility that in addition to having a nuclear targeting activity, BDV N also has a nuclear export activity. Analysis of subcellular distribution of GFP-N fusion proteins revealed that a segment of N corresponding to amino acids 128 to 145 was sufficient to mediate the cytoplasmic accumulation of the GFP chimeric protein (Kobayashi et al., 2001). This N segment contained a leucine-rich motif (L^{128}TELEISSIFSHCC^{141}) similar to those found in other well-characterized nuclear export signals (NES). Mutations of the L or I positions within this putative NES eliminated the nuclear export activity of N. Proteins containing a leucine-rich NES use CRM1/exportin 1 as the export receptor to travel through the nucleopore complex (NPC) (Nakielny and Dreyfuss, 1999). The cell-permeating fungal metabolite leptomycin B specifically inhibits the interaction between the cargo and CRM1. Leptomycin B treatment eliminated the nuclear exclusion of GFP containing the NES of N, indicating that a CRM1-dependent pathway mediates nuclear export of N (Nakielny and Dreyfuss, 1999). Thus, BDV N exhibits the behavior of a bona fide nucleocytoplasmic shuttling protein and likely contributes to the nucleocytoplasmic transport of the BDV RNP.

The biological implications of the existence of two N isoforms with different subcellular targeting properties remain to be determined. Np38 also colocalized with P in the nuclei of cells cotransfected with the Np38 and P expression plasmids, suggesting a P-Np38 interaction (Kobayashi et al., 2001; Kobayashi et al., 1998; Pyper and Gartner, 1997). In vitro binding studies have suggested that two regions of N (amino acids 56 to 100 and 131 to 155) are involved in binding to P (Berg et al., 1998). Hence, it seems likely that Np38 lacking an NLS can be transported into the nucleus from the cytoplasm through heterodimerization with N or P. Interestingly, Np38 was retained in the nuclei of cells cotransfected with Np38 and P. This retention could be due to the overlap between the NES of Np38 and one of its P binding sites, which might result in masking of the Np38 NES. Therefore, it is possible that by interacting with Np40 and P, Np38 might play a role in the control of the bidirectional trafficking of BDV RNP.

Nucleocytoplasmic Transport of BDV P

BDV P and P' can be detected in the cytoplasm and nucleus of BDV-infected cells (Bause-Niedrig et al., 1991; Thierer et al., 1992) and both P and P' are found in the nucleus of cells transfected with the corresponding expression plasmids (Bause-Niedrig et al., 1991; Kobayashi et al., 2000; Shoya et al., 1998). Inspection of the ORF II amino acid sequence identified a basic-amino-acid-rich sequence, $R^{22}RKRSGSPRPRK^{33}$, as a good candidate for being the NLS of P. Analysis of carboxy- and amino-terminal truncation mutants of P showed that amino acids 20 to 37 were sufficient to promote efficient nuclear accumulation of a P-GFP fusion protein (Schwemmle et al., 1998). This NLS comprised of amino acids 20 to 37 of P appeared to have a bipartite structure consisting of two basic amino acid-rich sequences, $R^{22}RER^{25}$ and $R^{30}PRKIPR^{36}$, separated by four nonbasic amino acids, $S^{26}GSP^{29}$. There is evidence that proline at position 29 may be also part of this NLS (Shoya et al., 1998). P' lacks the first 55 amino acid residues of P, which include the N-terminal NLS. However, P' was capable of translocation into the nucleus, indicating the existence of an additional NLS within P/P' with the capability of operating independently of the N-terminal NLS. Results from subcellular localization of a variety of P mutants and chimeric proteins consisting of various portions of P fused to β-galactosidase provided evidence of the existence of an additional independent NLS ($P^{181}PRIYPQLPSAPT^{193}$) located in the in the carboxy-terminal region of P (Shoya et al., 1998). Unlike other previously described NLSs, frequently rich in basic amino acids, both P NLSs are proline-rich instead. P was also found to bind to serpin and pendulin (karyopherin alpha/importin-60), proteins implicated in NLS binding during nuclear import, providing additional support of the nuclear targeting activity of P. N-P complexes have been found in the nuclei of infected cells, and mutational analysis of P showed that its C terminus (amino acids 197 to 201) contains an N-binding site. Therefore, nucleocytoplasmic transport of P could be also mediated by its interaction with N.

Nucleocytoplasmic Transport of BDV X

BDV X is detected in brain cells of naturally and experimentally infected animals (Wehner et al., 1997). Immunofluorescence analyses of BDV-infected cells using a rabbit polyclonal serum specific to X showed that X is present in the nucleus and cytoplasm of infected cells both in cultured cells and infected animals (Malik et al., 1999; Wehner et al., 1997). However, inspection of the amino acid sequence of the X ORF failed to reveal the presence of a motif similar to previously identified NLSs of nuclear proteins. Moreover, in X-transfected cells, X protein was detected predominantly in the cytoplasm. Results from the yeast two-hybrid system have failed to show any interaction of X with serpin or pendulin, further suggesting that the nuclear localization of X is dependent on its interaction with other viral proteins. X was found in the nuclei of cells co-transfected with X and P, and coimmunoprecipitation studies indicated that X forms a complex with P. Direct interaction between X and P, but not between X and N, has been also demonstrated in the yeast two-hybrid system and in in vitro binding assays using Ni-agarose-bound N (Schwemmle et al., 1998; Wolff et al., 2000). In contrast to these findings, immunofluorescence studies documented a nuclear colocalization of X and N in cells cotransfected with X and N expression plasmids (Malik et al., 1999). Furthermore, in vitro protein-protein interaction studies on solid-phase-bound N showed a direct interaction between X and N (Malik et al., 1999). Currently available evidence is conflicting and does not permit us to reach a final conclusion on whether there is a direct interaction between X and N proteins. Subcellular localization studies showed colocalization of X with P′ in BDV-infected cells. Whether this finding reflects a direct X-P′ interaction remains to be clarified. Results from coimmunoprecipitation studies supported a direct interaction between X and P′ (Kobayashi et al., 2000). However, binding of P to X has been mapped to amino acids 33 to 115 of P (Malik et al., 2000). This domain is likely to be disrupted in P′ because the 55 N-terminal amino acid residues of P are not present in P′.

BDV X protein contains an amino-terminal short peptide motif that is similar to those previously characterized as bona fide NES in the Rev protein of human immunodeficiency virus type 1 and the NEP/NS2 proteins of influenza virus, as well as the cellular cyclic AMP-dependent protein kinase inhibitor. This finding led to the proposal that X could play a role in nuclear export of BDV proteins and RNP (Schwemmle et al., 1998). However, recent studies of X-P interaction demonstrated that an amino-terminal motif of X rich in leucine, S^2SDLRLTLLELVRRL^{16}, mediates the X-P interaction, and that S^2 and L^{16} are important for this interaction (Malik et al., 2000; Schwemmle et al., 1998). Therefore, the putative NES of X would overlap with the P-binding site, S^2SDLRLTLLELVRRL^{16}, which could interfere with the predicted nuclear export activity of X. Moreover, an X mutant lacking this putative NES was also predominantly found in the cytoplasm (Malik et al., 2000), suggesting that this putative NES may not play an important role in localizing the X protein to the cytoplasm. Further studies will be needed to elucidate the nuclear export activity and the regulatory function(s) of X.

Nuclear Transport of BDV L

Transcription and replication of the BDV genome take place in the nucleus. Therefore, BDV L protein, the predicted viral RNA-dependent RNA polymerase, should be present also in the nucleus. Within the BDV L, amino acid sequence motifs (V^{189}SKNAKWPPV^{197} and W^{943}YKVRKVT^{950}) are present that resemble those proposed to mediate nuclear import of the L protein of the plant nucleorhabdovirus sonchus yellow neat virus. However, it is unknown whether these sequences actually mediate nuclear targeting of BDV L. Immunofluorescence analyses with antisera specific to synthetic L peptides demonstrated that, in the absence of other viral proteins, the L protein is predominantly present in the nuclei of cells transfected with the eukaryotic L expression plasmid (Walker et al., 2000). This suggests that the L protein may possess a functional NLS and is actively translocated to the nucleus after its synthesis in the cytoplasm.

As with other NNS RNA viruses, BDV P and L are expected to interact during the formation of the virus polymerase complex. Coimmunoprecipitation experiments provided evidence for such an interaction. In addition, P and L appear to colocalize in the nucleus of BDV-infected cells (Walker et al., 2000). Unexpectedly, when L and P were cotransfected in cells, L was found in the cytoplasm, whereas P was found in the cytoplasm and the nucleus. It was proposed that overexpression of L and P might have contributed to the observed phenomenon. However, this finding could also reflect our currently limited knowledge about the mechanisms involved in nucleocytoplasmic transport of BDV proteins.

A model for the nucleocytoplasmic trafficking of BDV RNP has been proposed based on the NLS and NES signals, as well as interacting domains, identified in BDV proteins (Kobayashi et al., 2001). This model proposes that relative levels of Np40, Np38, and P may play a key role determining the directionality of BDV RNP movement. Increased levels of nuclear P could reduce nuclear export mediated by the NES of N, due to an overlap between the NES present in N and one of the N binding sites for P'. On the other hand increased levels of Np38 could result in a net increase in the density of NES in Np40/p38 complexes. This, in turn, could enhance nuclear export over retention. Although very attractive, this model does not satisfactorily explain the observation that BDV RNPs that contain the virus genome RNA accumulate in the nucleus and are barely detectable in the cytoplasm at any stage of infection. In addition, there is little evidence supporting significant changes in the N/P ratio during the first 96 h following BDV infection of a variety of susceptible cell lines. However, during this time the virus is able to complete its life cycle as determined by a steady-state increase in the number of infected cells.

PERSPECTIVES

BDV is the prototypic member of a new family of RNA animal viruses. Therefore, the investigation of its molecular and cellular biology may uncover new aspects of the biology of these infectious agents. These investigations will greatly benefit from the establishment of a reverse genetic system similar to those already developed for several NNS RNA viruses. Such a system will allow a detailed analysis of the virus RNA cis-acting signals and viral trans-acting factors required for BDV replication and transcription, as well as assembly and budding of infectious particles. Furthermore, the possibilities of generating predetermined specific mutations within the BDV genome and analyzing their phenotypic expression in animal models will significantly contribute to the elucidation of the molecular mechanisms underlying BDV-host interactions, including BDV persistence and associated disease. BDV also provides an excellent system for the investigation of the steps governing the nucleocytoplasmic transport of cellular mRNAs and proteins, a subject of major importance and wide interest.

Evidence indicates that BDV might infect humans. However, the prevalence of BDV in humans and its possible association with certain neuropsychiatric disorders remains to be solved. Increased knowledge about the molecular and cellular biology of BDV should help in the development of standardized sensitive and reliable serological and nucleic acid diagnostic tests to address this pressing question.

REFERENCES

Barksdale, S., and C. C. Baker. 1995. Differentiation-specific alternative splicing of bovine papillomavirus late mRNAs. J. Virol. 69:6553–6556.

Bause-Niedrig, I., G. Pauli, and H. Ludwig. 1991. Borna disease virus-specific antigens: two different proteins identified by monoclonal antibodies. Vet. Immunol. Immunopathol. 91:293–301.

Berg, M., C. Ehrenborg, J. Blomberg, R. Pipkorn, and A. L. Berg. 1998. Two domains of the Borna disease virus p40 protein are required for interaction with the p23 protein. J. Gen. Virol. 79:2957–2963.

Berget, S. M. 1995. Exon recognition in vertebrate splicing. J. Biol. Chem. 270:2411–2414.

Boulikas, T. 1993. Nuclear localization signals (NLS). Crit. Rev. Eukaryot. Gene Expr. 3:193–227.

Briese, T., J. C. de la Torre, A. Lewis, H. Ludwig, and W. I. Lipkin. 1992. Borna disease virus, a negative-strand RNA virus, transcribes in the nucleus of infected cells. *Proc. Natl. Acad. Sci. USA* **92:**11486–11489.

Carbone, K. M., C. S. Duchala, J. W. Griffin, A. L. Kincaid, and O. Narayan. 1987. Pathogenesis of Borna disease virus in rats: evidence that intra-axonal spread is the major route for dissemination and determinant for disease incubation. *J. Virol.* **61:**3431–3430.

Chabot, B. 1996. Directing alternative splicing: cast and scenarios. *Trends Genet.* **12:**472–478.

Compans, R. W., L. R. Melsen, and J. C. de la Torre. 1994. Virus-like particles in MDCK cells persistently infected with Borna disease virus. *Virus Res.* **94:**261–268.

Cubitt, B., and J. C. de la Torre. 1994. Borna disease virus (BDV), a nonsegmented RNA virus, replicates in the nuclei of infected cells where infectious BDV ribonucleoproteins are present. *J. Virol.* **68:**1371–1381.

Cubitt, B., C. Ly, and J. C. de La Torre. 2001. Identification and characterization of a new intron in Borna disease virus. *J. Gen. Virol.* **82:**641–646.

de la Torre, J. C. 1994. Molecular biology of Borna disease virus: prototype of a new group of animal viruses. *J. Virol.* **94:**7669–7675.

Etessami, R., K. K. Conzelmann, B. Fadai-Ghotbi, B. Natelson, H. Tsiang, and P. E. Ceccaldi. 2000. Spread and pathogenic characteristics of a G-deficient rabies virus recombinant: an in vitro and in vivo study. *J. Gen. Virol.* **81:**2147–2153.

Fearns, R., and P. L. Collins. 1999. Model for polymerase access to the overlapped L gene of respiratory syncytial virus. *J. Virol.* **73:**388–397.

Furrer, E., T. Bilzer, L. Stitz, and O. Planz. 2001. Neutralizing antibodies in persistent Borna disease virus infection: prophylactic effect of gp94-specific monoclonal antibodies in preventing encephalitis. *J. Virol.* **75:**943–951.

Gonzalez-Dunia, D., B. Cubitt, and J. C. de la Torre. 1998. Mechanism of Borna disease virus entry into cells. *J. Virol.* **72:**783–788.

Gonzalez-Dunia, D., B. Cubitt, F. A. Grasser, and J. C. de la Torre. 1997a. Characterization of Borna disease virus p56 protein, a surface glycoprotein involved in virus entry. *J. Virol.* **71:**3208–3218.

Gonzalez-Dunia, D., C. Sauder, and J. C. de la Torre. 1997b. Borna disease virus and the brain. *Brain Res.* **44:**647–664.

Gorlich, D. 1998. Transport into and out of the cell nucleus. *EMBO J* **17:**2721–2727.

Gosztonyi, G., B. Dietzschold, M. Kao, C. E. Rupprecht, H. Ludwig, and H. Koprowski. 1993. Rabies and borna disease. A comparative pathogenetic study of two neurovirulent agents. *Lab. Investig.* **93:**285–295.

Gosztonyi, G., and H. Ludwig. 1995. Borna disease—neuropathology and pathogenesis, p. 39–74. *In* H. Koprowski and W. I. Lipkin (ed.), *Borna Disease Virus.* Springer-Verlag, Berlin, Germany.

Haas, B., H. Becht, and R. Rott. 1986. Purification and properties of an intranuclear virus-specific antigen from tissue infected with Borna disease virus. *J. Gen. Virol.* **86:**235–241.

Hatalski, C. G., A. J. Lewis, and W. I. Lipkin. 1997. Borna disease. *Emerg. Infect. Dis.* **3:**129–135.

Hutchinson, L., C. Roop-Beauchamp, and D. C. Johnson. 1995. Herpes simplex virus glycoprotein K is known to influence fusion of infected cells, yet is not on the cell surface. *J. Virol.* **69:**4556–4563.

Jehle, C., W. I. Lipkin, P. Staehell, R. M. Marion, and M. Schwemmle. 2000. Authentic Borna disease virus transcripts are spliced less efficiently than cDNA-derived viral RNAs. *J. Gen. Virol.* **81:**1947–1954.

Kanopka, A., O. Muhlemann, S. Petersen-Mahrt, C. Estmer, C. Ohrmalm, and G. Akusjarvi. 1998. Regulation of adenovirus alternative RNA splicing by dephosphorylation of SR proteins. *Nature* **393:**185–187.

Kliche, S., T. Briese, A. H. Henschen, L. Stitz, and W. I. Lipkin. 1994. Characterization of a Borna disease virus glycoprotein, gp18. *J. Virol.* **94**:6918–6923.

Kobayashi, T., W. Kamitani, G. Zhang, M. Watanabe, K. Tomonaga, and K. Ikuta. 2001. Borna disease virus nucleoprotein requires both nuclear localization and export activities for viral nucleocytoplasmic shuttling. *J. Virol.* **75**:3404–3412.

Kobayashi, T., Y. Shoya, T. Koda, I. Takashima, P. K. Lai, K. Ikuta, M. Kakinuma, and K. Masahiko. 1998. Nuclear targeting activity associated with the amino terminal region of the Borna disease virus nucleoprotein. *Virology* **243**:188–197.

Kobayashi, T., M. Watanabe, W. Kamitani, K. Tomonaga, and K. Ikuta. 2000. Translation initiation of a bicistronic mRNA of Borna disease virus: a 16-kDa phosphoprotein is initiated at an internal start codon. *Virology* **277**:296–305.

Kohno, T., T. Goto, T. Takasaki, C. Morita, T. Nakaya, K. Ikuta, I. Kurane, K. Sano, and M. Nakai. 1999. Fine structure and morphogenesis of Borna disease virus. *J. Virol.* **73**:760–766.

Kraus, I., M. Eickmann, S. Kiermayer, H. Scheffczik, M. Fluess, J. A. Richt, and W. Garten. 2001. Open reading frame III of Borna disease virus encodes a nonglycosylated matrix protein. *J. Virol.* **75**:12098–12104.

Lamb, R. A., and D. Kolakofsky. 1996. Paramyxoviridae: the viruses and their replication, p. 1177–1204. *In* D. M. Knipe, B. N. Fields, P. M. Howley, R. M. Chanock, J. L. Melnick, T. P. Monath, B. Roizman, and S. E. Straus (ed.), *Fields Virology,* 3rd ed. Lippincott-Raven, Philadelphia, Pa.

Lamb, R. A., and C. M. Horvath. 1991. Diversity of coding strategies in influenza viruses. *Trends Genet.* **7**:261–266.

Lipkin, W. I., C. G. Hatalski, and T. Briese. 1997. Neurobiology of Borna disease virus. *J. Neurovirol.* **3**:S17–S20.

Lopez, A. J. 1998. Alternative splicing of pre-mRNA: developmental consequences and mechanisms of regulation. *Annu. Rev. Genet.* **32**:279–305.

Malik, T. H., M. Kishi, and P. K. Lai. 2000. Characterization of the P protein-binding domain on the 10-kilodalton protein of Borna disease virus. *J. Virol.* **74**:3413–3417.

Malik, T. H., T. Kobayashi, M. Ghosh, M. Kishi, and P. K. Lai. 1999. Nuclear localization of the protein from the open reading frame ×1 of the Borna disease virus was through interactions with the viral nucleoprotein. *Virology* **258**:65–72.

Nakielny, S., and G. Dreyfuss. 1999. Transport of proteins and RNAs in and out of the nucleus. *Cell* **99**:677–690.

Perez, M., M. Watanabe, M. A. Whitt, and J. C. de la Torre. 2001. N-terminal domain of Borna disease virus G (p56) protein is sufficient for virus receptor recognition and cell entry. *J. Virol.* **75**:7078–7085.

Peters, C. J., A. Sanchez, P. E. Rollin, T. G. Ksiazek, and F. A. Murphy. 1996. Filoviridae: Marburg and ebola viruses, p. 1161–1176. *In* D. M. Knipe, B. N. Fields, P. M. Howley, R. M. Chanock, J. L. Melnick, T. P. Monath, B. Roizman, and S. E. Straus (ed.), *Fields Virology,* 3rd ed. Lippincott-Raven, Philadelphia, Pa.

Pyper, J. M., J. E., Clements, and M. C. Zink. 1998. The nucleolus is the site of Borna disease virus RNA transcription and replication. *J. Virol.* **72**:7697–7702.

Pyper, J. M., and A. E. Gartner. 1997. Molecular basis for the differential subcellular localization of the 38- and 39-kilodalton structural proteins of Borna disease virus. *J. Virol.* **71**:5133–5139.

Richt, J. A., I. Pfeuffer, M. Christ, K. Frese, K. Bechter, and S. Herzog. 1997. Borna disease virus infection in animals and humans. *Emerg. Infect. Dis.* **3**:343–352.

Rott, R., and H. Becht. 1995. Natural and experimental Borna disease in animals, p. 17–30. *In* H. Koprowski and W. I. Lipkin (ed.), *Borna Disease.* Springer-Verlag, Berlin, Germany.

Sanchez, A., S. G. Trappier, B. W. Mahy, C. J. Peters, and S. T. Nichol. 1996. The virion glycoproteins of Ebola viruses are encoded in two reading frames and are expressed through transcriptional editing. *Proc. Natl. Acad. Sci. USA* **93**:3602–3607.

Schneemann, A., P. A. Schneider, S. Kim, and W. I. Lipkin. 1994. Identification of signal sequences that control transcription of Borna disease virus, a nonsegmented, negative-strand RNA virus. *J. Virol.* **94:**6514–6522.

Schneemann, A., P. A. Schneider, R. A. Lamb, and W. I. Lipkin. 1995. The remarkable coding strategy of borna disease virus: a new member of the nonsegmented negative strand RNA viruses. *Virology* **95:**1–8.

Schneider, P. A., R. Kim, and W. I. Lipkin. 1997. Evidence for translation of the Borna disease virus G protein by leaky ribosomal scanning and ribosomal reinitiation. *J. Virol.* **71:**5614–5619.

Schwemmle, M., B. De, L. Shi, A. Banerjee, and W. I. Lipkin. 1997. Borna disease virus P-protein is phosphorylated by protein kinase Cε and casein kinase II. *J. Biol. Chem.* **272:**21818–21823.

Schwemmle, M., M. Salvatore, L. Shi, J. Richt, C. H. Lee, and W. I. Lipkin. 1998. Interactions of the Borna disease virus P, N, and X proteins and their functional implications. *J. Biol. Chem.* **273:**9007–9012.

Shoya, Y., T. Kobayashi, T. Koda, K. Ikuta, M. Kakinuma, and M. Kishi. 1998. Two proline-rich nuclear localization signals in the amino- and carboxyl-terminal regions of the Borna disease virus phosphoprotein. *J. Virol.* **72:**9755–9762.

Sierra-Honigmann, A. M., S. A. Rubin, M. G. Estafanous, R. H. Yolken, and K. M. Carbone. 1993. Borna disease virus in peripheral blood mononuclear and bone marrow cells of neonatally and chronically infected rats. *J. Neuroimmunol.* **93:**31–32.

Smith, C. W., and J. Valcarcel. 2000. Alternative pre-mRNA splicing: the logic of combinatorial control. *Trends Biochem. Sci.* **25:**381–388.

Staeheli, P., C. Sauder, J. Hausmann, F. Ehrensperger, and M. Schwemmle. 2000. Epidemiology of Borna disease virus. *J. Gen. Virol.* **81:**2123–2135.

Thiedemann, N., P. Presek, R. Rott, and L. Stitz. 1992. Antigenic relationship and further characterization of two major Borna disease virus-specific proteins. *J. Gen. Virol.* **92:**1057–1064.

Thierer, J., H. Riehle, O. Grebenstein, T. Binz, S. Herzog, N. Thiedemann, L. Stitz, R. Rott, F. Lottspeich, and H. Niemann. 1992. The 24K protein of Borna disease virus. *J. Gen. Virol.* **92:**413–416.

Tomonaga, K., T. Kobayashi, B.-J. Lee, M. Watanabe, W. Kamitani, and K. Ikuta. 2000. Identification of alternative splicing and negative splicing activity of a nonsegmented negative-strand RNA virus. Borna disease virus. *Proc. Natl. Acad. Sci. USA* **97:**12788–12793.

Wagner, R. R., and J. K. Rose. 1996. Rhabdoviridae: the viruses and their replication, p. 1121–1135. *In* D. M. Knipe, B. N. Fields, P. M. Howley, R. M. Chanock, J. L. Melnick, T. P. Monath, B. Roizman, and S. E. Straus (ed.), *Fields Virology,* 3rd ed. Lippincott-Raven, Philadelphia, Pa.

Walker, M. P., I. Jordan, T. Briese, N. Fischer, and W. I. Lipkin. 2000. Expression and characterization of the Borna disease virus polymerase. *J. Virol.* **74:**3325–4428.

Wehner, T., A. Ruppert, C. Herden, K. Frese, H. Becht, and J. A. Richt. 1997. Detection of a novel Borna disease virus-encoded 10 kDa protein in infected cells and tissues. *J. Gen. Virol.* **78:**2459–2466.

Whittaker, G. R., and A. Helenius. 1998. Nuclear import and export of viruses and virus genomes. *Virology* **246:**1–23.

Wolff, T., R. Pfleger, T. Wehner, J. Reinhardt, and J. A. Richt. 2000. A short leucinerich sequence in the Borna disease virus p10 protein mediates association with the viral phospho- and nucleoproteins. *J. Gen. Virol.* **4:**939–947.

Zimmermann, W., H. Breter, M. Rudolph, and H. Ludwig. 1994. Borna disease virus: immunoelectron microscopic characterization of cell-free virus and further information about the genome. *J. Virol.* **68:**6755–6758.

.

Borna Disease Virus and Its Role in Neurobehavioral Disease
Edited by K. M. Carbone
© 2002 ASM Press, Washington, D.C.

Chapter 3

Laboratory Diagnosis

Christian Sauder, Tetsuya Mizutani, and Kazunari Yamaguchi

Laboratory diagnosis of Borna disease virus (BDV) has increasingly become a crucial issue in BDV research during the past 15 years. The methods of intra vitam diagnosis of BDV infection in animals that display neurological symptoms typical for Borna disease (BD) have gained general acceptance. However, the question whether latent BDV infections both in animals and humans can be proven unequivocally intra vitam using the currently available diagnostic tools has become the subject of a controversial debate, which is still ongoing. So far, definitive proof of BDV infection still requires postmortem analysis. Before we discuss the manifold specific problems inherent to BDV diagnosis, the various tools for BDV diagnosis currently in use will be presented.

SEROLOGY

Serology is still the most commonly used intra vitam detection method. As discussed in chapters 4 and 6, seroepidemiological studies employing diverse serological methods suggest a worldwide presence of BDV-reactive antibodies both in animals such as horses, sheep, cats, and cattle and in humans. Since the vast majority of animals identified as seropositive were healthy, these studies also imply that inapparent BDV infections occur much more frequently than previously thought. How-

Christian Sauder • Department of Virology, Institute for Medical Microbiology and Hygiene, University of Freiburg, Hermann-Herder-Strasse 11, 79104 Freiburg, Germany. **Kazunari Yamaguchi** • Blood Transfusion Service and Internal Medicine, Kumamoto University School of Medicine, Honjo 1-1-1, Kumamoto 860-8556, Japan. **Tetsuya Mizutani** • Laboratory of Public Health, Department of Environmental Veterinary Sciences, Graduate School of Veterinary Medicine, Hokkaido University, Kita-ku, Kita-18, Nishi-9, Sapporo 060-0818, Japan.

ever, alternatively, these findings might be due to the use of serological methods that lack sufficient specificity, thus yielding false-positive results. Serum and plasma samples were used in most cases in these studies. Cerebrospinal fluid (CSF) was also found to contain BDV-reactive antibodies in some studies. An intriguing feature of BDV serology is the finding that titers of BDV-reactive antibodies both in humans and naturally infected animals often are below 1:40. Therefore, highly sensitive, but also specific, serological techniques are required. The question of whether the currently used serological techniques meet both criteria is a central issue of BDV serology. In the following, these techniques will be described (Table 1). Later in this chapter (under "Difficulties Encountered in Diagnosis") their diagnostic values for BDV diagnosis will be critically evaluated.

IFA

Indirect immunofluorescence assay (IFA) is the most commonly used method for detection of anti-BDV antibodies in animals and humans. Various persistently infected cell lines are used as a source of BDV antigen, such as young rabbit brain cells, rabbit embryonic fibroblasts, rabbit kidney cells (RK-13), Madin-Darby canine kidney (MDCK) cells (Herzog and Rott, 1980; Rott et al., 1985; Waltrip et al., 1995; Kitze et al., 1996; Kubo et al., 1997), baby hamster kidney (BHK) cells (Kao et al., 1993), Vero cells, rat glioblastoma (C6) cells, or oligo cells (Katz et al., 1998; Allmang et al., 2001). In case of IFA employing MDCK cells, sera usually are diluted 1:10 in swine serum following adsorption with swine liver powder to eliminate nonspecific background staining (Rott et al., 1985). Sera then are added in twofold dilutions to both uninfected MDCK cells and persistently BDV-infected MDCK cells. Fluorescein (FL) isothiocyanate-conjugated antiserum to human or animal immunoglobulin is used as secondary antibody and bound antibody can be visualized by standard fluorescent mi-

Table 1. Serological methods to detect anti-BDV antibodies

IFA
WBA
ELISA techniques
  • Indirect ELISA
  • Capture ELISA
  • cELISA
  • RS-ELISA
IP
ECLIA

croscopy. A sample is determined to be seropositive when a typical intranuclear fluorescence can be identified in the persistently BDV-infected MDCK cells, but not in the uninfected control cells. BDV-specific antibodies generally exhibit a characteristic punctate fluorescence confined to the nuclei of infected cells. An example of a seropositive horse and human serum tested on infected and uninfected C6 cells is shown in Fig. 1.

Bode et al. (1992) developed a modified double-stain immunofluorescence test. They used BDV-infected young rabbit brain cells and performed IFA by incubation of cells with a mixture of test serum and a mouse monoclonal antibody (MAb) specific for BDV-p40 (nucleoprotein

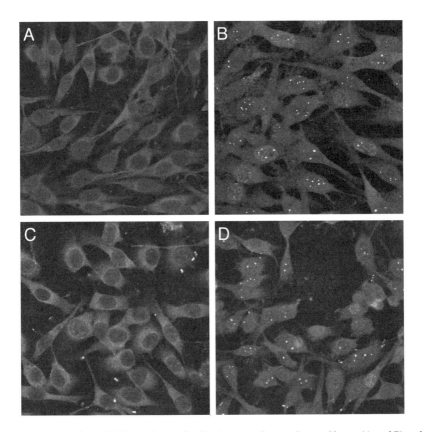

Figure 1. IFA to detect BDV-reactive antibodies in serum from a diseased horse (A and B) and a psychiatric patient (C and D), using C6 cells (A and C) and persistently BDV-infected C6 cells (B and D). Both sera contain BDV-reactive antibodies as judged by the punctate staining pattern in nuclei of infected cells. (Courtesy of Christian Billich.)

[N]). After applying two different anti-immunoglobulin (anti-Ig) species-specific antibodies linked to two different fluorescent molecules, sera were scored as positive when the immunofluorescent signal for the test sera revealed the same characteristic nuclear staining pattern as the immunofluorescent signal for the mouse monoclonal anti-BDV antibody.

WBA

In contrast to IFA, Western blot assay (WBA) allows discrimination between recognition of one, two, or more BDV proteins. The various WBAs that have been used by several research groups differ mainly in the source of antigens separated by sodium dodecyl sulfate-polyacrylamide gel electrophoresis. Both crude cell extracts and purified antigens have been used. Whole-cell extracts were prepared from persistently BDV-infected MDCK cells (Rott et al., 1991) or BDV-infected human neuroblastoma SK-N-SY5Y cell lines (Waltrip et al., 1995), as well as from insect cells expressing the BDV proteins N, p24 (phosphoprotein [P]), or p16 (matrix protein [M]), respectively, following infection with genetically modified baculoviruses carrying the respective BDV genes (Hsu et al., 1994; Sauder et al., 1996; Ogino et al., 1998). In some laboratories, the criterion for specificity of positive sera was evidence of successful competition of binding of test serum antibodies to immobilized BDV proteins by prior absorption of test sera with cell extracts from insect cells containing the respective BDV antigens (Sauder et al., 1996). Waltrip et al. (1995) introduced as a criterion for seropositivity the recognition of at least two BDV proteins by test sera.

Purified antigens for WBA were prepared from the following sources. BDV-infected cells (rabbit kidney cells [Fu et al., 1993]), BDV-infected rat brains (Kao et al., 1993) and bacteria which express BDV proteins fused to different tags: glutathione S-transferase (GST)-P (Kishi et al., 1995; Nakamura et al., 1995); GST-P and GST-N (Takahashi et al., 1997); and GST-N, -P, and -M (Nakaya et al., 1999). GST alone was always used as a negative control. In some studies, competition experiments were carried out to demonstrate specificity of WBA signals by preadsorption of sera with GST-N or GST-P (Nishino et al., 1999). Fukuda et al. (2001) generated bacterially expressed viral N and P proteins fused to GST that was subsequently cleaved off the viral proteins. These proteins were subjected to further purification by MonoQ column chromatography. BDV specificity of antibodies was evaluated by binding competition tests employing purified BDV antigens.

His-tagged BDV antigens (N, P, and M) were expressed in bacteria and purified, and subsequently the His tag was removed (Briese et al., 1995). BDV proteins N and P, each fused to intein, were expressed in bacteria, purified, and released from intein (Chen et al., 1999b). In the latter case, WBA included competition experiments, consisting of preadsorption of sera with crude cell extracts prepared from infected and noninfected MDCK cells.

ELISA

Several enzyme-linked immunosorbent assay (ELISA) techniques were developed with the intention to provide a rapid, sensitive screening method.

Classical ELISA

In classical ELISA, plates are coated with BDV antigens and then incubated with test sera. The various laboratories employed different proteins as follows:

1. Weisman et al. (1994) and Briese et al. (1995) used bacterially expressed His-tagged BDV N, P, and M. Proteins were purified following removal of the His tag. In these two studies, no unrelated control protein was used as a control.
2. Evengård et al. (1999) improved this method by including bacterially expressed purified β-galactosidase as an unrelated protein for a negative control. More-stringent criteria for seropositivity were introduced, i.e., recognition of two or more BDV proteins.
3. Reeves et al. (1998) used purified His-tagged P protein for the analysis of cat sera. Preadsorption of sera with *Escherichia coli* proteins was required because of high amounts of antibodies against *E. coli* in cat sera. No unrelated proteins were used as a negative control.
4. Purified GST-P and GST as a negative control were used (Kishi et al., 1995; Kitani et al., 1996; Takahashi et al., 1997). Purified GST-N, GST-P, GST-M, and GST (negative control) were used by Berg et al. (1999).

Capture ELISA

Tsujimura et al. (1999) developed a capture ELISA based on detection of antibodies against BDV N to investigate the prevalence of BDV infection among wild rats. The plates are coated with MAbs against BDV N (which do not cross-react with P) and are subsequently incubated with re-combinant N antigen. The latter is secreted by insect cells following infec-tion with a recombinant baculovirus (Hsu et al., 1994). After addition of serum samples, bound antibodies can be visualized with horseradish per-oxidase-labeled anti-rat IgG. This capture ELISA was found to be specific and sensitive when rat sera were analyzed.

cELISA

Katz et al. (1998) analyzed sera of ponies experimentally infected with BDV for presence of BDV antibodies using competitive ELISA (cELISA). BDV N antigen, secreted by insect cells infected with an N recombinant baculovirus, was spread onto a 96-well plate. Test sera and negative con-trol sera (here, preinoculation serum) then were placed in duplicate wells. Without removing test or control sera, a defined amount of a mouse anti-N MAb was added to each well as a competitor. Bound anti-N MAb was detected using a goat origin anti-mouse IgG conjugated to peroxidase. Test sera were evaluated to their end points. The end point was defined as the greatest test serum dilution producing more than 40% inhibition of the optical density at 405 nm relative to the respective negative control (preinoculation) serum cELISA optical density at 405 nm. Sera from dif-ferent species can be screened without need for species-specific secondary antibodies in this assay. Nevertheless, instead of using an anti-N MAb, polyclonal rabbit anti-N serum might be preferred, since antibodies in test sera most likely also recognize epitopes on N other than the one recog-nized by a MAb. Polyclonal N serum, rather than an N MAb, likely will be more able to compete with test sera for binding to these epitopes.

RS-ELISA

Horimoto et al. (1997) established a reverse-type sandwich ELISA (RS-ELISA) to detect specific antibodies to BDV. Microplate wells were coated with purified BDV N antigen (bacterially expressed as GST-N; GST was cleaved off). Bacterial proteins, present at a low level in the N prepa-rations as contaminants, also bind to the wells. Next, test samples were added at a low dilution, with hopes that the BDV-specific antibodies would bind to N with only one side of the molecule. In a similar manner, serum antibodies specific for bacterial proteins would also bind. More-over, nonspecific binding of antibodies (both sides of the molecule) to the solid phase of wells can occur when samples are used at low dilutions. To block binding sites of antibodies to bacterial proteins, wells were incu-bated with E. coli lysates. Next, wells were incubated with biotinylated N antigen, which can be captured by the remaining free binding site of bound N-specific antibodies. A preformed complex of streptavidin and horseradish peroxidase-conjugated biotin and an enzyme substrate were then used to measure the captured biotinylated N. The RS-ELISA was designed with the aim to specifically detect anti-BDV antibodies without nonspecific signals. In addition, RS-ELISA allows detection of antibodies from different species using the same assay, without the requirement for antibodies with specificity for different immunoglobulin classes and species. Thus, BDV serological studies are possible even in species where suitable reagents are not yet available.

IP

Bode et al. (1992) performed immunoprecipitation (IP) to detect BDV-reactive human antibodies using cell lysates prepared from persistently BDV-infected and uninfected Vero cells, respectively. The cell lysates were ultracentrifuged, and the supernatants were used for IP. Human sera were incubated with anti-species IgG-agarose beads. After the beads were washed, lysate and control lysate, respectively, were added. After boiling, the precipitates were separated by sodium dodecyl sulfate-polyacrylamide gel electrophoresis and blotted onto nitrocellulose. The immunostaining was carried out using BDV rabbit immune serum and normal rabbit serum, respectively. VandeWoude et al. (1990) generated, by in vitro translation, [35S]methionine-labeled BDV P protein, which was subjected to IP using human sera.

ECLIA

Yamaguchi et al. (1999) developed an electrochemiluminescence immunoassay (ECLIA) for detection of BDV antibodies against BDV N and P proteins with the aim to provide a rapid, sensitive, and specific serological screening method to detect BDV antibodies. Full-length BDV N and P proteins fused to GST were bacterially expressed and released from GST by cleavage with factor Xa following binding on glutathione-Sepharose. To remove contaminating proteins derived from *E. coli*, possibly present in the preparations, recombinant proteins were additionally purified by ion-exchange chromatography using Mono Q followed by affinity chromatography using Sepharose 4B that was loaded with rabbit anti-*E. coli* IgG. Recombinant proteins were mixed and subsequently used to coat microbeads, and the washed recombinant protein-coated beads were incubated with test sera, diluted 1:10 in normal rabbit serum. After being washed, the beads then were mixed with the second antibody, anti-species specific (anti-human, anti-horse, etc.) rabbit IgG monoclonal or polyclonal antibodies coupled with ruthenium (II) Tris (bipyridyl)-N-hydroxysuccin-imide ester [Ru(bpy)$_3^{2+}$]. After washing, the beads were conducted into the electrode, and the photons (wavelength: 620 nm) emitted from Ru(bpy)$_3^{2+}$ coupled with the second antibody were counted by the photomultiplier tube. This ECLIA procedure can be carried out in an automatic ECLIA an-alyzer. A sample is considered positive if the ECLIA counts are higher than the cutoff counts, i.e., in case of human sera, the mean plus 3 standard deviations of the ECLIA counts measured in 200 human blood donor sam-ples as controls. A competitive inhibition test was introduced as an addi-tional criterion for specificity of ECLIA-positive samples. The inhibition test was carried out by preincubation of serum samples with 10 volumes of normal rabbit serum containing 1 μg each of both recombinant proteins or, as a control, with normal rabbit serum alone. Samples were then sub-jected to ECLIA. The sera were finally scored as antibody positive if the ECLIA counts were reduced by more than 50% compared to those mea-sured in the controls.

Recently, Yamaguchi et al. (2001) also developed an ECLIA for detec-tion of BDV specific antibodies based on three synthetic peptides corre-sponding to amino acid (aa) 3 to 20 and aa 338 to 358 of BDV N and to aa 59 to 79 of BDV P. These peptides were found to be selectively bound by sera of several rabbits immunized with recombinant full-length BDV P or N proteins. It was concluded that these peptides represented the main BDV N and P epitopes. Analysis of sera derived from experimentally in-fected rats and horses as well as of uninfected control animals and natu-rally infected horses suggests a good sensitivity and specificity of this ECLIA.

VIRUS ANTIGEN DETECTION

To directly demonstrate infection with BDV, several methods to de-tect BDV antigens are in use (Table 2). For obvious reasons, most of these techniques can only be applied for postmortem diagnosis.

IHC

Immunohistochemistry (IHC) is the most commonly used technique for postmortem confirmation of BDV infection in animals, using frozen brain sections or, more frequently, sections from paraffin-embedded, for-malin-fixed brains. Antigens have been detected employing polyclonal an-

Table 2. Virus antigen and RNA detection methods for BDV diagnosis

Methods
Antigen detection
IHC
WBA
Antigen capture ELISA
FACS analysis
RNA detection
Northern hybridization
RT-PCR (one tube or two tube)
RT-nested PCR
RT-PCR-EIA
ISH

tibodies (Gosztonyi and Ludwig, 1984; Caplazi and Ehrensperger, 1998; de la Torre et al., 1996) or MAbs specific for BDV antigens N, P, M, gp94 (envelope protein [G]), and p10 (X) (Herzog et al., 1994; Weissenböck et al., 1998; Lundgren et al., 1995a; Bilzer et al., 1995; Herden et al., 1999; Wehner et al., 1997). Bound antibodies can be visualized using standard methods such as the IFA technique or streptavidin-biotin-horseradish peroxidase, peroxidase-anti-peroxidase, or alkaline phosphatase-antialkaline phosphatase (Degiorgis et al., 2000) techniques with diaminobenzidine, 3-amino-9-ethylcarbazole (Lundgren et al., 1995a) or fast red as chromogen substrates. BDV antigens usually are predominantly present in neurons but are also present in astrocytes and ependymal cells (Carbone et al., 1989; Bilzer et al., 1995; Bilzer et al., 1996).

WBA

As an alternative to IHC, WBA is also commonly used to detect viral antigen in tissues. In addition to postmortem analysis of homogenates derived from different brain regions and peripheral organs, saliva, nasal secretions, conjunctival fluid, and CSF have been subjected to WBA analysis (Herzog et al., 1994; Bilzer et al., 1995; Lebelt and Hagenau, 1996). Studies employing postmortem tissues of horses, sheep, and donkeys with BD suggested that IHC and WBA analyses display comparable reliability (Bilzer et al., 1996; Herden et al., 1999).

BDV antigen is usually detectable in brains of naturally or experimentally infected animals. However, limited information is available regarding detection rates of antigen in peripheral organs of naturally infected animals by means of WBA or IHC. In experimentally BDV-infected newborn rats and adult, immunosuppressed, BDV-infected rats, BDV antigen was detected in the peripheral and autonomic nervous systems and also in nonneural peripheral tissues (Herzog et al., 1984; Stitz et al., 1991, 1998). In contrast to previous studies that failed to demonstrate BDV antigens in peripheral tissues of adult BDV-infected, immunocompetent rats (Herzog et al., 1984; Stitz et al., 1991), other studies suggest the presence of BDV antigens in peripheral nerves and nerve fibers or ganglion cells of the autonomic nervous system in virtually all tissues investigated (Carbone et al., 1987; Stitz et al., 1998). The discrepancies between the studies might be related to the time postinfection when animals were euthanized; e.g., Stitz et al. (1998) found antigen in the peripheral nervous system only after day 21 postinfection.

BDV antigen seems to be only very rarely detected in peripheral organs in natural infections (Herzog et al., 1994; Bilzer et al., 1995; Lebelt and Hagenau, 1996). Therefore, diagnosis of BDV infection by IHC and WBA should be primarily focused on brain material.

Even though BDV antigen usually can easily be detected in the infected brain, there are exceptions. For instance, only a low amount of BDV N antigen was detectable in a few neurons in the brain of a sheep displaying typical neurological signs and strong inflammation (Caplazi and Ehrensperger, 1998). Similarly, BDV-specific antigen was only present in a few cells in brains of cats with BD-like meningoencephalitis (staggering disease) (Lundgren et al, 1995a). Studies employing IHC and/or WBA clearly showed that the detection rates and distribution of BDV antigens in brains could vary considerably, e.g., depending on the MAb used. In animals with BD, viral antigen is reported most often in the hippocampus, consistent with the known affinity of the virus for limbic structures. In one study, expression of BDV M antigen in horse brains was found to be strong and widespread, whereas localization of N antigen in the same brains was mainly confined to the hippocampus (Bilzer et al., 1995; Lebelt and Hagenau, 1996). Another study, employing MAbs specific for BDV proteins N, P, X, and G, found positive immunoreactivity against BDV proteins N, P, and X in all 28 horse brains analyzed, whereas detection of the viral glycoprotein G succeeded only in 43% of cases (Herden et al., 1999). These discrepancies likely are both related to the sensitivity and specificity of the respective antibodies used as well as to the specific biology of the virus. Interestingly, when analyzing the brain of one diseased horse by IHC and WBA, Herzog et al. (1994, 1997) could easily detect BDV proteins P and N using sera from infected rats but failed to detect BDV N antigen using a MAb (Bo18) specific for this protein. This example suggests the existence of BDV variants, which may not be detected using certain MAbs. Taken as a whole, these data suggest that detection of BDV antigen should not exclusively rely on use of only one monospecific serum but rather should employ polyclonal sera or a combination of different MAbs (Herden et al., 1999). Results thus far show the possibility of considerable variability both in the amount and distribution of antigen in brain and in the existence of BDV variants, considerations that have to be taken into account for diagnosis of BDV by means of IHC and WBA.

Antigen Capture ELISA

In addition to these techniques, an antigen capture ELISA for BDV antigen detection has been developed (Lundgren et al., 1995b; Dürrwald, 1993). This assay is based on the principle of a sandwich ELISA. Briefly, a cocktail of MAbs against BDV P and N is bound to an ELISA plate via goat anti-mouse antiserum. Following incubation of plates with test material, bound antigens then can be detected using heterologous hyperimmune sera against BDV N or P, preferentially of rabbit origin. Rabbit IgG is monitored in the ELISA by anti-rabbit Ig antibodies conjugated with alkaline phosphatase. This assay has been used to detect BDV antigen in brain homogenates of diverse animals, such as horses, cattle, and cats, and also in homogenates of peripheral organs of these animals, such as spleen, liver, and kidney (Dürrwald, 1993; Bode et al., 1994a; Lundgren et al., 1995b). BDV antigen could be detected in these organs from several diseased horses and cattle when, in comparable studies, IHC or WBA techniques (Bilzer et al., 1995; Lebelt and Hagenau, 1996) failed to detect BDV antigen in these organs in virtually all cases analyzed. Thus, the antigen capture ELISA appears to display a higher sensitivity than WBA or IHC. The antigen capture ELISA has been used to provide evidence for presence of BDV antigen in CSF and blood samples both of human and animal origin (Deuschle et al., 1998; Bode and Ludwig, 1997). Intriguingly, BDV antigen was detected in 66% of CSF samples ($n = 30$) obtained from horses with BD (Dürrwald, 1993). In contrast, however, none of the 11 CSF samples from diseased horses scored positive by WBA analysis employing monoclonal anti-BDV N and -BDV P antibodies (Lebelt and Hagenau, 1996). Again, these discrepant findings might be due to differences in assay sensitivities. Alternatively, it cannot be excluded that a poor specificity of the antigen ELISA accounts for divergent findings. Since no experimental data are available so far regarding a direct comparison of this assay with the traditional IHC or WBA techniques using aliquots of the same samples, a test of the relative specificity and sensitivity of these assays is needed.

FACS

Since CSF and blood are amenable to intra vitam diagnosis techniques, the question of whether BDV antigen can be detected in these compartments in BDV-infected individuals is of considerable importance for epidemiological studies. In particular, this question also relates to studies that screened peripheral blood mononuclear cells (PBMCs) of humans and animals for the presence of BDV antigens by means of fluorescence-activated cell sorting (FACS) analysis employing MAbs against BDV N and P proteins (Bode et al., 1994b, Bode et al., 1995; Bode, 1995). Astonishingly, BDV antigens were reported in a subpopulation (15 to 17%) of monocytes, or 1% of total PBMCs, in as much as 40 to 50% of psychiatric patients ($n = 140$). Unfortunately, the antigen detection rate using this technique in a healthy control cohort is unknown. Moreover, although BDV antigen-positive monocytes also were reported to be present in naturally or experimentally infected animals, the prevalence rates for antigen in these animals were not published, and this information is needed to evaluate the specificity of this assay. Moreover, other researchers' findings with experimental animals have failed to support the hypothesis of the presence of large numbers of BDV-infected, circulating monocytes. Data resulting from studies using experimentally infected rats indicate that the number of infected PBMCs is extremely low, less than one in several million PBMCs (Sierra-Honigmann et al., 1993; Rubin et al., 1995; Sauder et al., 1998). Therefore, detection of infected PBMCs in animals required the highly sensitive reverse transcription (RT)–nested-PCR methodology to capture evidence of viral RNA in these cells (see below and chapter 5). Narayan et al. (1983) also failed to demonstrate infectivity and antigen in cultures of macrophages derived from the peripheral blood of adult infected rats. Likewise, by means of IFA, Rubin et al. (1995) could show that BDV-infected cells in PBMCs of newborn infected rats were not macrophages, but possibly circulating fibroblastic stromal cell precursors in the peripheral blood. Finally, in vitro infection studies suggest that rabbit macrophages are resistant to infection with BDV (Herzog and Rott, 1980). Although caution is warranted when extrapolating these findings to human tissue, the animal data are in contrast to the reported presence of BDV antigens in human monocytes (Bode et al., 1994b). Even under the assumption that the viral load per cell is very low, detection of BDV RNA in 1% of human PBMCs should not require the use of RT-nested PCR. While the reasons for these discrepancies are unknown, they raise concerns regarding the specificity of the FACS assay proposed by Bode et al. The BDV-related findings using this assay still await independent confirmations and the diagnostic value of this method remains to be defined.

In summary, IHC and WBA are reliable tools to detect BDV antigen in postmortem brain tissue and are indispensable for definitive proof of BDV infection.

VIRUS RNA DETECTION

Following the cloning and sequencing of the BDV genome in the early 1990s, (VandeWoude et al., 1990; Lipkin et al., 1990; Briese et al., 1994; Cubitt et al., 1994), the development of specific and sensitive methods for detection of BDV RNA in tissues of BDV-infected individuals became feasible. Several techniques to detect BDV RNA have since been established (Table 2), and this section provides an overview on the various techniques in use. Later (see "Difficulties Encountered in Diagnosis"), we will discuss the problems that were encountered when applying those methods for BDV diagnosis.

Generally, BDV can be detected in postmortem tissues and also in tissues amenable to intra vitam diagnosis such as blood and body secretions. Either BDV sequences are identified in RNA prepared from these tissues, or virus can more directly be detected in tissue sections via in situ hybridization (ISH). Most tissues are frozen at −80°C upon removal, and thus RNA can be extracted easily using traditional RNA extraction methods. For detection of BDV RNA in archival material and other formalin-fixed, paraffin-embedded tissues, Sorg et al. (1995) improved existing procedures, showing that deparaffinization of tissues with xylene, digestion with proteinase K, and extraction with guanidium thiocyanate, phenol, and chloroform, followed by RT-nested PCR, form a reliable approach. Using basically the same technology, BDV has been detected in formalin-fixed brain tissues of a dog (Weissenböck et al., 1998) and diverse zoo animals (Schüppel et al., 1995). Since mRNAs coding for the viral nucleoprotein (p40; N) and phosphoprotein (p24; P) are the most abundant viral transcripts in BDV-infected tissues and cells (Briese et al., 1994; Cubitt et al., 1994), almost all RNA detection studies have aimed to detect BDV N- or P-specific sequences.

Northern Hybridization

For in vitro experiments employing BDV-infected cell lines, Northern hybridization is a suitable tool to detect BDV RNA, due to the abundance of both viral genomic RNA and mRNA in these cells. Also, to prove BDV infection of the CNS of animals, such as rats and mice following experimental inoculation with BDV, Northern hybridization generally is sufficient. However, to detect BDV in the CNS of naturally infected animals, as well as in tissues amenable to intra vitam diagnosis, Northern hybridization often is not sensitive enough due to the low amount of RNA available, or due to low amounts of viral RNA present in tissue specimens. Instead, more-sensitive PCR-based techniques have been applied.

RT-PCR and RT-Nested PCR

Most epidemiological studies employed RT-PCR or RT-nested PCR methodology to trace viral RNA in biological tissues. Although an RT-nested PCR assay for BDV RNA was first developed as a research tool in 1993 (Sierra-Honigmann et al., 1993), a standardized RT-PCR protocol for detection of BDV RNA in biological specimens still does not exist. While the RT reaction and first-round PCR were carried out in separate tubes in some laboratories, others combined RT reaction and first-round PCR in a one-tube reaction. The sensitivity of traditional RT-PCR assays that use 20 to 40 PCR cycles could be increased up to 100-fold by adding a second round of PCR (20 to 40 cycles) that employs nested primer sets (Sierra-Honigmann et al., 1993; Zimmermann et al., 1994). Most two-tube RT-PCR assays used Moloney murine leukemia virus RT (e.g., Superscript II, Gibco-BRL Life Technologies) and *Taq* polymerase (Perkin-Elmer). One-tube RT-PCR assays employed commercially available kits such as the EZ r*Tth* RNA PCR kit (Perkin-Elmer) (Kishi et al., 1995) or the Titan one tube RT-PCR system (Roche Biochemicals) (Nowotny et al., 2000; Vahlenkamp et al., 2000; Chen et al., 1999a). As will be discussed below and in other chapters in more detail, since RT-nested PCR is a highly sensitive method, a major problem inherent to this technique is the risk of false-positive results due to contamination with plasmid DNA or PCR products handled in the laboratories. Therefore, to reduce the chance of DNA contamination, one-tube RT-PCR assays appear to be more favorable than the two-tube assays. It is thought that DNA contamination occurs most likely during transfer of the first round PCR product to the new reaction tube for the second-round PCR. Therefore, one-tube RT-PCR assays displaying the same sensitivity as one-tube RT-PCR combined with second-round PCR are desirable. Indeed, Mizutani et al. (1998) succeeded in developing such a system. A standard RT reaction is followed by a 70-cycle amplification step using AmpliTaqGold DNA Polymerase (Perkin-Elmer). This assay apparently is as sensitive as the ordinary RT-nested PCR methods, since as few as 10 copies of synthesized RNA could be amplified.

An alternative approach to reduce the risk of plasmid contamination took advantage of the mRNA selective PCR kit (TaKaRa Shuzo Corp.) that can only amplify cDNA synthesized from viral RNA, but not plasmid DNA encoding BDV genes (up to 5×10^7 molecules), by using deoxynucleoside triphosphate (dNTP) analogs (Mizutani et al., 1999). The dNTP analogs are incorporated first into the cDNA at the RT step. The resulting cDNA/mRNA hybrids, but not double-stranded DNA (dsDNA), can be denatured at 80°C, thereby ensuring selective amplification of the cDNA during the following PCR step. In the subsequent PCR cycles (in the presence of dNTP analogs and denaturation steps at 80°C), dsDNA molecules consisting of incorporated dNTP analogs on both DNA strands (referred to herein as "dsDNAmod") are generated. Only these dsDNAmod molecules, and not "normal" dsDNA-molecules, can be amplified in the PCR.

To confirm the specificity of RT-PCR products, RT-PCR or RT-nested PCR generally was followed in most studies by a BDV-specific confirmation method, e.g., Southern hybridization using BDV-specific probes radioactively or nonisotopically labeled. To simplify this procedure, a microplate hybridization method has been developed (Fujiwara et al., 1997). Following RT-nested PCR using BDV P-specific primers, the final PCR products are dispensed in wells of 96-well microplates (Maxisorp immunomodule; Nunc) and incubated at 37°C under conditions that allow denaturation and adsorption to the solid phase. After washing, bound DNA is hybridized with a mixture of three BDV P-specific FL-labeled oligonucleotides. The wells then are incubated with horseradish peroxidase-conjugated anti-FL antibody, and bound antibody is visualized by adding substrate. The color reaction is measured by the absorbance at 492 nm using a microplate reader. The sensitivity and specificity of this method were found to be comparable to those displayed by the traditional Southern blot hybridization technique. The major advantage of this procedure is the short time required for performance as well as the possibility to carry out the assay fully automated, allowing rapid diagnosis of a large number of biological specimens. The method was used to detect BDV-specific P RNA sequences in PBMCs of psychiatric patients.

RT-PCR-EIA

To detect BDV RNA in rat tissues and secretions, Sierra-Honigmann et al. (1993) took advantage of a technique which combines RT-nested PCR with an enzyme immunoassay (EIA). Briefly, BDV N-specific RT-PCR products are hybridized with a biotinylated BDV N-specific RNA probe. DNA-RNA hybrids then bind to goat antibiotin antibodies immobilized in wells of microtiter plates. Bound DNA-RNA hybrids are incubated with the Fab fragment of an enzyme-labeled MAb directed against DNA-RNA hybrids. Following addition of substrate, bound antibody is detected by measuring the amount of fluorescence using a microtiter plate fluorometer. This assay can detect viral RNA extracted from 0.001 C6BV cell. Using this assay, presence of BDV RNA in PBMCs of neonatally infected rats, and in adult inoculated rats in the chronic stage of infection, was first demonstrated (Sierra-Honigmann et al., 1993). This finding could only be replicated by others when highly sensitive RT-nested PCR was employed, thus indirectly confirming the high sensitivity and suitability of RT-PCR-EIA (Sauder et al., 1998; Furrer et al., 2001).

"Long" RT-PCR

Shoya et al. (1997) demonstrated that a full-length BDV cDNA could be amplified using a recombinant *Tth* DNA polymerase with proofreading activity, employing as little as 20 ng of total cellular RNA prepared from BDV-infected MDCK cells. Since the full-length genome is amplified by using primers encompassing the 5' and 3' genome ends and no internal sequences, this method should be a useful tool to study sequence variability between individual BDV genomes in more detail. Furthermore, it might be helpful to identify new BDV subtypes. Moreover, this technique might be instrumental in the generation of BDV-infectious clones. However, the suitability of this assay for epidemiological studies remains to be shown.

ISH

For histological diagnosis, viral RNA could be detected in sections of formalin-fixed, paraffin-embedded tissues using either radiolabeled or digoxigenin-labeled riboprobes (Carbone et al., 1991; de la Torre et al., 1996; Weissenböck et al., 1998; Stitz et al., 1998; Nakamura et al., 1999b). Although this method is likely more reliable than RT-PCR, since contamination of samples with few DNA molecules can be neglected, it is much less sensitive. So far, there has been no report that applied in situ RT-PCR technology for detection of BDV RNA in histological sections.

VIRUS INFECTIVITY

For analysis of virus infectivity, both in vitro and in vivo systems have been established. To determine infectivity in vitro, primary embryonal or young rabbit brain cells have been employed most often (Hirano et al., 1983; Herzog and Rott, 1980; Lebelt and Hagenau, 1996). In addition, MDCK cells, C6 cells (Katz et al., 1998), guinea pig cells (CRL 1405) (Stitz et al., 1998), or embryonic mink brain cells (Lundgren et al., 1995b) are suitable. Briefly, cells are infected with serial dilutions of cell ho-mogenates. Five to 14 days later, infected cells are detected using standard immunofluorescence methods. For in vivo analysis of infectivity, usually 10 to 20% (wt/vol) tissue homogenates (in phosphate-buffered saline) are injected intracerebrally into rabbits, newborn or adult rats, or newborn Mongolian gerbils (Gosztonyi and Ludwig, 1984; Hirano et al., 1983; Lundgren et al., 1995b; Nakamura et al., 2000).

To analyze the presence of infectious virus intra vitam, nasal secre-tions, conjunctival fluid, saliva, and PBMCs have been used. In naturally infected horses, infectious virus could only very rarely be found in the saliva and could not be found in other body fluids including blood (Lange et al., 1987; Richt et al., 1993; Lebelt and Hagenau, 1996; Herzog et al., 1994). Only in the case of experimentally BDV-infected newborn rats could infectious virus be consistently detected in tears, saliva, and urine, but infectious virus was not detected in the blood (Herzog et al., 1984; Morales et al., 1988). Thus, demonstration of infectious virus intra vitam in naturally infected animals is difficult. This method therefore is not suitable for sensitive detection of BDV, but when this method detects BDV, it can be helpful for confirmation of BDV infection.

For postmortem detection of infectious virus, both peripheral organs and brain tissue have been analyzed. Infectious virus in peripheral organs, such as pancreas, liver, spleen, and salivary and lacrimal glands, could only consistently be demonstrated in rats infected as newborns, in athymic homozygous nude Rowett rats infected at the age of 4 weeks, or in adult infected rats immunosuppressed by cyclosporine or cyclophosphamide treatment (Herzog et al., 1984; Stitz et al., 1991). Apart from being detected in the brain, infectious virus is only regularly detectable in the retina and nasal mucosa of adult infected immunocompetent rats (Narayan et al., 1983; Herzog et al., 1994; Morales et al., 1988).

In the case of naturally infected horses, the retina was shown to con-tain infectious virus in about 50 to 80% of analyzed animals (Gosztonyi and Ludwig, 1984; Bilzer et al., 1995; Lebelt and Hagenau, 1996; Herden et al., 1999). Infectious virus also was found in some cases to be present in the lacrimal gland, nasal mucosa, and olfactory epithelium of these horses (Herzog et al., 1994; Zimmermann et al., 1994; Bilzer et al., 1995). However, there is no evidence for the presence of infectious virus in other peripheral organs or the autonomous nerve system of naturally infected horses (Gosztonyi and Ludwig, 1984; Bilzer et al., 1996; Lebelt and Hagenau, 1996).

Importantly, even in brains of naturally infected animals, infectious virus could not always be detected, although BDV infection was con-firmed by antigen and/or RNA detection methods (Dürrwald, 1993; Zimmermann et al., 1994; Lange et al., 1987). For instance, infectious virus could only be detected in 75 out of 84 horse brains which were proven to be BDV infected based on BDV antigen detection methods (Herden et al., 1999). Consistent with the uneven distribution of viral antigen in brains of naturally infected animals (see above), infectious virus could not always be found in all regions of an infected brain (Gosztonyi and Ludwig, 1984). The failure to demonstrate infectious virus in every brain with proven BDV infection is most likely due to the fact that the sensitivity of the applied test systems is low compared to the more-sensitive RNA detection methods, such as RT-PCR. In addition, postmortem decomposition of tissue involving degradation of RNA might take place, which has been discussed to likely account for the failure to detect infectious virus at least in some cases (Herden et al., 1999). Thus, the interval between the death of the animal and the storage of frozen tissue is critical. Notably, determination of virus infectivity in vitro has been found to be less sensitive than that in in vivo systems. Thus, Katz et al. (1998) failed to demonstrate in vitro infectious virus in brains of ponies experimentally infected with BDV but were able to do so by infecting young adult rats with pony brain homogenates. Among the animals used for in vivo infectivity studies, newborn Mongolian gerbils have been suggested to be more susceptible to BDV infection than newborn rats (Nakamura et al., 1999a).

In conclusion, relying on the demonstration of infectious virus in postmortem brain tissue alone is not a reliable technique for diagnosis of BDV infection, since negative findings do not exclude the presence of infection.

DIFFICULTIES ENCOUNTERED IN DIAGNOSIS

Epidemiological studies largely depend on intra vitam diagnosis. However, unequivocal proof of BDV infection relying only on intra vitam diagnosis is difficult to achieve for several reasons. This is true not only for clinically overt infections in animals but also for inapparent infections believed to exist both in animals and humans.

The clinical signs displayed by infected horses and sheep may vary considerably, which is believed to be mainly due to differences in the localization of brain lesions (Rott and Becht, 1995; Richt et al., 2000). Clinical symptoms therefore cannot be regarded to be specific for BD and also occur in central nervous system infections with other pathogens. Analysis of CSF taken from horses during the acute and subacute phases of disease usually reveals pathological alterations, including increased protein concentrations and lymphomonocytic pleocytosis. Since they are not BDV specific but are typical for viral meningoencephalitis, these findings only support the clinical suspicions of diagnosis (Bilzer et al., 1996; Grabner and Fischer, 1991; Richt et al., 2000). Therefore, detection of BDV-specific antibodies in serum and/or CSF is mandatory. Although in many studies BDV serum and/or CSF antibodies were found in all cases where post-mortem analysis indicated BDV infection (Bilzer et al., 1996; Herden et al., 1999; Herzog et al., 1994), others have failed to confirm this finding, indicating that seronegative results do not necessarily prove a lack of BDV infection (Grabner and Fischer, 1991; Dürrwald, 1993; Caplazi and Ehrensperger, 1998; Zimmermann et al., 1994). Regarding the question of whether BDV antibodies can be detected more frequently in CSF than in serum, contradictory findings have been published (Grabner and Fischer, 1991; Herzog et al., 1994; Herden et al., 1999). The presence of neurological signs of disease and characteristic CSF alterations, together with seropositivity, generally is regarded to be sufficient for diagnosis of BD in animals. While this is certainly true for the vast majority of cases, a recent study indicates that caution is warranted. In this study, 148 horses that displayed diverse neurological disorders were subjected to BDV diagnostic testing (Herden et al., 1999). Among those, 89 were proven by postmortem diagnosis to be infected with BDV. In all 89 cases, the corresponding sera contained BDV antibodies. However, an additional 25 horses were found to be seropositive for BDV but suffered from neurological diseases other than typical equine BD, including idiopathic encephalitis. Whether these seropositive horses had previous contact with BDV but were able to clear the virus from the central nervous system is unknown. Alternatively, the possibility that the serological assay system used (IFA) yielded false-positive results cannot be ruled out. The likelihood of obtaining diagnostic misinterpretations when using IFA will be discussed below.

In conclusion, even though intra vitam diagnosis of BD generally is considered to be reliable when animals show neurological symptoms, BDV-specific serum and/or CSF antibodies, and characteristic CSF alterations, given current technologies, unequivocal proof of BDV infection is possible only by postmortem analysis using histopathological, immuno-histochemical, and virological tests. In brains of animals naturally infected with BD, variable degrees of a mononuclear cell encephalomyelitis can be diagnosed histopathologically (Gosztonyi and Ludwig, 1995; Bilzer et al., 1995; Caplazi and Ehrensperger, 1998). Both perivascular and parenchymal infiltration, predominantly consisting of CD4 and CD8 T cells, respectively, plus macrophages, usually can be observed (Bilzer et al., 1995; Caplazi and Ehrensperger, 1998). In 1909 Joest and Degen described the presence of inclusion bodies in the nuclei of neurons in hippocampi of horses with BD. These Joest-Degen inclusion bodies were used as diagnostic markers for BD (Gosztonyi and Ludwig, 1995). However, they cannot consistently be observed in brains of diseased animals (Grabner and Fischer, 1991; Richt and Rott, 2001). Detection of viral antigen in brains of naturally infected animals by WBA or IHC proves to be the most reliable method for postmortem diagnosis of BDV. In contrast, demonstration of viral RNA and virus infectivity in brains of diseased animals does not always yield positive results (see below).

As outlined above (see "Virus Antigen Detection" and "Virus RNA Detection"), and as will be further discussed below, the methods for detection of viral antigen and viral RNA in body secretions and blood are not reliable for intra vitam diagnosis of BDV infection. Thus, so far, serology represents the most important intra vitam diagnostic tool in the case of diseased animals, and in the case of inapparent BDV infections, intra vitam diagnosis still relies exclusively on serological methods.

One of the most intriguing features of BDV serology is the finding that antibody titers in animals and humans frequently are below 1:40. This includes titers in animals with BDV infection that was clearly proven postmortem (Bilzer et al., 1996; Katz et al., 1998; Caplazi and Ehrensperger, 1998), as well as reported latent infection of animals and humans based on positive serological findings (reviewed by Staeheli et al. [2000] and in chapters 4 and 6). Thus, serological tests for BDV-specific antibodies have to exhibit high sensitivity. However, reliable diagnostic tests also require high specificity. Therefore, knowledge of the sensitivity and specificity of the assay systems used for diagnosis of BDV infection is a critical issue.

As discussed in more detail in chapters 4 and 6, the questions of the frequency of inapparent BDV infections in animals and of whether BDV infects humans and contributes to psychiatric disease are subjects of a controversial and still-ongoing debate. Besides BDV and/or RNA contamination concerns and differences in clinical populations and geographic regions, differences in sensitivity and specificity of the assay systems used for BDV detection likely account for the controversial findings. To date, there is no consensus on a standardized reliable method for detection of BDV antibodies that adequately meets the criteria of both specificity and sensitivity. Likewise, a general agreement on a standardized, sensitive method for detection of BDV RNA is lacking.

A recent multicenter study involving several German laboratories and one Austrian laboratory engaged in BDV research attempted to evaluate the sensitivity, specificity, and reproducibility of different test systems for detection of BDV antibodies and BDV RNA (C. M. Nübling, J. Löwer, R. Kurth, and the Bornavirus Study Group, *Abstr. Jahrestag. Gesellschaft Virol.*, abstr. 2P1, 1999). Sera and PBMCs from both naturally and experimentally infected animals, as well as from humans, were subjected to the different test methods. The study revealed considerable discrepancies in test results among the different laboratories, especially regarding the detection of RNA in PBMCs but also with respect to serology. Thus, this study confirmed that the controversy regarding the above-mentioned issues is likely due to the lack of standardized methods for detection of anti-BDV antibodies and RNA. In the following sections, the suitability of currently available diagnostic test systems to detect BDV antibodies and RNA will be critically evaluated.

Serology

IFA

IFA in general is accepted to be a rapid, inexpensive, and relatively sensitive diagnostic tool. Since the native conformation of BDV antigens remains conserved in IFAs, antibodies that only recognize conformational epitopes are expected to be detectable by IFA but not by WBA. This advantage of IFA should not be overlooked.

However, several caveats concerning this method for BDV serology have to be considered. First of all, IFA is inherently subjective, and evaluation of IFA slides requires significant training. For example, since the criterion for BDV seropositivity in IFA is a specific type of punctate staining in the nucleus of infected cells (Fig. 1), interpretation of IFA slides can be complicated. Since the low titers of anti-BDV in sera often require testing at very low dilutions (1:5 or 1:10), nonspecific binding of antibodies may occur. Accordingly, Bechter et al. (1987) noticed that the IFA technique displays only a poor reliability and reproducibility when low-titer samples, such as human samples, are tested. Likewise, examination of sera derived from healthy humans employing both single IFA as well as double-labeling IFA by Waltrip et al. (1995) suggested a limited specificity of IFA. Kitze et al. (1996) observed that about 3% of sera from healthy individuals displayed nonspecific binding in IFA when tested on uninfected MDCK cells. Unfortunately, it is unclear whether these sera displayed the classic punctate nuclear or a diffuse staining in the uninfected control cells. In this study, no evidence of an association between multiple sclerosis and BDV infection was found. In contrast, using double-labeling IFA, Bode et al. (1992) reported a BDV seroprevalence of 13.2% among multiple sclerosis patients. Since the assay used by Bode et al. does not include uninfected cells as a negative control and since test sera were not preadsorbed against swine liver powder or lysates from uninfected cells (as done by Kitze et al.), it appears that the reported association of anti-BDV antibodies with multiple sclerosis was due to false-positive results, i.e., that nonspecifically bound antibodies sometimes are scored as positive (Kitze et al., 1996). The German-Austrian multicenter study also revealed that differences in the sensitivities between IFAs in different laboratories may be due to the use of different cell lines as the source of antigens (Nübling et al., *Abstr. Jahrestag. Gesellschaft Virol.*). Thus, sera positive for anti-BDV antibody seem to display higher titers of antibody when tested on BDV-infected rabbit embryonic fibroblasts or BDV-infected MDCK cells compared to those displayed when tested on BDV-infected C6, Vero, or Oligo cells (Allmang et al., 2001; P. Staeheli [Freiburg, Germany], personal communication). These examples demonstrate the need for a standardized reliable IFA method. Another essential drawback of IFA is that it does not allow determination of which antigen(s) is specifically recognized by a BDV-reactive serum. Thus, the question of whether BDV antibodies are directed against one or more antigens cannot be answered using IFA. Moreover, there remains the remote possibility that BDV infection of cells induces upregulation, stabilization, or rearrangement of cellular proteins, which then react with autoantibodies in test sera, thus resulting in false-positive signals. Especially with respect to the question of an association between BDV and psychiatric disorders, it appears that autoantibodies against nuclear structures frequently are observed in the sera of patients with such disorders (Legros et al., 1985; Sirota et al., 1991).

WBA

In contrast to the IFA, analysis of sera by WBA allows identification of the antigens that are recognized by serum antibodies. Therefore, the WBA should, in theory, display a higher specificity than IFA. Sera from animals with confirmed BDV infection usually recognize several BDV antigens (predominantly N, P, and M [Rott et al., 1991; Briese et al., 1995]). Curiously enough, in numerous studies that analyzed sera from humans and animals lacking neurological symptoms, sera that only recognized one viral protein were observed much more frequently than sera that were reactive with two or more antigens (Rott et al., 1991, Fu et al., 1993; Waltrip et al., 1995; Sauder et al., 1996; Takahashi et al., 1997; Chen et al., 1999b; Nakaya et al., 1999; Fukuda et al., 2001). Similar observations were also made when human and/or animal sera were analyzed by IP (Bode et al., 1992; Richt et al., 1992), ELISA (Berg et al., 1999) or ECLIA (Yamaguchi et al., 1999; Fukuda et al., 2001). Moreover, whereas some studies predominantly found reactivity against N, others more frequently found reactivity toward P. While the reason for antibody recognition of one versus multiple BDV antigens is not understood, differences in the sensitivities of the various WBAs might be a possible explanation. Accordingly, employing IFA, Ogino et al. (1998) showed that sera from rats immunized with either BDV N or P antigens readily recognized N or P expressed in insect cells, although anti-BDV N titers were much higher than anti-BDV P titers. In contrast, when tested by WBA, the same sera displayed reactivity against the N antigen but not against the P antigen, indicating that the sensitivities of WBA and IFA differed for different BDV antigens. Similarly, when tested by WBA (using purified BDV N, P, and M), sera derived from BDV-infected rats during the acute phase of disease reacted only with N and P, not with M. However, when tested by ELISA the sera recognized all three antigens, though titers of M were very low (Briese et al., 1995). Thus, it appears likely that the affinity of antibodies for BDV antigens used in WBA can vary, perhaps depending upon the source of the antigens used for WBA (e.g., bacterially expressed or whole-cell extracts, etc.)

Fu et al. (1993) discussed that cross-reactivity might explain a result in which reactivity against only one viral antigen is seen. For example, antibodies not generated originally against a BDV protein but produced in response to a protein of another pathogen, or against a host cellular protein, may share epitopes in common with or similar to those of BDV antigens. Finally, the possibility of nonspecific interactions between large amounts of BDV proteins and antibodies in sera at low dilutions on the blotting membranes cannot be completely ruled out, particularly when purified proteins are employed in the WBA.

To increase the specificity of WBA, more-stringent criteria for seropositivity have been introduced. For instance, Waltrip et al. (1995) scored as positive only those sera that reacted with two or more BDV antigens based upon similar problems initially encountered in human immunodeficiency virus (HIV) serology. Therefore, it may be assumed that WBAs formulated with only one BDV protein (Kishi et al., 1995; Nakamura et al., 1995) have a lower specificity than those which allow detection of reactivity against several antigens. However, more comprehensive studies employing sera from experimentally infected animals as well as from animals with proven natural infections are required to clarify these issues. Competition experiments were performed by some investigators (Sauder et al., 1996; Nishino et al., 1999; Fukuda et al., 2001) to increase the specificity of the WBA. Test sera were preadsorbed either with cell lysates prepared from BDV-infected cells or from cells expressing individual BDV antigens or with purified BDV antigens. Comparing the prevalence of anti-BDV N and P antibodies from human sera in WBAs with or without the performance of competitive inhibition tests, Fukuda et al. (2001) clearly showed that seroprevalence was reduced when inhibition tests were performed. If one presumes that competition tests result in the invalidation of false-positive results due to nonspecific antibody binding, the subsequent reduction in seropositivity provides evidence of the improvement in specificity added by the use of this additional step. Some studies employed a WBA that was based on purified GST and GST-BDV P fusion protein (Kishi et al., 1995; Nakamura et al., 1995). Sera that only reacted with GST-P but not with GST were scored as positive; however, the possibility that the GST-P fusion protein reacted with antibodies that might not react with GST or P alone cannot be ruled out. In this case, competition experiments using purified BDV P, rather than purified GST-P, might be helpful to increase specificity. In conclusion, the development of WBA that appear to be more specific than IFA may have been achieved at the expense of reduced sensitivity. Results from the German-Austrian multicenter study came to similar conclusions. Since WBA is rather time-consuming, it is not well suited for the large-scale screening of sera.

ELISAs

The major advantages of ELISA are that it is inexpensive and rapid. Moreover, it is probably the most sensitive technique compared to IFA and WBA. Briese et al. (1995) compared an ELISA based on BDV proteins N, P, and M with IFA or WBA, using sera from BDV-infected rats. This study suggested that ELISA is a more sensitive method for BDV serology than IFA and WBA. However, this study also showed that 100% specificity of the assay could only be reached when rat sera were used at dilutions of 1:500 or higher. Since the majority of sera from humans and naturally infected animals display much lower BDV antibody titers than do sera from experimentally infected rats or rabbits, the suitability of this assay for the analysis of low-dilution sera of humans and animals remains to be determined.

ELISA may provide greater sensitivity at the expense of specificity. Given the ubiquitous experience with *E. coli* in animals, one cannot completely rule out the possibility that positive signals in the ELISA are due to antibody reactions with contaminating *E. coli* proteins, which still might be present in the purified recombinant antigens produced by this bacterium. In addition, ELISAs employing purified GST-BDV proteins and GST as a control can give valid results only under the assumption that *E. coli*-contaminated GST-BDV and purified GST are quantitatively and qualitatively the same. The introduction of stringent criteria for seropositivity, such as reactivity against more than one BDV antigen, might increase ELISA specificity. However, Evengård et al. (1999) showed that even though numerous sera from chronic fatigue syndrome (CFS) patients reacted with more than two BDV antigens in an ELISA apparently identical in nature to the one described by Briese et al. (1995), these sera also all reacted with β-galactosidase in the ELISA, indicating that binding of sera was not specific.

Thus, while ELISA likely is a powerful technique for detection of high-titer anti-BDV antibodies, its suitability for analysis of sera at low dilutions, especially human sera, is unclear. To overcome these problems, some modified ELISA techniques have been developed that might significantly increase specificity. As already outlined for improvement of WBA serology, competition inhibition tests seem to be mandatory to reduce the risk of false-positive results. The efficacy of competition steps in increasing the specificity of the assay has been shown for the related ECLIA (see below) (Yamaguchi et al., 1999).

Horimoto et al. (1997) compared the reactivity of human sera in an indirect ELISA with their reactivity in an RS-ELISA using purified bacterially expressed N, and compared these results to results generated by IFA. While human sera scored as positive in both IFA and indirect ELISA, they were found to be negative in the RS-ELISA. It therefore was argued that positive results likely reflected nonspecific binding of antibodies, and it was concluded that RS-ELISA is highly specific. However, comparison of results obtained with sera from experimentally BDV-infected rabbits revealed that two out of four sera tested displayed reduced titers compared to those obtained by IFA and indirect ELISA. Thus, it appears that the increase of specificity was achieved at the expense of sensitivity. This notion was further supported when RS-ELISA was compared with other serological methods within the scope of the German-Austrian multicenter study (Nübling et al. *Abstr. Jahrestag. Gesellschaft Virol.*).

The capture ELISA (Tsujimura et al., 1999) seems to meet the criteria of both sensitivity and specificity. However, so far this test has only been evaluated using rat sera. Hence, it still remains to be determined whether this assay and its related tests (indirect ELISA and cELISA) are suitable for serology in farm animals and humans, when sera low with dilutions of antibody need to be tested. Due to the low BDV antibody titers and the lack of defined positive or negative reference sera in the case of humans and several animal species, evaluation of the specificity of the different ELISA systems is a challenging task.

IP

The suitability of IP for large-scale screening of samples for the presence of BDV antibodies is questionable, since it is time-consuming and expensive. Moreover, using human sera, Bode et al. (1992) could only immunoprecipitate detectable amounts of BDV antigens using sera displaying anti-BDV antibody titers of at least 1:320. Since most human sera exhibit considerably lower titers, the practical utility of this test for detection of human BDV infection is doubtful.

ECLIA

The ECLIA method was developed to provide higher sensitivity, a wider dynamic range, improved precision, and a shorter testing time compared to other conventional immunoassay methods. The specificity and sensitivity of an ECLIA that used N- and P-derived peptides (see "Virus Antigen Detection" above) were evaluated using a series of sera from experimentally BDV-infected as well as uninfected rats and horses (Yamaguchi et al., 2001). In rats the ECLIA detected anti-BDV antibodies in eight of nine infected rats, whereas all 11 uninfected rats were scored as negative by ECLIA. Seven out of the eight sera positive by ECLIA also were positive in the IFA. The ECLIA was able to identify 3 experimentally BDV-infected horses out of 13 horses, in accordance with the results from WBA and IFA. Notably, while four serum samples from additional horses were scored as seropositive by ECLIA and WBA, only one of these four serum samples was also found to be positive using IFA. Since defined negative horse sera do not exist, it is possible that the four healthy horses were latently or transiently infected with BDV. Assuming specificity of these four reactivities, these data would suggest that ECLIA is more sensitive than IFA. However, the possibility that the four positive reactions were nonspecific cannot be excluded. Thus, whereas in the rat system a high degree of specificity was achieved, determination of specificity in the horse system is more complicated due to the lack of negative reference sera.

ECLIA analysis of sera from HIV-infected patients and patients with CFS revealed that some of these sera had counts higher than the cutoff levels at the first screening; all but one were judged to be negative when the specific competitive inhibition test was performed (see "Serology") (Yamaguchi et al., 1999). Similar competition experiments were not consistently performed in studies that employed ELISA or WBA based on GST-BDV N and/or -BDV P fusion proteins and GST as controls (Auwanit et al., 1996; Kitani et al., 1996; Nakaya et al., 1996). Auwanit et al. (1996) reported an unusually high seroprevalence of BDV in HIV-infected patients by ELISA using GST-P fusion protein. Nakaya et al. (1996) and Kitani et al. (1996) reported 32 and 33.7%, respectively, of sera from CFS patients to be seropositive for P when analyzed by WBA or ELISA, respectively, employing GST-P and GST. Thus, discrepant findings regarding the prevalence of BDV antibodies among HIV-infected individuals and CFS patients might be due to these experimental differences (Evengård et al. [1999]). The specificity of ELISA and WBA systems based on GST-P and GST remains unclear due to the possibility of contamination of *E. coli* components and use of GST-P fusion protein instead of purified P released from GST (as discussed for WBA and ELISA). These findings suggest that confirmation tests, such as the inhibition test by soluble antigen, are needed to reduce the likelihood of false-positive results due to nonspecific reactions.

ECLIA analysis of human sera revealed differences in the profiles of BDV antibodies between patients with psychiatric disorders and blood donors (Yamaguchi et al., 1999). Although P-reactive antibodies were found more frequently than N-reactive antibodies in most cases, in some psychosis patients, antibody profiles showed reactivity against N only. The reason for this variable seroreactivity is unknown. Even though N and P are unrelated in amino acid sequence, thus presumably lacking common epitopes, the cross-reactivity of anti-N and anti-P sera in ELISA against P or N, respectively, has been described (Kliche et al. 1996), with monospecific sera and monoclonal antibodies to N found to cross-react with one discontinuous epitope located at the amino terminus of P.

In conclusion, ECLIA appears to exhibit high sensitivity and reasonable specificity, thus providing a serological screening tool potentially suitable for the measurement of anti-BDV N and anti-BDV P antibodies in studies aiming to evaluate the role of BDV in humans and animals. In particular, this rapid, economical technique might prove useful for the large-scale screening required for epidemiological studies of BDV in humans.

For the time being, utilizing an initial screening of sera by sensitive ECLIA, capture ELISA, or IFA methods, followed by confirmation of seropositive results employing more specific tests, such as WBA, might be an approach to ensure reasonable degrees of sensitivity and specificity.

Virus RNA Detection

The application of PCR techniques to BDV research yielded a wealth of information regarding sequence variability and diagnosis of BDV infection. Before discussing the manifold problems that arose when these techniques were applied to BDV diagnosis, below is a brief summary of the findings that have been obtained using these techniques for post-mortem and intra vitam diagnosis. Using RT-PCR to detect virus RNA in brains of animals (horses, donkeys, and sheep) with BD, the majority of studies could detect RNA in all cases analyzed (Zimmermann et al., 1994; Lebelt and Hagenau, 1996; Bilzer et al., 1995; Katz et al., 1998). However, two studies only detected BDV RNA in 80% (n = 10 and 19, respectively) of brains analyzed by RT-PCR (Herzog et al., 1994; Herden et al., 1999). It has been argued that the failure to detect viral RNA in some cases most likely is attributable to postmortem decomposition of the RNA, a problem often encountered in the processing of field cases. Limited information is available regarding detection rates of BDV RNA in brain tissue using ISH (Herden et al., 1999; Bilzer et al., 1996). In a single study, it was reported that ISH successfully detected BDV RNA in 100% of brains ($n = 17$) of horses with BD. Although this single study suggested a good reliability of the assay, this result has to be confirmed in more-comprehensive studies, since, in practice, ISH is considered to be much less sensitive than RT-PCR.

Notably, in agreement with the uneven distribution of antigen in infected brains, RNA is rarely found in all brain regions analyzed. Only in the hippocampus is BDV RNA detected in nearly 100% of cases (Zimmermann et al., 1994; Bilzer et al., 1995; Lebelt and Hagenau, 1996). Similarly, using RT-nested PCR and/or ISH, BDV RNA was reported to be present only in some brain regions of two healthy humans (Haga et al., 1997), one schizophrenic patient (Nakamura et al., 2000), and four Japanese horses that displayed locomotor disease (Hagiwara et al., 1997b). BDV RNA has also been detected in parotid gland, nasal mucosa (olfactory epithelium), retina, liver, kidney, lung, heart, and ovary tissue with variable prevalence rates, depending on the tissues analyzed (Zimmermann et al., 1994; Lebelt and Hagenau, 1996; Bilzer et al., 1996). Thus, BDV RNA appears to be present at a higher frequency in peripheral organs than would be assumed based on analysis of antigen and infectious virus. This is likely due to the fact that the sensitivity of RT-PCR is higher than those of the other detection methods. Notably, BDV RNA could also be detected in several peripheral tissues of immunocompetent adult BDV-infected rats (Shankar et al., 1992; Stitz et al., 1998). In these tissues, BDV RNA was confined to peripheral nerves of the autonomic nervous system, which is also likely to be the case in naturally infected animals.

In summary, diagnosis of BDV infection in postmortem brain tissues using RT-PCR and/or ISH techniques appears to display a reliability similar to that of detection of virus antigen. However, it should be kept in mind that contamination of tissue preparations or reagents with RNA or plasmid DNA can easily occur in some RT-PCRs and, more likely, in RT-nested PCR, complicating the interpretation of data (see below). Therefore, definitive confirmatory postmortem diagnosis of BDV infection should not exclusively rely on RT-PCR. Instead, it is advisable to combine this method with antigen detection procedures such as IHC or WBA (see above).

Intra vitam, viral RNA could be detected in conjunctival fluid and/or nasal secretions and/or the saliva of 2 out of 20 diseased ungulates (Lebelt and Hagenau, 1996), as well as in the respective secretions from 12 out of 77 healthy horses, which were suspected to be BDV-infected due to presence of BDV-reactive antibodies in their sera (Richt et al., 1993).

Sierra-Honigmann et al. (1993) first demonstrated that BDV-RNA could be detected in the blood of BDV-infected animals, namely, in PBMCs isolated from rats infected as newborns (designated "PTI-NB"), as well as in rats infected as adults during the chronic phase of disease, using RT-nested PCR-EIA. These findings were later confirmed by others (Sauder et al., 1998; Vahlenkamp et al., 2000; Furrer et al., 2001). Intriguingly, although detectable by highly sensitive assays, only a tiny percentage of cells in the peripheral blood are found to carry BDV, with a prevalence of only one BDV-infected cell in 1×10^5 to 5×10^6 PBMCs from PTI-NB rats (Rubin et al., 1995; Sauder et al., 1998). BDV could only rarely be detected in PBMCs isolated from adult-infected rats during the acute phase of disease (Sierra-Honigmann et al., 1993; Lieb et al., 1997; Sauder et al., 1998; Furrer et al., 2001) despite the presence of viral loads in the brains of these rats similar to those in the brains of PTI-NB rats. This indicates that the level of BDV RNA in blood does not necessarily reflect the viral load in the brain. Although caution is warranted when extrapolating these findings to other species, they may be helpful for interpretation of studies using PBMCs of these species.

Since the initial report by Sierra-Honigmann et al. (1993), a considerable number of studies have been undertaken to detect BDV RNA in PBMCs of animals and humans. Employing diverse RT-PCR or RT–nested-PCR methods (see above), numerous studies apparently succeeded in detecting BDV RNA in PBMCs from various healthy and diseased ungulates, healthy humans, and patients with diverse psychiatric diseases (Staeheli et al., 2000) (see chapters 4 and 6). Nevertheless, other studies were not able to confirm these findings, arguing that the discrepant results might be due to laboratory artifacts (e.g., contamination) resulting from the extremely high sensitivity of RT-nested PCR. Thus, the issue of whether BDV RNA is present in PBMCs of naturally infected animals, as well as in humans, with or without associated clinical disease, has become the subject of an ongoing controversial debate. Using RT-nested PCR or modified one-tube RT-PCR, even small numbers of BDV mRNA molecules can be detected (Sauder et al., 1998; Mizutani et al., 1998; Vahlenkamp et al., 2000). Therefore, extreme caution must be undertaken to avoid contamination of samples with BDV plasmid DNA or BDV RNA from infected cells handled in the respective laboratories. A recent report by Schwemmle et al. (1999) suggested that in some of the studies that provided evidence of BDV RNA in human PBMCs, sample contamination might indeed have taken place. Based on these findings and the high risk of sample contamination, RT-nested PCR appears not to be a suitable tool for routine laboratory diagnosis of BDV infection. Discrepant findings in some cases might also be related to different sensitivities of the various

RT-PCR and RT–nested-PCR techniques used. Thus, differences in the amount of blood used to prepare PBMCs (Sauder et al., 1998), the method of RNA preparation, the amount of RNA used for RT, as well as the nature of primers and enzymes used for RT and PCR vary between laboratories. Hence, similar to the situation for serology, there is no agreement on a standardized RT-PCR method, a situation that hampers the interpretation of results obtained in different laboratories.

In order to achieve an agreement between the various laboratories engaged in BDV diagnostics, it has been suggested that multicenter studies should be organized in which pre-RT-PCR handling of samples is performed by an independent laboratory with no history of experimental or diagnostic work on BDV. In addition strict precautions should be taken, and the highest PCR standards need to be observed, to avoid contamination. Thus, it is mandatory that "minus-RT" negative control reactions, which omit the RT enzyme, be carried out using aliquots of test samples.

Furthermore, RNA prepared from BDV-infected cell lines should not be employed as a positive control for the assays. Numerous studies routinely used these RNAs as positive controls for RT-PCR, which likely has been one source of sample contamination (Schwemmle et al., 1999). To circumvent this problem, and to be able to standardize RT-PCR techniques, the use of internal or external RNA standards which can clearly be distinguished from the wild-type BDV RNA has been recommended. BDV N and P RNA molecules which contain non-BDV-related sequences (Sauder et al., 1998; Czygan et al., 1999; Legay et al., 2000) or deletions in the BDV N molecules have been designed for these purposes (Vahlenkamp et al., 2000). In addition, as mentioned above (see "Virus RNA Detection"), the application of modified RT-PCR methods (mRNA selective PCR system) which do not allow amplification of plasmid DNA-containing BDV sequences has been suggested (Mizutani et al., 1999). So far, nucleic acid sequence-based amplification has not been applied to detect BDV RNA, but this might be an alternative approach to minimize the risk of DNA contamination, since it is a sensitive RNA detection method which does not include dsDNA amplification steps.

Furthermore, one-tube RT-PCR assays combined with a second PCR round (Kishi et al., 1995; Chen et al., 1999a; Nowotny et al., 2000; Vahlenkamp et al., 2000) or, preferably, modified one-tube RT-PCRs which do not require a second PCR round due to high sensitivity (Mizutani et al., 1998), can reduce the risk of contamination (see "Virus RNA Detection" above). Nevertheless, these assays still require the same precautions needed when performing traditional RT-nested PCR, since PCR end products themselves, as well as cell line-derived RNA, can be a source of contamination when handled in the same environment where RT-PCR is performed.

Sequencing of the RT-PCR or RT–nested-PCR products might help to define whether PCR products were amplified from laboratory BDV plasmids or contaminating BDV RNA or whether they represent new BDV strains. Intriguingly, Schwemmle et al. (1999) could show that most BDV sequences derived from human PBMC samples were very closely related to the respective BDV strains used in the respective laboratories. Thus, knowledge of the exact sequences of the BDV strains used in the respective laboratories seems to be mandatory (Schwemmle et al., 1999; Staeheli et al., 2000). In cases of PCR products derived from human or animal PBMCs which display 100% identity to the sequences of the laboratory strains, interpretation of the findings is difficult.

Despite the fact that BDV is an RNA virus, there is a considerably high degree of sequence conservation among BDV sequences derived from naturally infected horses from different geographic areas and separated by several years, as well as for BDV sequences derived from naturally infected animals of different species, a hitherto-unresolved mystery in BDV research (Schneider et al., 1994; Binz et al., 1994; Formella et al., 2000; Staeheli et al., 2000). Therefore, the interpretation of sequencing data is complicated and caution is warranted to avoid wrong conclusions. Notably, the fact that BDV sequences deduced from human tissues display a remarkably high sequence conservation relative to BDV isolates from animals also could be related, at least in part, to the nature of the primers selected for RT-PCR. Thus, until recently, the currently used RT-PCR protocols employed primers which were designed based on the available sequences of the prototype BDV strains V, He/80, WT-1, and MDCK, which are closely related, differing by less than 5% (Schneider et al., 1994; Staeheli et al., 2000). The close relationship between the sequences of the different PCR fragments might be due to a PCR primer-based selection, thereby excluding the detection of new BDV variants. The existence of such variants has recently been shown by Nowotny et al. (2000), who isolated a new BDV variant, named No/98, from an Austrian pony stallion. The nucleotide sequence of No/98 differs from the above-mentioned prototype BDV strains by more than 15% and was difficult to detect using standard RT-PCR or RT–nested-PCR methods (Nowotny et al., 2000). This new finding complicates the design of sensitive RT–nested-PCR assays, since a novel subtype of BDV may escape detection by RT-nested PCR using primers that have been commonly used for diagnosis.

Many RT-PCR methods used in the past for detection of BDV RNA in PBMCs of animals or humans are not suitable for deducing proper sequence information from PCR products. For the correct synthesis of PCR products, high-fidelity DNA amplification is achieved by employing a polymerase that exhibits proofreading activity and by using low concentrations of dNTPs and polymerase, a buffer system that ensures stable maintenance of pH 6 throughout the PCR cycles, and short synthesis times (Eckert and Kunkel, 1991). In addition, PCR buffers should not contain manganese, since it significantly reduces the fidelity of the polymerase in the PCR step. This should be kept in mind when employing one-tube RT-PCR assays that are based on buffers containing manganese, which is needed during the RT reaction (Sauder et al., 1996). Sequences of PCR products generated using inappropriate conditions and strategies might artifactually differ considerably from the known BDV strains, an additional complication for proper interpretation of sequences. Finally, there is some evidence that *E. coli* can bias the results of molecular cloning by means of incorporation of mutations in PCR fragments during the cloning procedure, additionally complicating the study of viral heterogeneity (Forns et al., 1997).

Recently, Legay et al. (2000) pointed out that RNA extracted from nervous tissue, but not from blood, has an inhibitory effect on the detection of BDV RNA by RT-PCR. In addition, as mentioned, decomposition of brain tissue (and RNA) during the time between removal and storage likely takes place in some cases (Herden et al., 1999). Thus, despite the highly sensitive assay characteristic, false-negative RT-PCR results might occasionally occur. To control the quality of RNA samples, the use of internal BDV RNA standards has been suggested. In addition, RT-PCRs should be designed that allow detection of genes that are expressed at only low levels in the brain, such as the porphobilinogen deaminase gene (Salvatore et al., 1997; Czygan et al., 1999).

One common theme in virtually all studies that have aimed to detect both BDV RNA in animal and human PBMCs, as well as serum BDV antibodies, is that there was a lack of strict correlation between seropositivity and detection of BDV RNA in the PBMCs. Absence of antibodies in the presence of RNA, and vice versa, was observed more frequently than coincident positivity of both parameters (Kishi et al., 1995; Nakaya et al., 1996; Sauder et al., 1996; Nakamura et al., 1995). While the reasons for this finding are unknown, it represents an additional serious complication in the intra vitam diagnosis of BDV infections. Seropositive but BDV RNA-negative cases might theoretically represent BDV infections that have been cleared by the host immune response. However, clearance of natural BDV infections by the host's immune response has not yet been demonstrated. Hagiwara et al. (1997a) observed that BDV RNA was more prevalent in the blood of lambs than in that of adult sheep, whereas the latter had higher seroprevalence than lambs, suggesting that raising an immune response to BDV reduced the level of RNA in blood. In the case of adult BDV-infected rats, the presence of BDV RNA in blood was proposed to trigger the generation of neutralizing antibodies (Furrer et al., 2001). Nevertheless, in this case, RNA was still detectable in blood in the presence of neutralizing antibodies, arguing against a role of antibodies in the clearance of BDV from the blood (Furrer et al., 2001). Presence of RNA in the absence of BDV antibodies might be indicative of recent infections with delayed humoral immune responses. However, another explanation might be that RNA-positive samples were due to laboratory artifacts (see discussion above).

FUTURE DIRECTIONS

The overall difficulty in recovery of BDV from the blood of humans and animals carries with it some significant risk of false-positive and false-negative results, most likely due to the manifold problems inherent to RT-PCR technologies as discussed above. For the foreseeable future and certainly for mass screening attempts serological assays, therefore, are likely to remain the major tests for intra vitam BDV diagnosis. However, currently there is no agreement on a sensitive and specific test to detect BDV antibodies. Since BDV antibody titers both in humans and animals usually are very low, the majority of the currently used serological assays have been optimized for highest sensitivity, most likely at the expense of specificity, and serological assays used by the various BDV laboratories vary considerably with respect to sensitivity and specificity (Nübling et al., *Abstr. Jahrestag. Gesellschaft Virol.*). Regarding the possible infection of humans, there still is no indisputable proof of BDV infection (Staeheli et al., 2000) (see chapter 6). Thus, there is a lack of human reference serum samples containing antibodies which have been definitively raised following contact with BDV. This represents a major problem in the evaluation of sensitivity and specificity of serological tests designed to detect antibodies in humans. Similarly, in cases of serological studies to detect BDV antibodies in healthy horses, sheep, and cattle, defined negative reference samples are difficult to obtain. Despite these problems, and however detected, the presence of serum antibodies in the blood of humans and healthy animals is taken as strong evidence for BDV infection by some researchers (Bode et al., 1992; Bechter et al., 1992). However, it remains unknown whether the presence of reactive antibodies indicates a persistent or previous infection with BDV or, alternatively, whether these antibodies represent false-positive results (e.g., cross-reactive antibodies originally raised against another pathogen or a cellular protein).

There is some evidence that nonsymptomatic BDV carriers do exist, at least temporarily, on farms with sporadic BDV cases (Staeheli et al., 2000), but there is no incontrovertible evidence that transient natural infections do occur. Long-term studies employing a herd consisting of both experimentally infected and uninfected ungulate species (horses, sheep, or cattle), kept under controlled conditions, might be the key to solving these problems.

Recently, it was shown that a collection of human sera ($n = 25$) which had been judged to be BDV seropositive based on reactivity in IFA displayed only low avidity when subjected to treatment with 3 M urea in the washing step (Allmang et al., 2001). In contrast, BDV-reactive immunoglobulins in sera of experimentally or naturally infected animals were shown to bind with high avidity under the same conditions. The authors concluded from this investigation that BDV-reactive antibodies in human sera were probably not induced by BDV but rather were generated originally following infection with an antigenically related microorganism or following exposure to other related immunogens. The study by Allmang et al. (2001) seriously questions the diagnostic values of human BDV-reactive antibodies. However, the possibility should be considered that the observed anomalies in human serum antibody responses might reflect our limited understanding of human BDV infections, which were suggested to involve only low levels of viral antigen (de la Torre et al., 1996; Nakamura et al., 2000). It is tempting to speculate that this might result in less robust antibody responses. Therefore to clarify this issue, more-comprehensive serum avidity studies, which also should include sera from animals with suspected inapparent infections, are urgently needed. Identification of BDV antigen epitopes, recognized by human and animal sera using arrays consisting of overlapping BDV protein-derived peptides, might prove crucial in elucidating the true nature of BDV-reactive antibodies.

REFERENCES

Allmang, U., M. Hofer, S. Herzog, K. Bechter, and P. Staeheli. 2001. Low avidity of human serum antibodies for Borna disease virus antigens questions their diagnostic value. *Mol. Psychiatry* 6:329–333.

Auwanit, W., P. I. Ayuthaya, T. Nakaya, S. Fujiwara, T. Kurata, K. Yamanishi, and K. Ikuta. 1996. Unusually high seroprevalence of Borna disease virus in clade E human immunodeficiency virus type 1-infected patients with sexually transmitted diseases in Thailand. *Clin. Diagn. Lab. Immunol.* 3:590–593.

Bechter, K., S. Herzog, B. Fleischer, R. Schüttler, and R. Rott. 1987. Kernspintomographische Befunde bei psychiatrischen Patienten mit und ohne Serum-Antikörper gegen das Virus der Bornaschen Krankheit. *Nervenarzt* 58:617–624.

Bechter, K., S. Herzog, and R. Schüttler. 1992. Possible significance of Borna disease for humans. *Neurol. Psychiat. Brain Res.* **1**:23–29.

Berg, A. L., R. Dörries, and M. Berg. 1999. Borna disease virus infection in racing horses with behavioral and movement disorders. *Arch. Virol.* **144**:547–559.

Bilzer, T., A. Grabner, and L. Stitz. 1996. Immunpathologie der Borna-Krankheit beim Pferd: klinische, virologische und neuropathologische Befunde. *Tierarztl. Prax.* **24**:567–576.

Bilzer, T., O. Planz, W. I. Lipkin, and L. Stitz. 1995. Presence of CD4+ and CD8+ T cells and expression of MHC class I and MHC class II antigen in horses with Borna disease virus-induced encephalitis. *Brain Pathol.* **5**:223–230.

Binz, T., J. Lebelt, H. Niemann, and K. Hagenau. 1994. Sequence analysis of the p24 gene of Borna disease virus in naturally infected horse, donkey and sheep. *Virus Res.* **34**:281–289.

Bode, L. 1995. Human infections with Borna disease virus and potential pathogenic implications, p. 103–130. *In* H. Koprowski and W. I. Lipkin (ed.), *Borna Disease.* Springer, Berlin, Germany.

Bode, L., R. Dürrwald, and H. Ludwig. 1994a. Borna virus infections in cattle associated with fatal neurological disease. *Vet. Rec.* **135**:283–284.

Bode, L., and H. Ludwig. 1997. Clinical similarities and close genetic relationship of human and animal Borna disease virus. *Arch. Virol.* **13**(Suppl.):167–182.

Bode, L., S. Riegel, W. Lange, and H. Ludwig. 1992. Human infections with Borna disease virus: seroprevalence in patients with chronic diseases and healthy individuals. *J. Med. Virol.* **36**:309–315.

Bode, L., F. Steinbach, and H. Ludwig. 1994b. A novel marker for Borna disease virus infection. *Lancet* **343**:297–298.

Bode, L., W. Zimmermann, R. Ferszt, F. Steinbach, and H. Ludwig. 1995. Borna disease virus genome transcribed and expressed in psychiatric patients. *Nat. Med.* **1**:232–236.

Briese, T., C. G. Hatalski, S. Kliche, Y. S. Park, and W. I. Lipkin. 1995. Enzyme-linked immunosorbent assay for detecting antibodies to Borna disease virus-specific proteins. *J. Clin. Microbiol.* **33**:348–351.

Briese, T., A. Schneemann, A. J. Lewis, Y. S. Park, S. Kim, H. Ludwig, and W. I. Lipkin. 1994. Genomic organization of Borna disease virus. *Proc. Natl. Acad. Sci. USA* **91**:4362–4366.

Caplazi, P., and F. Ehrensperger. 1998. Spontaneous Borna disease in sheep and horses: immunophenotyping of inflammatory cells and detection of MHC-I and MHC-II antigen expression in Borna encephalitis lesions. *Vet. Immunol. Immunopathol.* **61**:203–220.

Carbone, K. M., C. S. Duchala, J. W. Griffin, A. L. Kincaid, and O. Narayan. 1987. Pathogenesis of Borna disease in rats: evidence that intra-axonal spread is the major route for virus dissemination and the determinant for disease incubation. *J. Virol.* **61**:3431–3440.

Carbone, K. M., B. D. Trapp, J. W. Griffin, C. S. Duchala, and O. Narayan. 1989. Astrocytes and schwann cells are virus-host cells in the nervous system of rats with Borna disease. *J. Neuropathol. Exp. Neurol.* **48**:631–644.

Carbone, K. M., T. R. Moench, and W. I. Lipkin. 1991. Borna disease virus replicates in astrocytes, Schwann cells and ependymal cells in persistently infected rats: location of viral genomic and messenger RNAs by in situ hybridization. *J. Neuropathol. Exp. Neurol.* **50**:205–214.

Chen, C. H., Y. L. Chiu, C. K. Shaw, M. T. Tsal, A. L. Hwang, and K. J. Hsiao. 1999a. Detection of Borna disease virus RNA from peripheral blood cells in schizophrenic patients and mental health workers. *Mol. Psychiatry* **4**:566–571.

Chen, C. H., Y. L. Chiu, F. C. Wei, F. J. Koong, H. C. Liu, C. K. Shaw, H. G. Hwu, and K. J. Hsiao. 1999b. High seroprevalence of Borna virus infection in schizophrenic patients, family members and mental health workers in Taiwan. *Mol. Psychiatry* **4**:33–38.

Cubitt, B., C. Oldstone, and J. C. de la Torre. 1994. Sequence and genome organization of Borna disease virus. *J. Virol.* **68**:1382–1396.

Czygan, M., W. Hallensleben, M. Hofer, S. Pollak, C. Sauder, T. Bilzer, I. Blümcke, P. Riederer, B. Bogerts, P. Falkai, M. J. Schwarz, E. Masliah, P. Staeheli, F. T. Hufert, and K. Lieb. 1999. Borna disease virus in human brains with a rare form of hippocampal degeneration but not in brains of patients with common neuropsychiatric disorders. *J. Infect. Dis.* **180**:1695–1699.

Degiorgis, M.-P., A.-L. Berg, C. Hård Af Segerstad, T. Mörner, M. Johansson, and M. Berg. 2000. Borna disease in a free-ranging lynx (*Lynx lynx*). *J. Clin. Microbiol.* **38**:3087–3091.

De la Torre, J. C., D. Gonzalez-Dunia, B. Cubitt, M. Mallory, N. Mueller-Lantzsch, F. A. Grässer, L. A. Hansen, and E. Masliah. 1996. Detection of Borna disease virus antigen and RNA in human autopsy brain samples from neuropsychiatric patients. *Virology* **223**:272–282.

Deuschle, M., L. Bode, I. Heuser, J. Schmider, and H. Ludwig. 1998. Borna disease virus proteins in cerebrospinal fluid of patients with recurrent depression and multiple sclerosis. *Lancet* **352**:1828–1829.

Dürrwald, R. 1993. Die natürliche Borna-Virus-Infektion der Einhufer und Schafe. Untersuchungen zur Epidemiologie, zu neueren diagnostischen Methoden (ELISA, PCR) und zur Antikörperkinetik bei Pferden nach Vakzination mit Lebendimpfstoff. Inaugural doctoral dissertation. Freie Universität Berlin, Berlin, Germany.

Eckert, K. A., and T. A. Kunkel. 1991. DNA polymerase fidelity and the polymerase chain reaction. *PCR Methods Appl.* **1**:17–24.

Evengård, B., T. Briese, G. Lindh, S. Lee, and W. I. Lipkin. 1999. Absence of evidence of Borna disease virus infection in Swedish patients with chronic fatigue syndrome. *J. Neurovirol.* **5**:495–499.

Formella, S., C. Jehle, C. Sauder, P. Staeheli, and M. Schwemmle. 2000. Resistance to superinfection can explain high sequence stability of Borna disease virus genomes in persistently infected cell cultures. *J. Virol.* **74**:7878–7883.

Forns, X., J. Bukh, R. H. Purcell, and S. U. Emerson. 1997. How Escherichia coli can bias the results of molecular cloning: preferential selection of defective genomes of hepatitis C virus during the cloning procedure. *Proc. Natl. Acad. Sci. USA* **94**:13909–13914.

Fu, Z. F., J. D. Amsterdam, M. Kao, V. Shankar, H. Koprowski, and B. Dietzschold. 1993. Detection of Borna disease virus-reactive antibodies from patients with affective disorders by Western immunoblot technique. *J. Affect. Disord.* **27**:61–68.

Fujiwara, S., H. Takahashi, T. Nakaya, Y. Nakamura, K. Nakamura, K. Iwahashi, H. Kazamatsuri, S. Iritani, N. Kuroki, K. Ikeda, and K. Ikuta. 1997. Microplate hybridization for Borna disease virus RNA in human peripheral blood mononuclear cells. *Clin. Diagn. Lab. Immunol.* **4**:387–391.

Fukuda, K., K. Takahashi, Y. Iwata, N. Mori, K. Gonda, T. Ogawa, K. Osonoe, M. Sato, S. Ogata, T. Horimoto, T. Sawada, M. Tashiro, K. Yamaguchi, S. Niwa, and S. Shigeta. 2001. Immunological and PCR analyses for Borna disease virus in psychiatric patients and blood donors in Japan. *J. Clin. Microbiol.* **39**:419–429.

Furrer, E., T. Bilzer, L. Stitz, and O. Planz. 2001. Neutralizing antibodies in persistent Borna disease virus infection: prophylactic effect of gp94-specific monoclonal antibodies in preventing encephalitis. *J. Virol.* **75**:943–951.

Gosztonyi, G., and H. Ludwig. 1984. Borna disease of horses. An immunohistological and virological study of naturally infected animals. *Acta Neuropathol.* (Berlin) **64**:213–221.

Gosztonyi, G., and H. Ludwig. 1995. Borna disease—neuropathology and pathogenesis, p. 39–73. *In* H. Koprowski and W. I. Lipkin (ed.), *Borna Disease.* Springer, Berlin, Germany.

Grabner, A., and A. Fischer. 1991. Symptomatologie und Diagnostik der Borna-Enzephalitis des Pferdes. Eine Fallanalyse der letzten 13 Jahre. *Tierarztl. Prax.* **19**:68–73.

Haga, S., M. Yoshimura, Y. Motol, K. Arima, T. Aizawa, K. Ikuta, M. Tashiro, and K. Ikeda. 1997. Detection of Borna disease virus genome in normal human brain tissue. *Brain Res.* **770:**307–309.

Hagiwara, K., S. Kawamoto, H. Takahashi, Y. Nakamura, T. Nakaya, T. Hiramune, C. Ishihara, and K. Ikuta. 1997a. High prevalence of Borna disease virus infection in healthy sheep in Japan. *Clin. Diagn. Lab. Immunol.* **4:**339–344.

Hagiwara, K., N. Momiyama, H. Taniyama, T. Nakaya, N. Tsunoda, C. Ishihara, and K. Ikuta. 1997b. Demonstration of Borna disease virus (BDV) in specific regions of the brain from horses positive for serum antibodies to BDV but negative for BDV RNA in the blood and internal organs. *Med. Microbiol. Immunol.* **186:**19–24.

Herden, C., S. Herzog, T. Wehner, C. Zink, J. A. Richt, and K. Frese. 1999. Comparison of different methods of diagnosing Borna disease in horses post mortem. *Eq. Infect. Dis.* **8:**286–290.

Herzog, S., K. Frese, and R. Rott. 1994. Ein Beltrag zur Epizootiologie der Bornaschen Krankheit beim Pferd. *Wien. Tierarztl. Monschr.* **81:**374–379.

Herzog, S., C. Kompter, K. Frese, and R. Rott. 1984. Replication of Borna disease virus in rats: age-dependent differences in tissue distribution. *Med. Microbiol. Immunol.* **173:**171–177.

Herzog, S., I. Pfeuffer, K. Haberzettl, H. Feldmann, K. Frese, K. Bechter, and J. A. Richt. 1997. Molecular characterization of Borna disease virus from naturally infected animals and possible links to human disorders. *Arch. Virol.* **13**(Suppl.):183–190.

Herzog, S., and R. Rott. 1980. Replication of Borna disease virus in cell cultures. *Med. Microbiol. Immunol.* **168:**153–158.

Hirano, N., M. Kao, and H. Ludwig. 1983. Persistent tolerant or subacute infection in Borna disease virus-infected rats. *J. Gen. Virol.* **64:**1521–1530.

Horimoto, T., H. Takahashi, M. Sakaguchi, K. Horikoshi, S. Iritani, H. Kazamatsuri, K. Ikeda, and M. Tashiro. 1997. A reverse-type sandwich enzyme-linked immunosorbent assay for detecting antibodies to Borna disease virus. *J. Clin. Microbiol.* **35:**1661–1666.

Hsu, T., K. M. Carbone, S. A. Rubin, S. L. Vonderfecht, and J. J. Eiden. 1994. Borna disease virus p24 and p38/40 synthesized in a baculovirus expression system: virus protein interactions in insect and mammalian cells. *Virology* **204:**854–859.

Joest, E., and K. Degen. 1909. Über eigentümliche Kerneinschlüsse der Ganglienzellen bei der enzootischen Gehirn-Rückenmarksentzündung der Pferde. *Z. Infektkrankh. Haustiere* **6:**348–356.

Kao, M., A. N. Hamir, C. E. Rupprecht, Z. F. Fu, V. Shankar, H. Koprowski, and B. Dietzschold. 1993. Detection of antibodies against Borna disease virus in sera and cerebrospinal fluid of horses in the USA. *Vet. Rec.* **132:**241–244.

Katz, J. B., D. Alstad, A. L. Jenny, K. M. Carbone, S. A. Rubin, and R. W. Waltrip II. 1998. Clinical, serologic, and histopathologic characterization of experimental Borna disease in ponies. *J. Vet. Diagn. Investig.* **10:**338–343.

Kishi, M., T. Nakaya, Y. Nakamura, Q. Zhong, K. Ikeda, M. Senjo, M. Kakinuma, S. Kato, and K. Ikuta. 1995. Demonstration of human Borna disease virus RNA in human peripheral blood mononuclear cells. *FEBS Lett.* **364:**293–297.

Kitani, T., H. Kuratsune, I. Fuke, Y. Nakamura, T. Nakaya, S. Asahi, M. Tobiume, K. Yamaguti, T. Machil, R. Inagi, K. Yamanishi, and K. Ikuta. 1996. Possible correlation between Borna disease virus infection and Japanese patients with chronic fatigue syndrome. *Microbiol. Immunol.* **40:**459–462.

Kitze, B., S. Herzog, P. Rieckmann, S. Poser, and J. A. Richt. 1996. No evidence of Borna disease virus specific antibodies in multiple sclerosis patients in Germany. *Neurology* **234:**660–661.

Kliche, S., L. Stitz, H. Mangalam, L. Shi, T. Binz, H. Niemann, T. Briese, and W. I. Lipkin. 1996. Characterization of the Borna disease virus phosphoprotein, p23. *J. Virol.* **70**:8133–8137.

Kubo, K., T. Fujiyoshi, M. M. Yokoyama, K. Kamei, J. A. Richt, B. Kitze, S. Herzog, M. Takigawa, and S. Sonoda. 1997. Lack of association of Borna disease virus and human T-cell leukemia virus type 1 infections with psychiatric disorders among Japanese patients. *Clin. Diagn. Lab. Immunol.* **4**:189–194.

Lange, H., S. Herzog, W. Herbst, and T. Schliesser. 1987. Seroepidemiologische Untersuchungen zur Bornaschen Krankheit (Ansteckende Gehirn-Rückenmarkentzündung) der Pferde. *Tierarztl. Umschau* **42**:938–946.

Lebelt, J., and K. Hagenau. 1996. Die Verteilung des Bornavirus in naturlich infizierten Tieren mit klinischer Erkrankung. *Berl. Munch. Tierarztl. Wochenschr.* **109**:178–183.

Legay, V., C. Sailleau, G. Dauphin, and S. Zientara. 2000. Construction of an internal standard used in RT nested PCR for Borna disease virus RNA detection in biological samples. *Vet. Res.* **31**:565–572.

Legros, S., J. Mendlewicz, and J. Wybran. 1985. Immunoglobulins, autoantibodies and other serum fractions in psychiatric disorders. *Eur. Arch. Psychiatry Neurol. Sci.* **235**:9–11.

Lieb, K., W. Hallensleben, M. Czygan, L. Stitz, P. Staeheli, and the Bornavirus Study Group. 1997. No Borna disease virus-specific RNA detected in blood from psychiatric patients in different regions of Germany. *Lancet* **350**:1002.

Lipkin, W. I., G. H. Travis, K. M. Carbone, and M. C. Wilson. 1990. Isolation and characterization of Borna disease agent cDNA clones. *Proc. Natl. Acad. Sci. USA* **87**:4184–4188.

Lundgren, A. L., R. Lindberg, H. Ludwig, and G. Gosztonyi. 1995a. Immunoreactivity of the central nervous system in cats with a Borna disease-like meningoencephalomyelitis (staggering disease). *Acta Neuropathol.* (Berlin) **90**:184–193.

Lundgren, A. L., W. Zimmermann, L. Bode, G. Czech, G. Gosztonyi, R. Lindberg, and H. Ludwig. 1995b. Staggering disease in cats: isolation and characterization of the feline Borna disease virus. *J. Gen. Virol.* **76**:2215–2222.

Mizutani, T., Y. Nishino, H. Kariwa, and I. Takashima. 1999. Reverse transcription-nested polymerase chain reaction for detecting p40 RNA of Borna disease virus without risk of plasmid contamination. *J. Vet. Med. Sci.* **61**:77–80.

Mizutani, T., M. Ogino, Y. Nishino, T. Kimura, H. Kariwa, K. Tsujimura, H. Inagaki, and I. Takashima. 1998. A single-tube RT-PCR method for the detection of Borna disease viral genomic RNA. *Jpn. J. Vet. Res.* **46**:73–81.

Morales, J. A., S. Herzog, C. Kompter, K. Frese, and R. Rott. 1988. Axonal transport of Borna disease virus along olfactory pathways in spontaneously and experimentally infected rats. *Med. Microbiol. Immunol.* **177**:51–68.

Nakamura, K., H. Takahashi, Y. Shoya, T. Nakaya, M. Watanabe, K. Tomonaga, K. Iwahashi, K. Ameno, N. Momiyama, H. Taniyama, T. Sata, T. Kurata, J. C. de la Torre, and K. Ikuta. 2000. Isolation of Borna disease virus from human brain. *J. Virol.* **74**:4601–4611.

Nakamura, Y., M. Kishi, T. Nakaya, S. Asahi, H. Tanaka, H. Sentsui, K. Ikeda, and K. Ikuta. 1995. Demonstration of Borna disease virus RNA in peripheral blood mononuclear cells from healthy horses in Japan. *Vaccine* **13**:1076–1079.

Nakamura, Y., T. Nakaya, K. Hagiwara, N. Momiyama, Y. Kagawa, H. Taniyama, C. Ishihara, T. Sata, T. Kurata, and K. Ikuta. 1999a. High susceptibility of Mongolian gerbil (Meriones unguiculatus) to Borna disease virus. *Vaccine* **17**:480–489.

Nakamura, Y., M. Watanabe, W. Kamitani, H. Taniyama, T. Nakaya, Y. Nishimura, H. Tsujimoto, S. Machida, and K. Ikuta. 1999b. High prevalence of Borna disease virus in domestic cats with neurological disorders in Japan. *Vet. Microbiol.* **70**:153–169.

Nakaya, T., H. Takahashi, Y. Nakamur, H. Kuratsune, T. Kitani, T. Machii, K. Yamanishi, and K. Ikuta. 1999. Borna disease virus infection in two family clusters of patients with chronic fatigue syndrome. *Microbiol. Immunol.* **43:**679–689.

Nakaya, T., H. Takahashi, Y. Nakamura, S. Asahi, M. Tobiume, H. Kuratsune, T. Kitani, K. Yamanishi, and K. Ikuta. 1996. Demonstration of Borna disease virus RNA in peripheral blood mononuclear cells derived from Japanese patients with chronic fatigue syndrome. *FEBS Lett.* **378:**145–149.

Narayan, O., S. Herzog, K. Frese, H. Scheefers, and R. Rott. 1983. Pathogenesis of Borna disease in rats: immune-mediated viral ophthalmoencephalopathy causing blindness and behavioral abnormalities. *J. Infect. Dis.* **148:**305–315.

Nishino, Y., M. Funaba, R. Fukushima, T. Mizutani, T. Kimura, R. Iizuka, H. Hirami, and M. Hara. 1999. Borna disease virus infection in domestic cats: evaluation by RNA and antibody detection. *J. Vet. Med. Sci.* **61:**1167–1170.

Nowotny, N., J. Kolodziejek, C. O. Jehle, A. Suchy, P. Staeheli, and M. Schwemmle. 2000. Isolation and characterization of a new subtype of Borna disease virus. *J. Virol.* **74:**5655–5658.

Ogino, M., K. Yoshimatsu, K. Tsujimura, T. Mizutani, J. Arikawa, and I. Takashima. 1998. Evaluation of serological diagnosis of Borna disease virus infection using recombinant proteins in experimentally infected rats. *J. Vet. Med. Sci.* **60:**531–534.

Reeves, N. A., C. R. Helps, D. A. Gunn-Moore, C. Blundell, P. L. Finnemore, G. R. Pearson, and D. A. Harbour. 1998. Natural Borna disease virus infection in cats in the United Kingdom. *Vet. Rec.* **143:**523–526.

Richt, J. A., A. Grabner, and S. Herzog. 2000. Borna disease in horses. *Vet. Clin. N. Am. Eq. Pract.* **16:**579–595.

Richt, J. A., S. Herzog, K. Haberzettl, and R. Rott. 1993. Demonstration of Borna disease virus-specific RNA in secretions of naturally infected horses by the polymerase chain reaction. *Med. Microbiol. Immunol.* **182:**293–304.

Richt, J. A., and R. Rott. 2001. Borna disease virus: a mystery as an emerging zoonotic pathogen. *Vet. J.* **161:**24–40.

Richt, J. A., S. VandeWoude, M. C. Zink, J. E. Clements, S. Herzog, L. Stitz, R. Rott, and O. Narayan. 1992. Infection with Borna disease virus: molecular and immunobiological characterization of the agent. *Clin. Infect. Dis.* **14:**1240–1250.

Rott, R., and H. Becht. 1995. Natural and experimental Borna disease in animals, p. 17–30. *In* H. Koprowski and W. I. Lipkin (ed.), *Borna Disease.* Springer, Berlin, Germany.

Rott, R., S. Herzog, K. Bechter, and K. Frese. 1991. Borna disease, a possible hazard for man? *Arch. Virol.* **118:**143–149.

Rott, R., S. Herzog, B. Fleischer, A. Winokur, J. Amsterdam, W. Dyson, and H. Koprowski. 1985. Detection of serum antibodies to Borna disease virus in patients with psychiatric disorders. *Science* **228:**755–756.

Rubin, S. A., A. M. Sierra-Honigmann, H. M. Lederman, R. W. Waltrip II, J. J. Eiden, and K. M. Carbone. 1995. Hematologic consequences of Borna disease virus infection of rat bone marrow and thymus stromal cells. *Blood* **85:**2762–2769.

Salvatore, M., S. Morzunow, M. Schwemmle, W. I. Lipkin, and the Bornavirus Study Group. 1997. Borna disease virus in brains of North American and European people with schizophrenia and bipolar disorder. *Lancet* **349:**1813–1814.

Sauder, C., and J. C. de la Torre. 1998. Sensitivity and reproducibility of RT-PCR to detect Borna disease virus (BDV) RNA in blood: implications for BDV epidemiology. *J. Virol. Methods* **71:**229–245.

Sauder, C., A. Müller, B. Cubitt, J. Mayer, J. Steinmetz, W. Trabert, B. Ziegler, K. Wanke, N. Mueller-Lantzsch, J.C. de la Torre, and F. A. Grässer. 1996. Detection of Borna disease virus (BDV) antibodies and BDV RNA in psychiatric patients: evidence for high sequence conservation of human blood-derived BDV RNA. *J. Virol.* **70:**7713–7724.

Schneider, P. A., T. Briese, W. Zimmermann, H. Ludwig, and W. I. Lipkin. 1994. Sequence conservation in field and experimental isolates of Borna disease virus. *J. Virol.* **68:**63–68.

Schüppel, K. F., M. Reinacher, J. Lebelt, and D. Kulka. 1995. Bornasche Krankheit bei Primaten, p. 115–120. *In Erkrankungen der Zootiere: Verhandlungsbericht des 37. Internationalen Symposiums.*

Schwemmle, M., C. Jehle, S. Formella, and P. Staeheli. 1999. Sequence similarities between human bornavirus isolates and laboratory strains question human origin. *Lancet* **354:**1973–1974.

Shankar, V., M. Kao, A. N. Hamir, H. Sheng, H. Koprowski, and B. Dietzschold. 1992. Kinetics of virus spread and changes in levels of several cytokine mRNAs in the brain after intranasal infection of rats with Borna disease virus. *J. Virol.* **66:**992–998.

Shoya, Y., T. Kobayashi, T. Koda, P. K. Lai, H. Tanaka, T. Koyama, K. Ikuta, M. Kakinuma, and M. Kishi. 1997. Amplification of a full-length Borna disease virus (BDV) cDNA from total RNA of cells persistently infected with BDV *Microbiol. Immunol.* **41:**481–486.

Sierra-Honigmann, A. M., S. A. Rubin, M. G. Estafanous, R. H. Yolken, and K. M. Carbone. 1993. Borna disease virus in peripheral blood mononuclear and bone marrow cells of neonatally and chronically infected rats. *J. Neuroimmunol.* **45:**31–36.

Sirota, P., K. Schild, M. Firer, A. Tanay, A. Elizur, D. Meytes, and H. Slor. 1991. Autoantibodies to DNA in multicase families with schizophrenia. *Biol. Psychiatry* **29:**2715.

Sorg, I., and A. Metzler. 1995. Detection of Borna disease virus RNA in formalin-fixed, paraffin-embedded brain tissues by nested PCR. *J. Clin. Microbiol.* **33:**821–823.

Staeheli, P., C. Sauder, J. Hausmann, F. Ehrensperger, and M. Schwemmle. 2000. Epidemiology of Borna disease virus. *J. Gen. Virol.* **81:**2123–2135.

Stitz, L., K. Nöske, O. Planz, E. Furrer, W. I. Lipkin, and T. Bilzer. 1998. A functional role for neutralizing antibodies in Borna disease: influence on virus tropism outside the central nervous system. *J. Virol.* **72:**8884–8892.

Stitz, L., D. Schilken, and K. Frese. 1991. Atypical dissemination of the highly neurotropic Borna disease virus during persistent infection in cyclosporine A-treated, immunosuppressed rats. *J. Virol.* **65:**457–460.

Takahashi, H., T. Nakaya, Y. Nakamura, S. Asahi, Y. Onishi, K. Ikebuchi, T. A. Takahashi, T. Katoh, S. Sekiguchi, M. Takazawa, H. Tanaka, and K. Ikuta. 1997. Higher prevalence of Borna disease virus infection in blood donors living near thoroughbred horse farms. *J. Med. Virol.* **52:**330–335.

Tsujimura, K., T. Mizutani, H. Kariwa, K. Yoshimatsu, M. Ogino, Y. Morii, H. Inagaki, J. Arikawa, and I. Takashima. 1999. A serosurvey of Borna disease virus infection in wild rats by a capture ELISA. *J. Vet. Med. Sci.* **61:**113–117.

Vahlenkamp, T. W., H. K. Enbergs, and H. Muller. 2000. Experimental and natural borna disease virus infections: presence of viral RNA in cells of the peripheral blood. *Vet. Microbiol.* **76:**229–244.

VandeWoude, S., J. A. Richt, M. C. Zink, R. Rott, O. Narayan, and J. E. Clements. 1990. A Borna virus cDNA encoding a protein recognized by antibodies in humans with behavioral diseases. *Science* **250:**1278–1281.

Waltrip, R. W., II, R. W. Buchanan, A. Summerfelt, A. Breier, W. T. Carpenter, Jr., N. L. Bryant, S. A. Rubin, and K. M. Carbone. 1995. Borna disease virus and schizophrenia. *Psychiatry Res.* **56:**33–44.

Wehner, T., A. Ruppert, C. Herden, K. Frese, H. Becht, and J. A. Richt. 1997. Detection of a novel Borna disease virus encoded 10 kDa protein in infected cells and tissues. *J. Gen. Virol.* **78:**2459–2466.

Weisman, Y., D. Huminer, M. Malkinson, R. Meir, S. Kliche, W. I. Lipkin, and S. Pitlik. 1994. Borna disease virus antibodies among workers exposed to infected ostriches. *Lancet* **344:**1232–1233.

Weissenböck, H., N. Nowotny, P. Caplazi, J. Kolodziejek, and F. Ehrensperger. 1998. Borna disease in a dog with lethal meningoencephalitis. *J. Clin. Microbiol.* **36:**2127–2130.

Yamaguchi, K., T. Sawada, T. Naraki, R. Igata-Yi, H. Shiraki, Y. Horii, T. Ishii, K. Ikeda, N. Asou, H. Okabe, M. Mochizuki, K. Takahashi, S. Yamada, K. Kubo, S. Yashiki, R. W. Waltrip II, and K. M. Carbone. 1999. Detection of borna disease virus-reactive antibodies from patients with psychiatric disorders and from horses by electrochemiluminescence immunoassay. *Clin. Diagn. Lab. Immunol.* **6:**696–700.

Yamaguchi, K., T. Sawada, S. Yamane, S. Haga, K. Ikeda, R. Igata-Yi, K. Yoshiki, M. Matsuoka, H. Okabe, Y. Horii, H. Nawa, R. W. Waltrip II, and K. M. Carbone. 2001. Synthetic peptide-based electrochemiluminescence immunoassay for anti-Borna disease virus p40 and p24 antibodies in rat and horse serum. *Ann. Clin. Biochem.* **38:**348–355.

Zimmermann, W., R. Dürrwald, and H. Ludwig. 1994. Detection of Borna disease virus RNA in naturally infected animals by a nested polymerase chain reaction. *J. Virol. Methods* **46:**133–143.

Chapter 4

Epidemiology and Infection of Natural Animal Hosts

*Kazuyoshi Ikuta, Katsuro Hagiwara, Hiroyuki Taniyama,
and Norbert Nowotny*

Borna disease, a usually fatal acute nonsuppurative encephalitis of horses, was first described as *hitzige Kopfkrankheit* (acute head disease) in the late 18th century in southeastern Germany (von Sind, 1767). The name refers to the city of Borna in Saxony, Germany, where many horses died during an epidemic between 1894 and 1896. Experimental transmission of the disease to animals using brain homogenates from diseased horses together with filtration studies demonstrated a viral etiology for Borna disease (Zwick et al., 1927; Nicolau and Galloway, 1928). The main natural hosts of Borna disease virus (BDV) are horses and sheep. Natural Borna disease was also diagnosed in donkeys, goats, cattle, rabbits, and dogs. Borna disease in these animals was mainly restricted to areas of endemicity in central Europe, e.g., Germany, Switzerland, Austria, and Liechtenstein (Metzler et al., 1976; Metzler et al., 1979; Ludwig et al., 1985; Waelchli et al., 1985; Lange et al., 1987; Grabner and Fischer, 1991; Dürrwald, 1993; Herzog et al., 1994; Bilzer and Stitz, 1996; Dürrwald and Ludwig, 1997; Suchy et al., 1997; Suchy et al., 2000; Weissenböck et al., 1998b; Caplazi et al., 1999; Nowotny et al., 2000). At a lower prevalence, sporadic cases of Borna disease have also been found outside the areas of endemicity (Nowotny

Kazuyoshi Ikuta • Department of Virology, Research Institute for Microbial Diseases, Osaka University, Suita, Osaka 565-0871, Japan.   **Katsuro Hagiwara** • Department of Veterinary Microbiology, Faculty of Veterinary Medicine, Rakuno Gakuen University, Ebetsu, Hokkaido 069-8501, Japan.   **Hiroyuki Taniyama** • Department of Pathology, Faculty of Veterinary Medicine, Rakuno Gakuen University, Ebetsu, Hokkaido 069-8501, Japan.   **Norbert Nowotny** • Clinical Virology Group, Institute of Virology, University of Veterinary Sciences, Vienna, A-1210 Vienna, Austria, and Department of Medical Microbiology, Faculty of Medicine and Health Sciences, United Arab Emirates University, P.O. Box 17666, Al Ain, United Arab Emirates.

et al., 2000). Furthermore, a variety of warm-blooded animals, including deer and zoo animals such as monkeys, sloths, llamas, alpacas, and pygmy hippopotamuses, are known to be natural hosts of BDV (Ernst and Hahn, 1927; Zwick, 1939; Heinig, 1969). A Borna-like disease was reported in cats and ostriches (Lundgren, 1992; Malkinson et al., 1993). Over the last 2 decades, infection with BDV or a related agent in the absence of typical disease has been reported in a wide variety of animal species worldwide.

In this chapter, we present the current knowledge available on classical and subclinical cases of natural Borna disease and cases of Borna-like disease in several animal species in different geographical regions.

GEOGRAPHICAL LOCATION OF NATURAL BORNA DISEASE IN HORSES AND SHEEP

A syndrome of progressive meningoencephalitis of horses and sheep was recognized 100 years before the disease received its name, Borna disease, from an epidemic near the town of Borna, Germany. Around 1900, the incidence of fatal Borna disease in horses in this area was fairly high (about 1%, based on a total number of about 150,000 horses) (Bode and Ludwig, 1997). Although severe cases of Borna disease still occur in this area, their incidence has remarkably decreased (Bode and Ludwig, 1997; Richt and Rott, 2001). Extensive studies on BDV infections, mostly from Germany, showed that a seasonal accumulation of cases is observed in spring and early summer, with a significant decrease in late autumn and winter (Wörz, 1858; Schmidt, 1912, 1952; Ludwig et al., 1985; Grabner and Fischer, 1991; Dürrwald and Ludwig, 1997; Richt et al., 2000). In sheep flocks, clinical Borna disease affects a large number of animals, while with horses usually only a few animals in a herd show clinical signs (Richt et al., 1997).

Clinically, histopathologically and virologically confirmed cases of Borna disease in horses and sheep have been mostly restricted to Germany, Switzerland, Austria, and Liechtenstein (Metzler et al., 1976; Metzler et al., 1979; Ludwig et al., 1985; Waelchli et al., 1985; Lange et al., 1987; Grabner and Fischer, 1991; Dürrwald, 1993; Herzog et al., 1994; Bilzer and Stitz, 1996; Dürrwald and Ludwig, 1997; Suchy et al., 1997; Suchy et al., 2000; Weissenböck et al., 1998b; Caplazi et al., 1999; Nowotny et al., 2000). Berg et al. (1999) reported Borna disease in Swedish horses; however, these horses had an atypical disease pattern such as diffuse mental and gait disturbances. Recently, two cases of horses with Borna disease were confirmed in Japan (Taniyama et al., 2001). In addition, BDV or a related agent was demonstrated at a high rate in restricted regions of the brain from Japanese horses with locomotor disease of unknown etiology (Hagiwara et al., 1997b). When these reports are taken together with the reports of subclinical cases of BDV infection in horses and sheep in many countries in the world, as will be described later, there seems to be a worldwide geographical distribution of BDV or a BDV-related agent. The reason why reports of Borna disease had mainly been described in the areas of endemicity in central Europe might be due to the fact that in areas of non-endemicity this disease is rather rare and outbreaks are usually sporadic and may go undiagnosed (Richt and Rott, 2001); alternatively, there may be certain cofactors present in the areas of endemicity that contribute to the development of clinical disease.

DISEASE MANIFESTATION IN HORSES AND SHEEP

The clinical manifestations and pathological findings in naturally BDV-infected horses and sheep are almost the same. However, most of the available data reviewed in this section are obtained mainly from horses. The clinical and pathological manifestations in these animals are summarized in Table 1, compared with those of other animals such as cattle, dogs, cats, and ostriches.

Table 1. Clinical and pathological manifestations of Borna disease in several natural animal species

Animal	Manifestations		References
	Clinical	Pathological	
Horse	Begins with excitability or depression; ends with severe hyperexcitability, aggressiveness, or lethargy; somnolence; and stupor	Encephalitis, meningitis	Zwick, 1939; Rott and Becht, 1995; Dürrwald and Ludwig, 1997; Taniyama et al., 2001
Sheep	Similar to those in horses	Encephalitis	Nicolau and Galloway, 1928; Ludwig et al., 1988
Cow	Reduced appetite, anxiety, ataxia, paresis, compulsive circling movements, and finally complete inability to move	Encephalitis	Caplazi et al., 1994; Okamoto et al., 2002a
Dog	Salivation, mydriasis, circling, and coma followed by death	Meningoencephalitis	Weissenböck et al., 1998a; Okamoto et al., 2002b
Cat	Hind leg ataxia, paresis, mental changes, anorexia, hypersensitivity, hyperaesthesia, and seizures	Meningoencephalomyelitis	Lundgren, 1992; Nowotny and Weissenböck, 1995
Ostrich	Clinical signs of incoordination followed by paresis	No specific lesions	Malkinson et al., 1993; Malkinson et al., 1995

Clinical Manifestations

BDV infection can result in peracute, acute, or subacute disease with meningoencephalitis. Typical clinical signs of Borna disease vary and can include loss of appetite, simultaneous or consecutive alterations in behavior, circling, ataxia, blindness, sometimes disturbances in fertility, obesity (rarely), and, in late stages, paralysis followed by death (Schmidt, 1912, 1952; Zwick et al., 1927; Zwick, 1939; Heinig, 1969; Ludwig et al., 1985; Rott and Becht, 1995; Dürrwald and Ludwig, 1997; Herden et al., 1999). Spontaneous recovery can occasionally occur despite a persistent infection in the central nervous system (CNS), and sometimes a recurrent course of the disease may be noticed (Schmidt, 1912; Mayr and Danner, 1974; Danner, 1982; Grabner and Fischer, 1991; Bode et al., 1994a).

Clinical manifestation of Borna disease is initiated by alterations in behavior and consciousness (Richt and Rott, 2001). Difficulties in swallowing and chewing (pipe-smoking syndrome) and recurrent fever are dominant (Grabner and Fischer, 1991; Dürrwald and Ludwig, 1997; Suchy et al., 2000). The neurological signs progress more gravely towards later stages of the disease with repetitive rhythmic motor activities; hyperexcitability; fearfulness and unusual aggressiveness; or lethargy, somnolence, and stupor. In addition, hypokinesia, abnormal postures, and decreased skin and deep sensory reactions are frequently found. In more-advanced stages of the disease, hyporeflexia of spinal reflexes, head tilt, and hypoesthesia with disturbances in proprioceptive sensory functions are characteristic. In this stage, ataxia, imbalance, and abnormal reaction towards exogenous stimuli and abnormal posture can be often observed. In addition, the following symptoms gradually develop: dysphagia and salivation (due to pharyngeal paralysis), decreased tongue tension and increased tongue movement, bruxism, trismus, and miosis. In the final stages of the disease, increased appearance of neurogenic torticollis, sometimes associated with compulsive circular walking, is noted. Also, slight tremor in the head area is usually followed by convulsions. Convulsions are regularly associated with head pressing, possibly the result of high cerebrospinal fluid (CSF) pressure caused by the inflammatory reaction in the CNS (Hiepe, 1960; Grabner and Fischer, 1991; Bilzer et al., 1996). Loss of the papillary reflex and strabismus are often found in this stage of the disease (Schmidt, 1912; Müller and Fritzsch, 1955), and affected animals can become comatose (Grabner and Fischer, 1991; Bilzer et al., 1996). Food intake can cease totally, and only few infected animals are able to swallow water. As a consequence, a fasting hyperbilirubinemia with icteric mucosal membranes is often seen (Grabner and Fischer, 1991; Dürrwald and Ludwig, 1997). Particularly in horses, paralysis is common.

Death usually occurs 1 to 4 weeks after the onset of initial signs in more than 80% of diseased animals (Schmidt, 1912, 1952; Ihlenburg, 1962; Danner, 1982; Grabner and Fischer, 1991; Dürrwald and Ludwig, 1997). If the animal survives the acute phase of the disease, alterations in behavior such as depression with apathy, somnolence, and fearfulness can be seen for the rest of the animal's life (Richt et al., 1997).

Blindness can be rarely observed in horses after the acute phase of the disease (Bilzer et al., 1996). Interestingly, the nonpurulent retinitis or chorioretinitis with degeneration of rods and cones in the retina that is often observed in experimentally infected rabbits and rats (Krey et al., 1979a; Krey et al., 1979b; Narayan et al., 1983; Kacza et al., 2000) does not occur in horses, despite occasional observation of clinical signs of blindness (Richt and Rott, 2001). Nevertheless, viral antigens and infectious BDV can be detected in the respective neuronal cell layers in most of the affected horses (Herden et al., 1999).

Pathological Findings

Generally, the pathological findings after BDV infection in naturally infected horses and sheep are similar to those in experimentally infected animals such as rats. They are usually restricted to the CNS (mainly in the gray matter), spinal cord, and retina. Histopathology reveals severe nonpurulent poliomeningoencephalomyelitis with massive perivascular cuffing consisting mainly of macrophages, CD3$^+$ T lymphocytes (CD4$^+$ and CD8$^+$) late in the infection (Fig. 1A), and some B lymphocytes and plasma cells, as well as expression of major histocompatibility complex (MHC) class I and II antigens on inflammatory cells (Deschl et al., 1990; Stitz et al.,

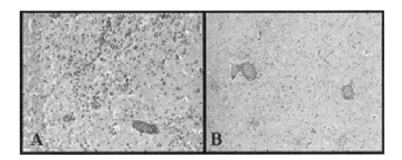

Figure 1. Nonsuppurative encephalitis in the olfactory bulb from a horse (A) and the frontal lobe from a bovine naturally infected with BDV (B). The neurological lesions are characterized by perivascular cuffing and mononuclear cell infiltration. Hematoxylin and eosin stain was used. Magnifications, ×12 (A) and ×6 (B).

1993; Stitz et al., 1995; Bilzer et al., 1995; Caplazi and Ehrensperger, 1998). The encephalitic reactions in the CNS in both experimentally infected rats and naturally infected horses and sheep were shown to be correlated to strong immune responses, especially $CD8^+$-T-cell-mediated immune response against one of the BDV major proteins, the nucleoprotein (N) (Caplazi and Ehrensperger, 1998; Berg et al., 1999; Planz and Stitz, 1999). A reactive astrocytosis can be regularly observed in all areas showing inflammatory lesions. Besides the olfactory bulb, basal cortex, caudate nucleus, thalamus, and hippocampus, periventricular areas mainly in the medulla oblongata can be also affected. No significant lesions are apparent in the cerebellum, and alterations in the spinal cord are rather inconsistent. In naturally infected horses, eosinophilic inclusion bodies (Joest-Degen bodies) are occasionally found in neurons, especially in the hippocampus, but are not always found in affected brains (Stitz et al., 1993; Gonzalez-Dunia et al., 1997; Weissenböck et al., 1998b).

Specific anti-BDV antibodies were demonstrated in the CNS of horses with clinical symptoms (Ludwig and Thein, 1977; Taniyama et al., 2001). Such antibodies were shown to be locally produced in the infected CNS, and the titer of immunoglobulins in the CSF is higher than that in the serum (Ludwig and Thein, 1977).

The presence of BDV N gene RNA was first demonstrated in the brains from naturally diseased animals by reverse transcription (RT)-PCR (Zimmermann et al., 1994). Samples from a total of 36 diseased animals (32 horses, one donkey, and three sheep), collected between 1991 and 1992 in Saxony, Thuringia, and Saxony-Anhalt, Germany, were all positive for BDV RNA, whereas samples from the control group (three healthy horses and four horses with an anamnestic report of lameness) gave no specific amplification. Subsequently, detailed immunohistological analyses of paraffin-embedded brain sections by immunohistochemistry (IHC) (Color Plate 1 [see color insert]) as well as in situ hybridization (ISH) (Color Plate 2 [see color insert]) have been used to understand BDV-induced pathogenicity in the brain from horses with Borna disease (see Nowotny et al., 2000; Weissenböck et al., 1998b; Gosztonyi and Ludwig, 1984; and Taniyama et al., 2001). Interestingly, the findings in these reports differ in respect to virus distribution in the brain.

Gosztonyi and Ludwig (1984) examined the brains of eight horses that had suffered from natural Borna disease. All neuronal compartments in different brain regions contained BDV antigens, though not always simultaneously. The largest amounts of antigens were found in the nuclei. They appeared deep brown in color, indicating a high concentration of the antigens. In larger neurons, often one or two relatively large (diameter, 2 to 4 μm) spherical accumulations were seen; in others, a finer distribution of antigens was characteristic. The nucleolus was always characterized by its distinct negativity for antigens. Infrequently, a rather diffuse intranuclear antigen distribution was noted. The distribution pattern of the intranuclear antigens was very similar to that of the Joest-Degen inclusion bodies. The cytoplasm and dendrites showed a more inconsistent presence of antigens than that in the nuclei. If the cytoplasm and dendrites were antigen positive, the reaction was always fainter, reflecting lower amounts of antigen than those found in the nucleus. Virus antigen was occasionally found to fill apical and basal dendrites extensively. In the hippocampus, a diffuse, slight positivity was found in the hilar region and in segments h1, h2, and h3, with rather sharp borders. Antigen-positive and -negative neurons occured frequently side by side; apart from the antigen content, these cells generally exhibited no morphological alterations. In some places antigen negativity of satellite glial cells contrasted sharply with the positivity of the neuronal cytoplasm. Axonal presence of antigens was obvious in the long tracts of the brain stem and in the hemispheral white matter. In the hippocampus, spherical structures with a diameter of 2 to 4 μm, resembling giant synaptic buttons, were occasionally seen to contain virus-specific antigens.

Gosztonyi and Ludwig (1984) estimated the overall amount of antigen in 10 brain areas, yielding a fair survey of antigen distribution. The regional distribution of antigen was compared with that of the inflammatory reaction. The highest amounts of antigen were found in the laterobasal cortex (including the piriform lobe) and in the hippocampus. The hypothalamus, mesencephalon, and pons contained a moderate amount of antigen, while the parasagittal cortex, basal ganglia, thalamus, and medulla oblongata contained a small amount. The cerebellum was distinguished by the almost-complete absence of antigen. Inflammatory cells and macrophages were also always negative for BDV-specific antigens.

The vulnerability of the retina in Borna disease is well known on the basis of clinical and pathological observations (Krey et al., 1979a; Krey et al., 1979b; Krey et al., 1982). Although BDV antigen is not frequently detected in the retina of naturally infected horses, the assessment of infectivity indicated beyond doubt that this part of the nervous system was not exempt from virus infection either.

Thus, the regional assessments of infectivity peak at the well-known preferred sites of the disease. Although the low titer in the cerebellum parallels strongly the lack or scarcity of histological changes and antigen, the titers in other brain areas were not strictly consistent in the three brains examined. A possible explanation for this divergence or variance is that the animals did not die or were not killed at the same phase of the disease; e.g., the virus titer could have been declining at a preferred site in one animal while still being high in another animal.

Taniyama et al. (2001) histopathologically examined the CNSs from two racing horses exhibiting pharyngeal paralysis, flaccid paresis, and motor incoordination. The animals were euthanized because of neural paralysis and submitted for postmortem analysis. Antibodies to BDV N protein were detected in serum and CSF from both animals.

Neuropathological lesions were characterized by a nonsuppurative encephalitis dominated by perivascular cuffs. Large pyramidal cells with satellitosis were frequently found in the neocortex of the parietal, temporal, and occipital lobes. Although these lesions were widespread in the cerebrum, cerebellum, and spinal cord, inflammatory changes were more predominant in the white matter than the gray matter. In areas without inflammatory lesions, shrunken neurons with strongly eosinophilic cytoplasm and pyknotic nuclei were frequently observed. The most severe lesions in the mare were localized in the olfactory bulbs, frontal and parietal white matter, diencephalons, corpus striatum, and mesencephalon. Mild lesions were found in the temporal lobe, occipital lobe, cerebellum, and spinal cord. In the stallion, severe lesions were found in the corpus striatum, diencephalons, and mesencephalon, and mild lesions were found in the pons, medulla oblongata, and cerebellum.

By IHC, strong immunoreactivity was diffusely distributed in the cytoplasm of small and large neurons and neuropils in areas with inflammatory changes, including the spinal cord. However, immunoreactivity was also recognized in areas without inflammatory changes. The N positivity predominantly appeared in shrunken neurons with strong eosinophilic cytoplasm and pyknotic nuclei. Large pyramidal cells in the brain neocortex frequently showed immunoreactivity in the neurites in addition to the cell bodies. Occasionally, astrocytes showing N immunopositivity were found in the gray matter. Some Purkinje cells in the cerebellum showed mild immunopositivity in their cell bodies. Strong immunopositivity was found in many neurons in gray matter of the spinal cord at all levels. The distributions of immunopositivity were similar in the two horses.

ISH revealed positive hybridization signals for sense and antisense riboprobes in the nuclei and cytoplasm of the neurons and occasionally astrocytes. The signals were evident in a large number of small and large neurons throughout the whole brain and spinal cord. Positive signals for the sense probe were mainly localized in the nuclei of the neurons, and signals for the antisense probe were found in the nuclei and cytoplasm. The distribution of positive hybridization signals was similar in both horses. Thus, the two horses were diagnosed as having Borna disease.

The distribution of inflammatory lesions differed from those in other cases described in horses. Borna disease lesions predominantly occur in the gray matter but also involve fiber tracts related to affected areas of the gray matter, while in the two horses described by Taniyama et al. (2001), inflammatory changes occurred predominantly in the diencephalon, corpus striatum, and mesencephalon rather than in the neocortex.

Neuronal degeneration and neuronophagia are frequently reported in BDV-infected horses (Lange et al., 1987; Dürrwald and Ludwig, 1997; Weissenböck et al., 1998b). Neuronophagia and satellitosis were frequently found in the cortical areas related to inflammatory lesions in the white matter. In the two thoroughbred horses discussed by Taniyama et al. (2001), eosinophilic Joest-Degen bodies were not detected in hippocampus neurons.

SUBCLINICAL INFECTION AND BDV PREVALENCE IN HORSES AND SHEEP

Asymptomatic infection in horses seems to be more frequent than expected, based on the detection of antiviral antibodies in sera as well as viral nucleic acid in tissue samples. The serological and molecular assays were mainly performed on the major BDV proteins N and/or phosphoprotein (P) and/or their RNAs, but the sensitivities of the assays differ significantly. In some naturally infected animals the specific signals are very low, and the data obtained regarding prevalence of BDV infection vary considerably among these studies. Although several groups have detected BDV nucleic acid in peripheral blood mononuclear cells (PBMCs) by nested RT-PCR, it is still not clear whether, during the course of infection in naturally BDV-infected animals, there is a period of viremia (Nowotny and Kolodziejek, 2000). Also, because of the high sensitivity of the testing method, laboratory contamination may occur during nested RT-PCR, as demonstrated by Schwemmle et al. (M. Schwemmle, C. Jehle, S. Formella, and P. Staeheli, Letter, *Lancet* **354**:1973–1974, 1999) for some published human BDV isolates and PCR amplification products.

BDV-specific antibodies or RNAs have been reported in apparently clinically healthy horses from Germany, Holland, Poland, Israel, North Africa, the United States, Iran, and Japan (Lange et al., 1987; Kao et al., 1993; Richt et al., 1993; Nakamura et al., 1995; Bahmani et al., 1996; Vahlenkamp et al., 2000). Prevalences of anti-BDV antibody or BDV RNA or protein in naturally infected horses and sheep are summarized in Tables 2 and 3, respectively, comparatively with those in other animal species.

Table 2. Anti-BDV antibodies in naturally infected animals in different geographic areas

| Animal | Country | % Prevalence (no. positive/total no. tested) | | Specimen(s) | Assay(s) | Reference |
		Disease	Subclinical infection			
Horse	Germany	28.6 (4/14)		Serum, CSF	CF[h]	Ludwig and Thein, 1977
			29 (29/100[f])	Serum	IF[i],WB[j]	Richt et al., 1993
	USA	100 (5/5)	28.6 (4/14)	Serum	IF	Vahlenkamp et al., 2000
			8.8 (26/295)	Serum	WB	Kao et al., 1993
			16.7 (5/30)	CSF	WB	Kao et al., 1993
			2.7 (8/295)	Serum	IF	Kao et al., 1993
			0 (0/30)	CSF	IF	Kao et al., 1993
	Japan		26.3 (15/57)	Serum	WB	Nakamura et al., 1995
		66.7 (4/6[a])		Serum	WB	Hagiwara et al., 1997b
			16.7 (9/54)	Serum	ELISA, WB	Takahashi et al., 1997
			17.8 (16/90)	Serum	ECLIA	Yamaguchi et al., 1999
		60.9 (28/46[a])	18.1 (13/72)	Serum	WB	Hagiwara et al., 2002
	Iran		24.5 (13/53)	Serum	WB	Bahmani et al., 1996
	Sweden	57.7 (15/26[b])	23.0 (11/48)	Serum	ELISA	Berg et al., 1999
	Bangladesh		75 (15/20)	Serum	ECLIA	Khan et al., 2000
	China			Serum	ELISA, WB	Hagiwara et al., 2001
Sheep	Japan		26.8 (85/317)	Serum	ELISA, WB	Hagiwara et al., 1997a
			21.8 (17/78)	Serum	ELISA	Hagiwara et al., 1997a
	Germany		16.0 (4/25)	Serum	IF	Vahlenkamp et al., 2000
	China		50.0 (10/20)	Serum	ELISA, WB	Hagiwara et al., 2001
Cattle	Japan		20.3 (15/74)	Serum	WB	Hagiwara et al., 1996
	China		0 (0/20)	Serum	ELISA, WB	Hagiwara et al., 2001

Cat	Sweden	45.8 (11/24)	16.7 (1/6)	Serum	IF	Lundgren et al., 1993
	Germany	12.5 (3/24[c])	6.9 (12/173)	Serum	IF	Lundgren et al., 1993
	Japan		8.4 (7/83)	Serum	WB	Nakamura et al., 1995
		66.7 (10/15[d])		Serum	WB	Nakamura et al., 1999
			18.8 (6/32)	Serum	WB	Nishino et al., 1999
	United Kingdom	35.3 (12/34[f])	5.9 (4/68[g])	Serum	ELISA	Reeves et al., 1998
Rodents	Japan		0 (0/106)	Serum	ELISA	Tsujimura et al., 1999
	China		0 (0/165)	Serum	ELISA, WB	Hagiwara et al., 2001

[a] Horses with locomotor disease.
[b] Horses with neurological signs.
[c] Cats with undefined neurological records.
[d] Cats with neurological signs.
[e] Cats with undiagnosed neurological signs.
[f] Horses with no clinical Borna disease but derived from stables with a history of at least one animal having clinical signs of Borna disease.
[g] Cats with clinical signs other than CNS signs.
[h] Complement fixation.
[i] IF, immunofluorescence.
[j] WB, Western blotting.

Table 3. BDV RNA or proteins in naturally infected animals in different geographic areas

Animal	Country	% Prevalence (no. positive/total no. tested)		Specimen(s)	BDV signal	Assay	Reference(s)
		Disease	Subclinical infection				
Horse	Germany	28.6 (4/14)		Brain	Virus	Infectivity test	Ludwig and Thein, 1977
			15.1 (8/53[f])	CF, NS, SA[f]	RNA	RT-PCR	Richt et al., 1993
		100 (9/9)		Brain	RNA	RT-PCR	Bilzer et al., 1995
		100 (9/9)		Brain	Protein	WB	Bilzer et al., 1995
		20.0 (1/5)	28.6 (4/14)	PBMCs	RNA	RT-PCR	Vahlenkamp et al., 2000
	Japan		29.8 (17/57)	PBMCs	RNA	RT-PCR	Nakamura et al., 1995
		66.7 (4/6[a])		Brain	RNA	RT-PCR	Hagiwara et al., 1997b
	Iran		23.6 (17/72)	PBMCs	RNA	RT-PCR	Bahmani et al., 1996
Sheep	Japan		17.9 (14/78)	PBMCs	RNA	RT-PCR	Hagiwara et al., 1997a
	Germany		4.0 (1/25)	PBMCs	RNA	RT-PCR	Vahlenkamp et al., 2000
Cattle	Japan		10.8 (8/74)	PBMCs	RNA	RT-PCR	Hagiwara et al., 1996
Cat	Japan		13.3 (11/83)	PBMCs	RNA	RT-PCR	Nakamura et al., 1996
			6.3 (2/32)	PBMCs	RNA	RT-PCR	Nakamura et al., 1999
		53.3 (8/15[b])		PBMCs	RNA	RT-PCR	Nishino et al., 1999
	United Kingdom	80.0 (4/5[b])	0 (0/5)	PBMCs	RNA	RT-PCR	Reeves et al., 1998
		33.3 (5/15[c])	33.3 (1/3[e])	Brain	RNA	RT-PCR	Reeves et al., 1998
Ostrich	Israel	53.8 (7/13)	10.0 (1/10)	Brain	Protein	ELISA	Malkinson et al., 1993, Malkinson et al., 1995

[a] Horses with locomotor disease.
[b] Cats with neurological signs.
[c] Cats with nervous signs.
[d] Horses with no clinical Borna disease but derived from stables with history that at least one animal had clinical signs of Borna disease.
[e] Cats with nonneurological signs.
[f] CF, conjunctival fluid; NS, nasal secretions; SA, saliva.

Serum samples from horses all over Germany were examined for BDV-specific antibodies to determine the prevalence of BDV infection (Richt et al., 1993). Among a total of 100 horses with no history of clinical Borna disease but housed in stables with a history of at least one animal having clinical signs of Borna disease, 29 were positive for anti-BDV antibodies. BDV RNA was also detected in some of these horses in their various secretions, such as saliva, nasal secretions, and conjunctival fluid, by RT-PCR (Richt et al., 1993). The assay proved to be highly sensitive, as 10 BDV RNA molecules were reproducibly amplified. A recent survey of horses in Germany showed the presence of both anti-BDV serum antibodies and BDV RNA in PBMCs in animals with Borna disease and healthy animals: BDV RNA was present in one of five seropositive horses with Borna disease, while anti-BDV antibodies and/or BDV RNA was present in 4 (among these 4, 2 were positive for both antibodies and RNA) of 14 healthy horses (Vahlenkamp et al., 2000). Notably, BDV-specific RNA was present in some cases in the absence of BDV-specific antibodies. However, vaccination of horses and sheep with live attenuated strains had been employed in Germany for half a century (Zwick and Witte, 1932; Möhlmann and Maas, 1960; Fechner, 1964; Danner, 1978; Dürrwald, 1993; Ludwig et al., 1993; Dürrwald and Ludwig, 1997). Therefore, such vaccination may contribute to some subclinical cases in those animals or be linked to evidence of BDV seropositivity in animals (e.g., vaccine seroconversion) without other evidence of natural infection (e.g., BDV RNA or infectious virus).

In the United States, Borna disease had been considered an exotic disease. A seroepidemiological study was performed on 295 horses in the United States with various diseases that were unrelated to the CNS (Kao et al., 1993). Immunofluorescence assay (IFA) and Western blot analysis revealed a 2.7% BDV seroprevalence by both assays and a 6.1% seroprevalence by Western blot analysis only. The indirect immunofluorescence titers of BDV antigens in infected baby hamster kidney cells ranged from 1:20 to 1:80. Western blotting was performed with the purified BDV-specific proteins isolated from infected rat brains. Information obtained from the owners about the history of the seropositive horses revealed that they were either clinically normal or had a diagnosis of a disease(s) unrelated to Borna disease.

In Japan, PBMCs derived from 57 healthy horses were examined by nested RT-PCR to determine the prevalence of BDV infection (Nakamura et al., 1995). Seventeen (29.8%) of the samples were positive for BDV RNA in PBMCs by RT-PCR, and 15 (26.3%) were seropositive by Western blotting. About 60% of BDV RNA-positive animals also showed seropositivity by Western blotting. Also, by using a newly developed electrochemiluminescence immunoassay (ECLIA), 16 out of 90 (17.8%) Japanese feral horses were found to be positive for BDV antibodies (Yamaguchi et al., 1999). There was no clinical evidence of neurological or behavioral disease observed in any of the horses. These horses had not been subjected to veterinary care, including vaccination or medication, for a long period of time. Furthermore, 112 out of 200 (56%) domestic horses in Japan showed antibodies to BDV, indicating that the BDV seroprevalence in domestic horses is apparently higher than in feral horses (Yamaguchi et al., 1999).

In Japan, BDV was also demonstrated at high rates in brains from horses with locomotor disease of unknown etiology (Hagiwara et al., 1997b). Horses from Hokkaido, Japan, were admitted to veterinary hospitals because of locomotor disease with dysbasia, i.e., superficial digital flexor tendonitis, cervical osteochondrosis, or osteochondritis dissecans of the stifle joint. All of these horses had no clinical signs characteristic for Borna disease, such as long-lasting behavioral changes, obesity syndrome, or paralysis with mortality. Also, these horses had no apparent histological abnormalities such as inflammation. Four out of six were positive for anti-BDV antibodies by Western blot analysis. BDV RNA was demonstrated in brain sections from seropositive, but not from seronegative, horses and was observed only in restricted regions such as the lateral ventricle, hippocampus, cerebellum, or spinal cord. All other organs tested, such as spleen, liver, kidney, and lymph nodes as well as PBMCs were negative. Another seroepidemiological study was performed on 125 culled racehorses in Hokkaido, Japan, to investigate the prevalence of BDV infection in different categories of diseases (Hagiwara et al., 2002). Antibodies to BDV N or P protein were detected in 19.2% (24 of 125) and 3.2% (4 of 125) of the horses, respectively. Antibodies to both proteins were detected in 24.8% (31 of 125). A total of 59 of 125 horses (47.2%) were positive for antibodies to BDV: 47.5% (28 of 59) with locomotory disorder, 22.0% (13 of 59) with digestive system disorder, and 13.5% (8 of 59) with nervous system disorder. Seropositivity in horses that did not match the above diagnosis, including retired horses, was 11.8% (7 of 59). There was no correlation between seropositivity and gender and age. Among the 31 horses positive for both N and P proteins, 24 were diagnosed as having locomotory or nervous system disorder. Thus, BDV may be associated with such disorders.

In another Asian country, Bangladesh, 23% (11 of 48) of normal horses were shown to be positive for anti-BDV antibody by ECLIA (Khan et al., 2000).

Seventy-two healthy racehorses (28 Arabian, 17 thoroughbred, and 27 crossbred) from Tehran, Iran, were examined for anti-BDV antibodies and BDV RNA (Bahmani et al., 1996). The prevalence of BDV antibodies and/or RNA was 41.2% in Arabian, 23.5% in thoroughbred, and 33.3% in crossbred horses, but only 17.9, 5.9, and 11.1% of them, respectively, showed positive signals for both BDV antibodies and RNA. Crossbred horses showed a higher prevalence for BDV RNA, detected only in females. In addition, a significantly higher prevalence for BDV RNA was observed in Arabian males and thoroughbred females. BDV prevalence did not increase with advancing age of the horses.

A similar investigation in two groups of Swedish racing horses, one clinically healthy and one including horses with diffuse neurological signs, revealed that BDV seroprevalence was 24.5% (13 of 53) and 57.5% (15 of 23), respectively (Berg et al., 1999). Thus, the BDV seroprevalence of healthy Swedish horses comes very close to that of Japanese horses (26.3%) (Nakamura et al., 1995) or Iranian horses (18.1%) (Bahmani et al., 1996). However, the seroprevalence of healthy horses in other countries is considerably lower: 11.5% (Herzog et al., 1994) and 12% (Lange et al., 1987) in Germany and 6.1% in the United States (Kao et al., 1993). Healthy farm horses, in which clinical cases of Borna disease had been observed, showed a seroprevalence of 33% (Herzog et al., 1994).

After experimental infection with BDV, ponies developed characteristic clinical signs as described for naturally occurring Borna disease, followed by death (two out of three ponies), about 1 month postinfection (Katz et al., 1998). In these ponies, seroconversion occurred only after the onset of clinical signs and only to weak IFA reactivity; high-titer antibodies (1:12,000) were found by IFA only in the convalescent animal. These results suggest that previously noted discrepancies in BDV seroprevalence in naturally infected animals could be due to differences in the stage of the disease at the time of serology testing.

Similar to horses, healthy sheep bred on Hokkaido Island, Japan, showed high rates of anti-BDV antibodies and BDV RNA in PBMCs (Hagiwara et al., 1997a). Initially, the sera from adult sheep collected in 1989 were examined by an enzyme-linked immunosorbent assay (ELISA) based on P protein, and 26.8% (85 of 317) of sheep were seropositive for BDV. During 1995 to 1996, blood samples from sheep were collected and the BDV infection prevalence, as tested by immunoblotting and/or RT-PCR, was 0% (0 of 19) in newborns (<1 month old), 51.7% (15 of 29) in lambs (1 to 6 months old), and 36.7% (11 of 30) in adults (>2 years old). Among animals positive for BDV, 60% of lambs and 45.5% of adults were positive for BDV RNA in their PBMCs, while BDV-specific antibodies were detected in 46.7% of lambs and 90.9% of adults. Thus, it is suggested that virus replication in blood, as observed in lambs, is later reduced in adulthood by immune responses raised to BDV. There is also one report on BDV prevalence in healthy sheep in Germany: 2 of 25 healthy sheep were seropositive and none were positive for BDV RNA in PBMCs. In this study, increasing age was associated with increased evidence of BDV infection: the results were shifted to four positive for anti-BDV antibodies and one positive for BDV RNA in PBMCs (Vahlenkamp et al., 2000).

GEOGRAPHICAL LOCATION OF NATURAL BORNA OR BORNA-LIKE DISEASE IN ANIMALS OTHER THAN HORSES AND SHEEP

Cattle

In cattle, a neurological disease resembling the classical Borna disease clinical course and neuropathology seen in horses and sheep had been reported long ago (Nicolau and Galloway, 1928; Frankhauser, 1961). Although there was no etiological proof for BDV infection in these cases, experimental infection of two calves with BDV has been reported (Matthias, 1954). Thus, it was suggested that cattle are susceptible to BDV infection. However, not until 1994 were the first confirmed cases of natural Borna disease in cattle reported, at approximately the same time in Germany and Switzerland (Bode et al., 1994b; Caplazi et al., 1994); the cases occurred in two areas in Germany: in the Nuremberg area in southern Germany, a region where Borna disease is endemic in horses and sheep, and in the Rostock area in northern Germany, a region where Borna disease is not endemic (Bode et al., 1994b). In addition, two bovine cases were demonstrated in an area in the eastern part of Switzerland where Borna disease is known to be endemic (Caplazi et al., 1994). Further, a case of Borna-like disease was recently found in cattle in Hokkaido, Japan (Okamoto et al., 2002a), where two cases of horses with Borna disease had been identified (Taniyama et al., 2001). In this area, BDV seropositivity had been demonstrated in apparently healthy animals of several species (Nakamura et al., 1995; Nakamura et al., 1996; Hagiwara et al., 1997a) including cattle (Hagiwara et al., 1996). In contrast, a retrospective examination of 51 Swiss cattle that were submitted for necropsy between 1985 and 1996 and exhibited nonsuppurative encephalomyelitis failed to demonstrate BDV antigen in the brain (Theil et al., 1998).

Dogs

For a long time, dogs were not suspected as a possible host species for BDV infection, and, therefore, there are no reports on serological and molecular surveys for BDV infection in dogs (Rott and Becht, 1995). Neither natural nor experimental Borna disease in a dog had ever been described until in 1998; the first case of a dog with Borna disease was reported from Vorarlberg, the westernmost state of Austria, an area where BDV infection is endemic (Weissenböck et al., 1998a). This case was verified by several laboratory methods, including histopathology, IHC, ISH, RT-PCR, and sequencing of the PCR amplification products. The second case of a dog with a similar syndrome was recently found in Japan (Okamoto et al., 2002b).

Cats

A group of neurological disorders in cats, histopathologically defined as nonsuppurative meningoencephalomyelitis, has been reported in many countries (Borland and McDonald, 1965; Vandevelde and Braund, 1979; Lundgren, 1992). In Sweden, a disease named "staggering disease" was first described by Kronevi et al. (1974). In the next report of this disorder (also called *vingelsjuka*) by Ström et al. (1992), based on a study carried out between 1988 and 1990, it was concluded that neither feline leukemia virus, feline immunodeficiency virus (FIV), feline infectious peritonitis virus, nor parasites such as *Toxoplasma gondii* and bacteria such as *Borrelia burgdorferi* were involved in the disease complex. Subsequent seroepidemiological investigations in cats with staggering disease from Uppsala in Sweden, Berlin in Germany (Lundgren et al., 1993), Austria (Weissenböck et al., 1994), the United Kingdom (Reeves et al., 1998), and Japan (Nakamura et al., 1999) exhibited a high prevalence of antibodies to BDV or a related agent. In addition, studies of a free-ranging lynx with abnormal behavior in the county of Gävleborg, Sweden, revealed a nonsuppurative meningoencephalitis with the evidence of BDV infection in the brain as demonstrated by ISH, IHC, and RT-PCR (Degiorgis et al., 2000).

Ostriches and Other Birds

BDV infection was reported to be responsible for paretic ostriches in Israel (Ashash et al., 1996; Malkinson et al., 1993; Malkinson et al., 1995). Young birds were imported from Africa in the early 1980s for breeding purposes, and by 1987 six breeding farms had been established (Malkinson et al., 1995). The paretic condition first appeared in young ostriches on several farms in 1988. Over a 5-year period (1989 to 1993), necropsy records and causes of mortality in ostriches up to 3 months old were published (Ashash et al., 1996). The annual mortality rates of all hatched ostriches over the 5-year period were 61, 58, 30, 29, and 16.6%, and the most significant cause of death was a paresis syndrome that accounted for 20, 11, 16, 10.1, and 2% mortality rates, respectively.

All attempts to identify a noninfectious cause were negative, including by biochemical, nutritional, genetic, ecological, and toxicological investigations. Also, no infectious agents commonly associated with nervous system diseases of birds were found. These included *Pasteurella* spp., *Chlamydia* spp., avian encephalomyelitis virus, Newcastle disease virus, turkey meningoencephalitis virus, and other arboviruses. Other less commonly encountered neurotropic viruses were also considered. Of special geographical interest was BDV. This agent had been isolated from the brains of wild birds caught in the Syrian countryside in the areas near farm animals suffering from an undiagnosed nervous system disease (Daubney and Mahlau, 1967). When brains were harvested from sick and healthy ostriches, BDV antigen was detected in 7 of the 13 sick ostriches and in only 1 of 10 healthy ostriches. Thus, the paresis syndrome was reported to be caused by an agent serologically related to BDV.

Other Animals

Spontaneous natural Borna disease has also been demonstrated in other animal species, such as several other equids, donkeys, goats, and rabbits (Metzler et al., 1978). Since geographical location, disease manifestation, and pathological findings in these animal species resemble classical Borna disease as described above, they are not described here in more detail.

DISEASE MANIFESTATION AND SUBCLINICAL PREVALENCE OF BDV OR A RELATED AGENT IN ANIMAL HOSTS OTHER THAN HORSES AND SHEEP

Cattle

Two cattle (Brown Swiss) diagnosed as having Borna disease in Switzerland (Caplazi et al., 1994) showed nonspecific neurological signs such as head tilt and deviation to the right, occasional circling to the right, refusal or inability to pick up food from the left, refusal to drink from the automated water supplies, mild proprioceptive deficits, and reduced response to the menace test (Caplazi et al., 1994). The most striking feature was a unique type of circling, like that of the hands of a clock, with the hindlimbs standing still in the center. The signs could not be attributed to any known bovine CNS disorder. Bode et al. (1994b) described about nine cattle of different breeds with Borna disease in Germany. The clinical symptoms had common features, with reduced appetite, anxiety, ataxia, paresis with paralytic symptoms, compulsive circling movements, and, finally, loss of appetite and complete inability to move. The duration of illness ranged between 1 and 6 weeks, with accelerated development of paresis inducing a quick death. In Japan, a 2-year-old Holstein-Friesian heifer initially showing sudden hyperesthesia and tremor 5 days later showed circling and posterior motor incoordination. This animal was diagnosed with Borna disease by pathological examination, which showed the brain tissue to be infected with BDV but not with bovine herpesvirus 1, *Chlamydia psittaci,* or listeriae (Okamoto et al., 2002a).

Serum antibodies to BDV have been detected in cattle by IFA (Caplazi et al., 1994) and ELISA (Bode et al., 1994b). Similar to horses with classical Borna disease, microscopic examination revealed a moderate to severe, nonpurulent meningoencephalitis in all brain sections evaluated (Caplazi et al., 1994; Okamoto et al., 2002a). Small intranuclear, eosinophilic inclusion bodies (Joest-Degen bodies) were detected frequently (Caplazi et al., 1994) or occasionally (Okamoto et al., 2002a) in neurons in the inflamed brain regions. Neuropathological lesions were characterized by a nonsuppurative encephalomyelitis dominated by thick perivascular cuffs consisting of lymphocytes, macrophages, and plasma cells (Fig. 1B). IHC examination for BDV antigen revealed that numerous neurons in different brain areas from all animals showed a strong positive reaction (Bode et al., 1994b; Caplazi et al., 1994; Okamoto et al., 2002a). BDV antigens were detected in neurons near inflammatory lesions, although neurons in areas without inflammatory lesions were also positive for BDV antigens (Okamoto et al., 2002a). Interestingly, viral antigens were also detected in the kidney, liver, spleen, thymus, tongue, salivary and lacrimal glands, tonsils, and nasal mucosa (Bode et al., 1994b). BDV RNA was also demonstrated in the nuclei and cytoplasm of neurons in the inflamed regions of the brain by ISH (Okamoto et al., 2002a).

There is one report of subclinical cases of BDV infection in cattle by Hagiwara et al. (1996), who reported a high BDV seropositivity rate (15 of 74 healthy cattle examined). BDV RNA in PBMCs was detected in eight cattle by PCR. Only two cases among these were positive for both anti-BDV antibodies and BDV RNA in PBMCs. Overall, 28.4% (21 of 74) were positive for BDV antibodies and/or RNA. Thus, these data suggest that BDV or a BDV-related infection may be widespread even among healthy-appearing cattle.

Although there have been only few publications on bovine Borna disease, the findings in Japanese cattle may suggest that the incidence of infection in cattle is higher than expected. Therefore, more effort is needed to accurately diagnose cattle with CNS disease as well as asymptomatic cases in order to assess the likely risk of BDV infection in cattle.

Dogs

There have been only two cases of Borna-like disease in dogs: one in Austria and the other in Japan. A 2-year-old female husky from Vorarlberg, Austria, with progressive neurological signs was diagnosed with BDV infection (Weissenböck et al., 1998a). Vorarlberg is the westernmost state of Austria, has endemic Borna disease in horses, and is near the area in eastern Switzerland in which Borna disease is endemic. The husky was subjected to a neuropathological examination, which revealed a severe nonsuppurative meningoencephalitis characterized by lymphocytic meningitis, perivascular lymphomonocytic cuffs, neuronal necrosis in the neocortex and hippocampus, subpial endothelial cell swelling, and focal gliosis. The lesions were most severe in the piriform lobe, rostral neocortex, periventricular gray matter, hippocampus, and mesencephalon, while minor changes were found in the occipital neocortex, medulla oblongata, and cerebellum. Some neurons contained single or multiple eosinophilic intranuclear Joest-Degen inclusion bodies. BDV antigen was found by IHC. In contrast, specimens from other dogs with nonsuppurative encephalitis of unresolved etiology in this area were negative for BDV antigens.

The second case of a dog with BDV infection was found in Japan (Okamoto et al., 2002b). A 3-year-old male Welsh corgi presented with a severe and acute progressive disorder in the CNS (hypoesthesia and tremor). Ten days later, the dog showed salivation, mydriasis, and circling and was suspected of having canine distemper. The dog fell into a coma and died, and a postmortem examination revealed neuropathological lesions characterized by a nonsuppurative encephalomyelitis with large, thick perivascular cuffs (lymphocytes [mainly $CD3^+$ T cells, macrophages, and plasma cells]), inflammatory cell infiltrates in the neural parenchyma, neuronophagia, and focal gliosis. Large pyramidal cells with satellitosis were frequently found in the neocortex of the frontal, parietal, temporal and occipital lobes. These lesions were widespread in the cerebrum, cerebellum, and spinal cord, and inflammatory changes were predominant in the gray matter. In areas without inflammatory lesions, shrunken neurons with strongly eosinophilic cytoplasm and pyknotic nuclei were frequently observed. However, eosinophilic Joest-Degen inclusion bodies were not found in this dog. MHC class I and II antigens were found by IHC on inflammatory cells in the perivascular cuffs and neural parenchyma and occasionally on neurons and astrocytes. Rare immunoglobulin G-positive cells were found in the perivascular cuffs. Strong IHC immunopositivity for BDV N was diffusely distributed in the cytoplasm of small and large neurons in areas with inflammatory changes, including the spinal cord. However, immunopositivity was also recognized in intact areas without inflammatory changes. BDV proteins were found distributed in many neurons in the gray matter of the spinal cord. Further, positive hybridization signals obtained by ISH with sense and antisense riboprobes were present in the nuclei and cytoplasm of small and large neurons throughout the whole brain and spinal cord. Positive hybridization signals were not detected in brain tissue samples from normal dogs when a BDV-specific probe was used. There have been no reports of subclinical BDV cases in dogs, but it is not clear how extensively this has been evaluated. Thus, although detected rarely, it is likely that BDV may be a CNS pathogen in dogs. Moreover, the finding of two diseased dogs that appear to have BDV infection in Austria and Japan suggests that BDV infection in dogs may be widespread albeit with low prevalence.

Cats

A neurological disorder in cats, commonly referred to as staggering disease, was observed in Sweden (Kronevi et al., 1974) and Austria (Weissenböck et al., 1994), and diseases resembling staggering disease were reported from Morocco (Martin and Hintermann, 1952), Australia (Borland and McDonald, 1965), the United States (Vandevelde and Braund, 1979), Switzerland (Hoff and Vandevelde, 1981), and Japan (Nakamura et al., 1999). Detailed neuropathological investigation of cats with staggering disease revealed mononuclear perivascular cuffing and gliosis throughout the brain and spinal cord consistent with a nonsuppurative meningoencephalomyelitis (Lundgren, 1992). The clinical manifestation of the disease included hindleg ataxia and paresis, inability to retract the claws, mental changes, anorexia, increased salivation, hypersensitivity to sound and light, hyperesthesia, impaired vision, and seizures (Kronevi et al., 1974; Ström et al., 1992).

Staggering disease was subsequently examined for association with BDV infection (Lundgren et al., 1993; Lundgren and Ludwig, 1993). The neuropathological examination of cats with this Borna-like disease revealed a marked inflammatory reaction in the cerebral leptomeninges as well as in the gray and white matter of the brain and spinal cord (Lundgren, 1992). The inflammatory reaction was most pronounced in the brain stem and the limbic system, although changes were present in other parts of the CNS as well.

In studies using selected groups of Swedish cats (Lundgren et al., 1993; Lundgren and Ludwig, 1993), the major clinical manifestations were a stiff, staggering gait, inability to jump normally, and incoordination of the hind legs. In addition to motor disturbances, mental changes were seen, including increased demonstrations of affection, mewing, or shyness. Aggressive behavior was rare. The disease progressed fatally (2 to 4 weeks) or continued to a chronic stage with residual neurological abnormalities. More than 44% of these diseased cats showed antibodies against BDV antigens, with titers in serum ranging from 1:10 to >1:2,000 (Lundgren and Ludwig, 1993); however, none of the sera exhibited BDV neutralizing activity.

These findings suggest that BDV or a related agent is not only present in cat populations but also is involved in the neurological disorder known as staggering disease. Although this proposed connection has stimulated some controversy, several analogies with Borna disease in horses reinforce this assumption, e.g., clinical findings in both diseases and limbic system as a preferred site for the inflammatory reactions in the CNS. When Lundgren et al. (1995b) tried to isolate BDV from the brain of a diseased cat, infectious virus could be demonstrated after three passages in embryonic mink brain cells, but the infectivity was lost in the next passage. This is quite different from horses and sheep with naturally acquired Borna disease, for which a persistent infection is readily established in rabbit brain cells in the first passage (Gosztonyi and Ludwig, 1984; Ludwig et al., 1993).

Infection of adult Wistar rats with feline brain tissue material did not result in clinical disease during a period of 5 months, nor did it result in growth of infectious virus in the rat brain. However, the brain suspension from a newborn rat inoculated with feline brain tissue material induced typical Borna disease in four adult rats. This indicates a possible adaptation of the cat virus to rats by passaging in rats. The amount of BDV RNA (measured by RT-PCR) and BDV antigen (evaluated by IHC and ELISA) in the CNS was lower in cats than in horses with Borna disease, providing further support for the notion that a distinct feline BDV strain exists. When four barrier-bred cats were inoculated intracerebrally with this newly isolated feline virus, one cat developed neurological signs and nonsuppurative encephalitis (Lundgren et al., 1997).

In contrast, an examination of Austrian cats with staggering disease showed that, despite the striking serological evidence for an infection of these cats with BDV or a related agent, all attempts to demonstrate BDV, viral antigen, or viral sequences in the feline brains failed (Nowotny and Weissenböck, 1995). Further, highly susceptible rabbits were inoculated intracerebrally with brain homogenates from the affected cats. During an observation period of 4 months, the rabbits remained clinically healthy; rectal temperature, blood cell counts, and differential blood cell counts were normal. In particular, and in sharp contrast to the picture seen after inoculation with BDV isolates from horses and sheep, the rabbits showed no signs of CNS disorders and no histological lesions. Nevertheless, the rabbits developed antibodies to BDV or a related agent (titers, 1:20 to 1:80), suggesting the presence of BDV or a related agent in the brains of cats with staggering disease. In the meantime, the Austrian cases of staggering disease have been reanalyzed by using several different highly sensitive RT-PCR and nested RT-PCR assays, again with clearly negative results.

The inflammatory cell composition and the expression of MHC antigens in the CNS of cats with staggering disease were investigated (Lundgren et al., 1995a). Lymphocytes were the predominating inflammatory cells within the adventitial space. There was a markedly increased MHC class II expression in cells morphologically resembling microglia. In several cats, BDV-specific antigen was detected, but only in a few cells, mainly of macrophage lineage. These findings indicate a long-standing inflammatory reaction in the CNS of cats with staggering disease, possibly triggered and sustained by a persistent viral infection, which may also lead to failure to isolate BDV from the brain of these cats.

Interestingly, in cats clinically showing muscle fasciculation and proprioceptive defects, numerous neurons were infected with BDV, despite the absence of encephalitis (Berg and Berg, 1998). The finding of BDV RNA in many neurons may point to a direct, virus-induced dysfunction of the CNS. An atypical disease pattern as in this case might be due to variation in the viral genome, or to host-specific factors such as age, breed, sex, and genetic makeup. Examination for BDV in cats in the United Kingdom also showed that BDV RNA was detected in buffy coat cells or in the brains of cats with neurological diseases as well as in cats with nonneurological disease (Reeves et al., 1998). Notably, the published partial nucleotide sequences of the feline virus were identical with a BDV laboratory strain (N. Nowotny, Letter, *Vet. Rec.* **144:**187, 1999). In a serosurvey, the incidence of BDV antibodies in cats with neurological disease was higher than in those with other types of disease (Reeves et al., 1998).

Even in a population taken randomly from cats in Germany, 7% of cases observed were seropositive, and in a preselected group of cats with undefined neurological disorders 13% were positive (Lundgren et al., 1993). Also, BDV RNA was demonstrated by nested RT-PCR in PBMCs from 11 of 83 (13.3%) randomly selected domestic cats in Hokkaido, Japan (Nakamura et al., 1996). None of the cats were positive for both BDV RNA and anti-BDV antibodies. Also, anti-BDV antibodies and/or BDV RNA was demonstrated in 7 out of 32 (21.9%) neurologically asymptomatic cats in Tokyo, Japan (Nishino et al., 1999). In addition, a total of 15 domestic Japanese cats with neurological disorders including epileptic seizure, circling, head tilt, ataxia, and tremor were examined for association with BDV (Nakamura et al., 1999). None, except for one with FIV, had detectable antibodies to FIV, feline leukemia virus, feline infectious peritonitis virus, and *T. gondii*. Serological and molecular epidemiological studies revealed a very high prevalence of BDV infection in these cats, with antibodies against BDV P and/or N proteins in 10 of 15 (66.7%), and P and/or N RNA in PBMCs in 8 of 15 (53.3%). Further, analyses of postmortem brain samples from one of the cats by IHC and ISH revealed BDV RNA and proteins predominantly in neuronal cells in restricted regions, such as the olfactory bulb and medulla of cerebrum and, faintly, in the medulla oblongata and cerebellum, while no apparent signals appeared in other regions such as pons and spinal cord. In contrast, hematoxylin-eosin staining showed axonal degeneration and loss of myelin in the medulla oblongata, pons, and spinal cord, while only mild lesions were seen in the medulla of the cerebrum with no apparent abnormalities in other regions, including the olfactory bulb. In this animal, there were no lesions and no BDV signals in the hippocampus, although this site is believed to be one of the major regions for inflammatory reactions in cats with staggering disease (Lundgren, 1992). Thus, the regions positive for BDV signals were different from those with histopathological abnormalities. The results reported on the detection of BDV signals in brains from cats with staggering disease have been inconsistent. One group demonstrated BDV RNA in brain samples by RT-PCR (Lundgren et al., 1995b, 1997), while another group's attempts to demonstrate BDV RNA and antigen in feline brains failed (Nowotny and Weissenböck, 1995). Some groups demonstrated BDV RNA in feline brain samples by nested RT-PCR, while other less sensitive techniques such as ISH and IHC failed to confirm the presence of BDV RNA and viral antigen, respectively (A.-L. Berg, Letter, *Vet. Rec.* **145:** 87, 1999). Thus, BDV may persist only in restricted brain regions in cats and at levels that seem to be extremely low compared with those in the brains from horses and sheep. The levels of BDV in the brains may be low by the time the neurological signs are clinically manifested. Alternatively, it is possible that the etiologic agent of staggering disease is not BDV itself but a BDV-related virus. In any case, evidence for BDV or a related infection in the cat—one of humankind's closest companions—has raised concern and interest, since the viral reservoir of possible human infections is still unknown.

Evidence of BDV infection was also found in wild felines. Histopathological examination of a free-ranging lynx revealed a nonsuppurative meningoencephalitis, with the presence of BDV in the brain detected by ISH, IHC, and RT-PCR analyses (Degiorgis et al., 2000).

Ostriches and Other Birds

BDV antigen was identified by ELISA in 7 out of 13 (53.8%) paretic ostriches in Israel and in 1 out of 10 (10%) healthy ostriches from a farm with diseased birds (Malkinson et al., 1993; Malkinson et al., 1995). Birds between 14 and 42 days old were mostly affected. In a minority of cases, clinical signs of incoordination were seen 1 to 3 days before paresis supervened. At this stage of the disease the birds could stand and move with difficulty if given external support. Mostly there was no forewarning of the disease. Appetite, vision, and hearing of the affected birds were normal, but secondary infections and infected pressure sores resulted in their demise within 1 to 3 weeks of sternal recumbency. About 1% of the ostriches seemed to recover when they were given intensive supportive care; however, they relapsed several months later.

No specific lesions were visible on gross necropsy other than that the cloaca was filled with a voluminous quantity of greenish-yellow liquid feces. In all field cases, lesions were confined to neurons located primarily in the central gray matter of the lumbosacral region of the spinal cord. The lesions ranged from degenerative changes accompanied by numerous infiltrating glial cells (satellitosis) and neuronophagia to the formation of glial nodules that replaced the neuronal remnants. In experimentally induced cases, perivascular cuffing was a notable feature.

Although the ostrich is the first natural avian host demonstrated to be affected clinically by the virus, chickens have been experimentally infected (Ludwig et al., 1988). In chickens, persistent infection resulted in ataxia over an extended period. The detection of BDV antigen in brains of paretic ostriches was the first step in identifying a viral etiology for the disease, followed by experimental infection of young ostriches. In field cases, the infection was suspected to occur via the oral-fecal route, while other factors, such as the presence of maternal immunity, was believed to govern the extended age incidence. The orally infected birds became sick at different times after exposure to the virus, which would indicate that the pathogenesis of the disease involves a replication site for the virus outside the CNS. Further work is required to determine whether this site is the gastrointestinal tract or the nasopharynx. Epidemiological findings, based on a comparison of the disease incidence among ostrich-rearing farms, indicated that the virus is not egg transmitted.

The gross and histopathological findings in avian species are substantially different from the mammalian experience. For example, perivascular cuffing was observed only in the spinal cords of experimentally infected birds, and no characteristic lesions have been seen in the brains of paretic ostriches. No Joest-Degen inclusion bodies have been identified so far.

All these data on BDV in ostriches have been derived from birds in Israel studied by only one group. Therefore, similar examinations involving a higher number of birds and additional investigations are needed to clarify the possible involvement of BDV in CNS diseases of this animal species.

ROUTE OF BDV TRANSMISSION

The vector(s) and reservoir(s) for natural BDV infection have not yet been identified, and the mode for intraspecies and interspecies transmission is unknown. Nonetheless, the number of horses imported from abroad, including horses from areas with endemic Borna disease, and the number of racing horses traveling around the world in general are increasing, thus enhancing the global risk of spreading Borna disease. Since the majority of natural host animals may experience subclinical infections—i.e., BDV infection has been found frequently in clinically healthy animals, and since such inapparently infected animals shed virus in various secretions and excretions (Herzog et al., 1994; Morales et al., 1998)—these animals might represent a virus reservoir and a potential source of infection (Richt et al., 1993).

The route of infection for BDV has never been unequivocally established, but many theories have been proposed. Natural infection of horses and sheep is typically sporadic, with the highest incidence of the disease between beginning of spring and beginning of summer. This period coincides with high insect activity, leading to considerations of insects as possible vectors (Rott and Becht, 1995; Dürrwald and Ludwig, 1997). An olfactory route of transmission has been proposed (Morales et al., 1998; Richt et al., 1993; Richt and Rott, 2001), because the virus is assumed to be excreted in salival, nasal, or conjunctival fluids and since BDV-specific RNA has been found in these excretions (Herzog et al., 1994; Becht and Richt, 1996; Lebelt and Hagenau, 1996; Richt et al., 1993; Richt et al., 1994). Following nasal uptake of BDV, the virus may infect olfactory nerve cells in the nasal mucosa and continue via intraneural transmission to the olfactory bulb and other brain regions (Nowotny and Kolodziejek, 2000). Another possible route for infection might follow oral exposure with transmission to brain via the trigeminal nerve (Bilzer et al., 1996). Animals may become infected by direct contact with secretions from infected subjects or, less likely, due to the friable nature of this enveloped virus, by exposure to contaminated food or water. In addition, recent reports on BDV nucleic acid and proteins in PBMCs also indicate a potential for hematogenous transmission.

Recently, vertical transmission of BDV in a pregnant mare has been reported (Hagiwara et al., 2000). A pregnant mare with pyrexia, reduced appetite, ataxia, and paresis was euthanized and examined for the presence of BDV. Her brain, with multiple sites of neuronal degeneration, necrosis, and hemorrhage, and the histologically normal brain of the fetus were both positive for BDV RNA. The BDV nucleotide sequences were identical in the mare and the fetus in the second open reading frame. Further, BDV RNA and proteins were also detected in placenta samples from three mares infected with BDV, supporting the likely potential of vertical transmission (M. Okamoto, W. Kamitani, K. Hagiwara, R. Kirisawa, H. Iwai, Y. Nakamura, K. Tomonaga, K. Ikuta, and H. Taniyama, unpublished data). Although it has been observed that BDV is not readily transmissible among cats, BDV- positive cases in several siblings indicate a possible vertical transmission (Berg et al., 1998).

The experimental data on rodents indicating that they can be persistently infected with BDV and excrete virus suggest that they have the potential to serve both as natural reservoirs and vectors for virus dissemination (Sierra-Honigmann et al., 1993; Rott and Becht, 1995; Hatalski et al., 1997; Berg et al., 1998; Boucher et al., 1999). However, studies on BDV infection in wild rodents in Japan (106 *Rattus norvegicus* rats in the Oshima district, Hokkaido) and the People's Republic of China (165 wild rodents of 18 species in Xinjiang) did not indicate natural infection (Tsujimura et al., 1999; Hagiwara et al., 2001). Thus, the significance of rodents as reservoir hosts for BDV remains to be proven.

There are several reports suggesting the possibility of BDV as a zoonotic agent. Farm workers exposed to infected paretic ostriches in Israel and a matched control group of blood donors (veterinarians and laboratory technicians) were compared with regard to BDV seroprevalence (Y. Weisman et al., Letter, *Lancet* **344**:1232–1233, 1994). Antibodies to BDV were detected in 46% of the farm workers versus 10% of the controls. Further, BDV seroprevalence and BDV RNA detection in PBMCs by nested RT-PCR were shown to be higher in blood donors originating from regions with many horses than in blood donors from urban areas (Takahashi et al., 1997). On the other hand, there is evidence for BDV or a related infection in house cats in several countries, although no human cases have been linked to these feline infections. Thus, even though BDV likely infects humans a number of questions regarding spread of BDV from animals to humans remain open.

VARIATION OF BDV DERIVED FROM DIFFERENT ANIMAL SPECIES

Comparison of the genetic variability of BDV isolates derived from natural host animals from different locations revealed very low divergence. Coding and noncoding sequences were analyzed from field and experimental isolates of BDV in Germany (Schneider et al., 1994). The highest variability in sequence (10%) was found in a 40-nucleotide stretch of genomic RNA between coding sequences for the N and P proteins. Thus, the authors concluded that the degree of sequence conservation in these isolates, passaged in various host species in vivo and in vitro over a period of 64 years, is unusually low for negative-strand RNA viruses. One report suggested a few antigenic variations in the N protein of BDV isolates from horses (Herzog et al., 1997), using brain material from horses with Borna disease screened by IHC and immunoblot analysis using various monoclonal antibodies.

In addition, viral sequences from several horse-derived PCR amplicons in the P protein gene region were compared with tissue culture-adapted isolates such as BDV-MDCK, strain V, and WT-1 (Binz et al., 1994). The results revealed that the homology among them was at least 96.2% at the nucleotide level and 97% at the amino acid level. Also, viral sequences from sheep, donkey, and horse were found to be as related to each other as were sequences from various infected horses. Phylogenetic analysis showed that a BDV isolate from a cat was closely related to other feline BDV sequences as well as to a BDV reference strain derived from a horse (C6BV) (Berg and Berg, 1998). Two amino acid substitutions in the P sequence of this feline virus could be regarded as major changes with potential functional implications for the phosphoprotein. The PCR amplicons in the N protein gene region from the Austrian dog also revealed high sequence conservation: 94 to 98% homology at the nucleotide level compared to published BDV sequences (Weissenböck et al., 1998a). In the case of the Swedish lynx variant, sequencing parts of the P gene identified 12 and 7 single-base changes, compared with the sequences of He/80 and V, respectively (Degiorgis et al., 2000). A comparison of the lynx sequence with two P sequences obtained from Swedish domestic cats with staggering disease revealed the presence of three and five amino acid substitutions, respectively. Also several amino acid substitutions were reported, compared to a BDV sequence obtained from a Swedish horse.

The CNS is unique in its response to viral infections, having no specialized lymphatic drainage and no apparent expression of MHC molecules by normal neurons and glial cells. This may explain the finding that the genetic variability of viruses from the CNS is extremely low, for example, as seen in human immunodeficiency virus (Korber et al., 1994; Monken et al., 1995). Recently, however, a BDV strain with a highly variant genome was isolated from a horse that was euthanized due to severe, incurable neurological disease (Nowotny et al., 2000). The diseased animal was a 7-year-old pony stallion, originating from the Austrian state of

Styria, where no cases of Borna disease had been previously recorded, and the animal had never been in any region of BDV endemicity. The animal's clinical and histopathological picture matched that of classical Borna disease. The nucleotide sequence of this new strain, named No/98, differs from the reference strains by more than 15%, and the subtype is difficult to detect using standard RT-PCR protocols. Due to these major differences in the nucleotide sequence of this strain, it has been proposed to belong to a new BDV subtype. However, the nucleotide changes of the novel BDV isolate have surprisingly little effect on the primary structures of most viral proteins, with the notable exception of the X protein, which is only 81% identical to its counterpart in reference strains. Thus, these data indicate that the BDV genome is far more variable than previously assumed and that naturally occurring subtypes may escape detection by currently used diagnostic assays. Thus, the isolation of BDV with a highly variant genome disproves the general opinion of high sequence conservation of all BDV isolates, and supports the hypothesis that further, yet unidentified, BDV subtypes do exist.

FUTURE DIRECTIONS

BDV is able to infect a wide variety of animal species, and it seems to be geographically more widespread than previously thought (including a significant number of subclinical cases). Additional and more-detailed information has to be obtained regarding the prevalence of BDV infection in various animal species in different geographical regions, since the limited data published so far suggest a significant role of BDV in CNS diseases of several animal species. A complicating factor in understanding the distribution of BDV in naturally infected animals around the world is to clarify the source of the virus in areas that have inoculated animals with live attenuated BDV vaccine strains. Two BDV live-virus vaccine strains (Zwick-vaccine and Dessau) derived from original equine isolates, both rabbit adapted, were employed for active immunization of horses and sheep in Germany for half a century (Zwick and Witte, 1932; Möhlmann and Maas, 1960; Fechner, 1964; Danner, 1978; Dürrwald, 1993; Ludwig et al., 1993; Dürrwald and Ludwig, 1997). The genome of the BDV sequence is highly conserved, with the exception of the recent isolate No/98 (Nowotny et al., 2000), and, therefore, at this time it is not possible to distinguish between wild-type and vaccine strains of BDV. Therefore, to solve this problem, sequence characteristics of the vaccine strains have to be identified and distinguished from those of natural, wild-type strains.

It is still poorly understood how the same infectious agent could play a role in the complex, varied CNS disorders seen in several different animal species when infected with BDV. This presentation of BDV-associated chronic illness or persistent BDV infection without illness also highlights our need to understand better the mechanisms of persistent BDV infection in nondividing neuronal cells.

Another issue is the specific role of immune responses to BDV in the pathogenicity in the CNS of naturally infected animals. BDV anti-N protein is the first virus-specific antigen expressed early after infection, is the predominant viral protein in infected cells, and is the major target for both humoral as well as cell-mediated immunities in infected animals. According to the data gained from experimentally infected rats, such immune responses against N are related to immune-mediated damage in the BDV-infected CNS. However, to complicate things further, the timing of the MHC class I-restricted cytotoxic T-cell response relative to time of infection can determine whether the infected animal's health status is improved by rapid and early elimination of virus-infected cells or, in the case of delayed immune responses where the virus is allowed to spread throughout the CNS, whether the later onset immune response proceeds to a severe, debilitating or fatal immunopathological disease (Nöske et al., 1998). Therefore, the timing of MHC class I-restricted recognition of BDV N protein may represent a key event in the different pathogenicity in naturally infected animals: immunopathology of Borna disease development or immunoprotection (Planz and Stitz, 1999). Variability in cytokine expression in the CNS during the course of Borna disease may also be important for modulation of the immune response (Jordan and Lipkin, 2001). The immunological and/or neurological stage of the host development at initial BDV infection may also be very important, affecting the subsequent course of the disease, in part, because BDV infection may proceed differently in mature and immature neuronal cells in the CNS. The identification of these and other conundrums and their clarification may lead to a better understanding of the variability in BDV-induced diseases in different animals, relative to differences in viral factors as well as host factors.

As discussed in chapter 3, a wide variety of assays (IFA, Western blotting, radioimmunoprecipitation, and ELISA) and antigen preparations (infected cells, infected cell extracts, and recombinant proteins produced in prokaryotic or baculovirus systems) have been used for BDV serological testing. Nevertheless, generally accepted standards for serological diagnosis of BDV infection have not been established yet. The situation is even worse regarding detection of BDV nucleic acid by RT-PCR and, particularly, nested RT-PCR, which is prone to artifacts because of the inadvertent introduction of template from laboratory isolates or cross-contamination of samples. Although nucleic acid amplification is mostly performed in the N and P protein gene region of BDV, individual laboratory techniques and approaches differ markedly. Thus, there is an urgent need for comparative multicenter assay validation studies, such as those initiated some time ago in central Europe as well as in Japan, to significantly reduce false-positive (and false-negative) results in future research. Given these and the many other unsolved BDV mysteries, there will be no lack of BDV research questions in the future.

Acknowledgments. We are grateful to Madiha S. Ibrahim (Department of Virology, Research Institute for Microbial Diseases, Osaka University) and Herbert Weissenböck (Institute of Pathology and Forensic Veterinary Medicine, University of Veterinary Sciences, Vienna, Austria) for valuable discussions.

REFERENCES

Ashash, E., M. Malkinson, R. Meir, S. Perl, and Y. Weisman. 1996. Causes of losses including a Borna disease paralytic syndrome affecting young ostriches of one breeding organization over a five-year period (1989–1993). *Avian Dis.* **40:**240–245.

Bahmani, M. K., I. Nowrouzian, T. Nakaya, Y. Nakamura, K. Hagiwara, H. Takahashi, M. A. Rad, and K. Ikuta. 1996. Varied prevalence of Borna disease virus infection in Arabic, thoroughbred and their cross-bred horses in Iran. *Virus Res.* **45:**1–13.

Becht, H., and J. A. Richt. 1996. Borna disease, p. 235–244. *In* M. J. Studdert (ed.), *Virus Infections of Equines.* Elsevier Science Publishers BV, Amsterdam, The Netherlands.

Beck, A., and H. Frohöse. 1926. Die enzootische Encephalitis des Schafes. Vergleichende experimentelle Untersuchungen üer die seuchenhafte Gehirnrückenmarksentzundung der Pferde und Schafe. *Schweiz. Arch. Tierheilkd.* **54:** 84–110.

Berg, A.-L., and M. Berg. 1998. A variant form of feline Borna disease. *J. Comp. Pathol.* **119:**323–331.

Berg, A.-L., R. Dorries, and M. Berg. 1999. Borna disease virus infection in racing horses with behavioral and movement disorders. *Arch. Virol.* **144:**547–559.

Berg, A.-L., R. Reid-Smith, M. Larsson, and B. Bonnett. 1998. Case control study of feline Borna disease in Sweden. *Vet. Rec.* **142:**715–717.

Bilzer, T., A. Grabner, and L. Stitz. 1996. Immunopathologie der Borna-Krankheit beim Pferd: klinische, virologische und neuropathologische Befunde. *Tieraerztl. Prax.* **24:**567–576.

Bilzer, T., O. Planz, W. I. Lipkin, and L. Stitz. 1995. Presence of CD4$^+$ and CD8$^+$ T cells and expression of MHC class I and MHC class II antigen in horses with Borna disease virus-induced encephalitis. *Brain Pathol.* **5:**223–230.

Bilzer, T., and L. Stitz. 1996. Immunopathogenesis of virus diseases affecting the central nervous system. *Crit. Rev. Immunol.* **16:**145–222.

Binz, T., J. Lebelt, H. Niemann, and K. Hagenau. 1994. Sequence analyses of the P gene of Borna disease virus in naturally infected horse, donkey and sheep. *Virus Res.* **34:**281–289.

Bode, L., R. Dürrwald, P. Koeppel, and H. Ludwig. 1994a. Neue Aspekte der equinen Borna-Virus-Infektion mit und ohne Krankheit. *Prakt. Tierarzt* **75:**1065–1068.

Bode, L., R. Dürrwald, and H. Ludwig. 1994b. Borna virus infections in cattle associated with fatal neurological disease. *Vet. Rec.* **135:**283–284.

Bode, L., and H. Ludwig. 1997. Clinical similarities and close genetic relationship of human and animal Borna disease virus. *Arch. Virol.* **13**(Suppl.):167–182.

Borland, R., and N. McDonald. 1965. Feline encephalomyelitis. *Br. Vet. J.* **121**:479–483.

Boucher, J.-M., E. Barbillon, and F. Cliquet. 1999. Borna disease: a possible emerging zoonosis. *Vet. Res.* **30**:549–557.

Caplazi, P., and F. Ehrensperger. 1998. Spontaneous Borna disease in sheep and horses: immunophenotyping of inflammatory cells and detection of MHC-I and MHC-II antigen expression in Borna encephalitis lesions. *Vet. Immunol. Immunopathol.* **61**:203–220.

Caplazi, P., K. Melzer, R. Goetzmann, A. Rohner-Cotti, V. Bracher, K. Zlinszky, and F. Ehrensperger. 1999. Borna disease in Switzerland and in the principality of Liechtenstein. *Schweiz. Arch. Tierheilkd.* **141**:521–527.

Caplazi, P., A. Waldvogel, L. Stitz, U. Braun, and F. Ehrensperger. 1994. Borna disease in naturally infected cattle. *J. Comp. Pathol.* **111**:65–72.

Danner, K. 1978. Bornasche Krankheit. *Prakt. Tierarzt* **59**:748–752.

Danner, K. 1982. *Borna-Virus und Borna-Infektionen: vom Miasma zum Modell.* Enke Copythek, Stuttgart, Germany.

Daubney, R., and E. A. Mahlau. 1967. Viral encephalomyelitis of equines and domestic ruminants in the Near East. I. *Res. Vet. Sci.* **8**:375–397.

Degiorgis, M.-P., A.-L. Berg, C. Hård Af Segerstad, T. Mörner, M. Johansson, and M. Berg. 2000. Borna disease in a free-ranging lynx (*Lynx lynx*). *J. Clin. Microbiol.* **38**:3087–3091.

Deschl, U., L. Stitz, S. Herzog, K. Frese, and R. Rott. 1990. Determination of immune cells and expression of major histocompatibility complex class II antigen in encephalitic lesions of experimental Borna disease. *Acta Neuropathol.* **81**:41–50.

Dürrwald, R. 1993. *Die natürliche Borna-Virus-Infektion der Einhufer und Schafe. Untersuchungen zur Epidemiologie, zu neueren diagnostischen Methoden (ELISA, PCR) und zur Antikörperkinetik bei Pferden nach Vakzination mit Lebendimpfstoff.* Inaugural dissertation. Freie Universität Berlin, Berlin, Germany.

Dürrwald, R., and H. Ludwig. 1997. Borna disease virus (BDV), a (zoonotic?) worldwide pathogen. A review of the history of the disease and the virus infection with comprehensive bibliography. *J. Vet. Med. B* **44**:147–184.

Ernst, W., and H. Hahn. 1927. Weitere Beiträge zur Borna'schen Krankheit der Pferde und zur Frage der Aetiologie des bösartgen Katarrhalfiebers der Rinder. *Muench. Tieraerztl. Wochenschr.* **78**:85–89.

Fechner, J. 1964. Impfung gegen die Bornasche Krankheit (Seuchenhafte Gehirn-Rückenmark-Entzündung), p. 208–214. *In* J. Fechner (ed.), *Schutzimpfungen bei Haustieren.* Hirzel, Leipzig, Germany.

Frankhouser, R. 1961. Sporadische Meningo-Encephalomyelitis beim Rind. *Schweiz. Arch. Tierheilkd.* **103**:225–235.

Gonzalez-Dunia, D., C. Sauder, and J. C. de la Torre. 1997. Borna disease virus and the brain. *Brain Res. Bull.* **44**:647–664.

Gosztonyi, G., and H. Ludwig. 1984. Borna disease of horse. An immunohistological and virological study of naturally infected animals. *Acta Neuropathol.* (Berlin) **64**:213–221.

Grabner, A., and A. Fischer. 1991. Symptomatology and diagnosis of Borna encephalitis of horses. A case analysis of the last 13 years. *Tieraerztl. Prax.* **19**:68–73.

Hagiwara, K., M. Asakawa, L. Liao, W. Jiang, S. Yan, J.-J. Chai, Y. Oku, K. Ikuta, and M. Ito. 2001. Seroprevalence of Borna disease virus in domestic animals in Xinjiang, China. *Vet. Microbiol.* **80**:383–389.

Hagiwara, K., W. Kamitani, S. Takamura, H. Taniyama, T. Nakaya, H. Tanaka, R. Kirisawa, H. Iwai, and K. Ikuta. 2000. Detection of Borna disease virus in a pregnant mare and her fetus. *Vet. Microbiol.* **72**:207–216.

Hagiwara, K., S. Kawamoto, H. Takahashi, Y. Nakamura, T. Nakaya, T. Hiramune, C. Ishihara, and K. Ikuta. 1997a. High prevalence of Borna disease virus infection in healthy sheep in Japan. *Clin. Diagn. Lab. Immunol.* **4:**339–344.

Hagiwara, K., N. Momiyama, H. Taniyama, T. Nakaya, N. Tsunoda, C. Ishihara, and K. Ikuta. 1997b. Demonstration of Borna disease virus (BDV) in specific regions of the brain from horses positive for serum antibodies to BDV but negative for BDV RNA in the blood and internal organs. *Med. Microbiol. Immunol.* **186:**19–24.

Hagiwara, K., T. Nakaya, Y. Nakamura, S. Asahi, H. Takahashi, C. Ishihara, and K. Ikuta. 1996. Borna disease virus RNA in peripheral blood mononuclear cells obtained from healthy dairy cattle. *Med. Microbiol. Immunol.* **185:**145–151.

Hagiwara, K., M. Okamoto, W. Kamitani, S. Takamura, H. Taniyama, N. Tsunoda, H. Tanaka, H. Iwai, and K. Ikuta. 2002. Nosological study of Borna disease virus infection in race horses. *Vet. Microbiol.* **84:**367–374.

Hatalski, C. G., A. L. Lewis, and W. I. Lipkin. 1997. Borna disease. *Emerg. Infect. Dis.* **3:**129–135.

Heinig, A. 1969. Die Bornasche Krankheit der Pferde und Schafe, p. 83–148. *In* H. Roehrer (ed.), *Handbuch der Virusinfektionen bei Tieren,* vol. 4. VEB Fischer Verlag, Jena, Germany.

Herden, C., S. Herzog, T. Wehner, C. Zink, J. A. Richt, and K. Frese. 1999. Comparison of different methods of diagnosing Borna disease in horses post mortem. *Equine Infect. Dis.* **8:**286–290.

Herzog, S., K. Frese, J. A. Richt, and R. Rott. 1994. Ein Beitrag zur Epizootiologie der Bornaschen Krankheit des Pferdes. *Wien. Tieraerztl. Monschr.* **81:**374–379.

Herzog, S., I. Pfeuffer, K. Haberzettl, H. Feldmann, K. Frese, K. Bechter, and J. A. Richt. 1997. Molecular characterization of Borna disease virus from naturally infected animals and possible links to human disorders. *Arch. Virol.* **13**(Suppl.)**:**183–190.

Hiepe, T. 1960. Die Bedeutung der Liquoruntersuchung für die Neurodiagnostik bei Pferd und Schaf. *Zentbl. Vetmed.* **7:**152–159.

Hoff, E. J., and M. Vandevelde. 1981. Non-suppurative encephalomyelitis in cats suggestive of a viral origin. *Vet. Pathol.* **18:**170–180.

Ihlenburg, H. 1962. Zur Therapie der Bornaschen Krankheit. *Monatsh. Vetmed.* **17:**151–156.

Jordan, I., and W. I. Lipkin. 2001. Borna disease virus. *Rev. Med. Virol.* **11:**37–57.

Kacza, J., T. W. Vahlenkamp, H. Enbergs, J. A. Richt, A. Germer, H. Kuhrt, A. Reichenbach, H. Müller, C. Herden, T. Stahl, and J. Seeger. 2000. Neuron-glia interactions in the rat retina infected by Borna disease virus. *Arch. Virol.* **145:**127–147.

Kao, M., A. N. Hamir, C. E. Rupprecht, Z. F. Fu, V. Shanker, H. Koprowski, and B. Dietzschold. 1993. Detection of antibodies against Borna disease virus in sera and cerebrospinal fluid of horses in the USA. *Vet. Rec.* **132:**241–244.

Katz, J. B., D. Alstad, A. L. Jenny, K. M. Carbone, S. A. Rubin, and R. W. Waltrip II. 1998. Clinical, serologic, and histopathologic characterization of experimental Borna disease in ponies. *J. Vet. Diagn. Investig.* **10:**338–343.

Khan, M. A., K. Yamaguchi, H. Miyata, A. Kazi, T. Kamahora, and S. Hino. 2000. Prevalence of anti-Borna disease virus antibody in horses and their caretakers in Bangladesh. *Yonago Acta Med.* **43:**59–67.

Korber, B. T., K. J. Kunstman, B. K. Patterson, M. Furtado, M. M. McEvilly, and R. Levy. 1994. Genetic differences between blood- and brain-derived viral sequences from human immunodeficiency virus type 1-infected patients: evidence of conserved elements in the V3 region of the envelope protein of brain-derived sequences. *J. Virol.* **68:**7467–7481.

Krey, H. F., H. Ludwig, and C. B. Boschek. 1979a. Multifocal retinopathy in Borna disease virus infected rabbits. *Am. J. Ophthalmol.* **87:**157–164.

Krey, H. F., H. Ludwig, and R. Rott. 1979b. Spread of infectious virus along the optic nerve into the retina in Borna disease virus-infected rabbits. *Arch. Virol.* **61:**283–288.

Krey, H. F., L. Stitz, and H. Ludwig. 1982. Virus-induced pigment epithelitis in rhesus monkeys. Clinical and histological findings. *Ophthalmologica* (Basel) **185:**205–213.

Kronevi, T., M. Nordström, W. Moreno, and P. O. Nilsson. 1974. Feline ataxia due to nonsuppurative meningoencephalomyelitis of unknown aetiology. *Nord. Vet. Med.* **26:**720–725.

Lange, H., S. Herzog, W. Herbst, and T. Schliesser. 1987. Seroepidemiologische Untersuchungen zur Bornaschen Krankheit (Ansteckende Gehirn-Rückenmarkentzündung) der Pferde. *Tieraerztl. Umsch.* **42:**938–946.

Lebelt, J., and K. Hagenau. 1996. Die Verteilung des Bornavirus in natürlich infizierten Tieren mit klinischer Erkrankung. *Berl. Muench. Tieraerztl. Wochenschr.* **109:**178–183.

Ludwig, H., L. Bode, and G. Gosztonyi. 1988. Borna disease: a persistent virus infection of the central nervous system. *Prog. Med. Virol.* **35:**107–151.

Ludwig, H., K. Furuya, L. Bode, N. Klein, and R. Dürrwald. 1993. Biology and neurobiology of Borna disease viruses (BDV), defined by antibodies, neutralizability and their pathogenic potential. *Arch. Virol.* **7**(Suppl.)**:**111–133.

Ludwig, H., W. Kraft, M. Kao, G. Gosztony, E. Dahme, and H. Krey. 1985. Borna-Virus-Infektion (Borna-Krankheit) bei natürlich und experimentell infizierten Tieren: ihre Bedeutung für Forschung und Praxis. *Tieraerztl. Prax.* **13:**421–453.

Ludwig, H., and P. Thein. 1977. Demonstration of specific antibodies in the central nervous system of horses naturally infected with Borna disease virus. *Med. Microbiol. Immunol.* **163:**215–226.

Lundgren, A.-L. 1992. Feline non-suppurative meningoencephalomyelitis: a clinical and pathological study. *J. Comp. Pathol.* **107:**411–425.

Lundgren, A.-L., G. Czech, L. Bode, and H. Ludwig. 1993. Natural Borna disease in domestic animals other than horses and sheep. *Zentbl. Vetmed. Reihe B* **40:**298–303.

Lundgren, A.-L., A. Johannisson, W. Zimmermann, L. Bode, B. Rozell, A. Muluneh, R. Lindberg, and H. Ludwig. 1997. Neurological disease and encephalitis in cats experimentally infected with Borna disease virus. *Acta Neuropathol.* (Berlin) **93:**391–401.

Lundgren, A.-L., R. Lindberg, H. Ludwig, and G. Gosztony. 1995a. Immunoreactivity of the central nervous system in cats with a Borna disease-like meningoencephalomyelitis (staggering disease). *Acta Neuropathol.* (Berlin) **90:**184–193.

Lundgren, A.-L., and H. Ludwig. 1993. Clinically diseased cats with non-suppurative meningoencephalomyelitis have Borna disease virus-specific antibodies. *Acta Vet. Scand.* **34:**101–103.

Lundgren, A.-L., W. Zimmermann, L. Bode, G. Czech, G. Gosztonyi, R. Lindberg, and H. Ludwig. 1995b. Staggering disease in cats: isolation and characterization of the feline Borna disease virus. *J. Gen. Virol.* **76:**2215–2222.

Malkinson, M., Y. Weisman, E. Ashash, L. Bode, and H. Ludwig. 1993. Borna disease in ostriches. *Vet. Rec.* **133:**304.

Malkinson, M., Y. Weisman, S. Perl, and E. Ashash. 1995. A Borna-like disease of ostriches in Israel. *Curr. Top. Microbiol. Immunol.* **190:**31–38.

Martin, L.-A., and J. Hintermann. 1952. Sur l'existence, au Maroc, d'une maladie contagieuse du chat, non encore décrite: la myélite infectieuse. *Bull. Acad. Vet. Fr.* **25:**387–392.

Matthias, D. 1954. Der Nachweis von latent infizierten Pferden, Schafen und Rindern und deren Bedeutung als Virusreservoir bei der Bornaschen Krankheit. *Arch. Exp. Vet. Med.* **8:**506–511.

Mayr, A., and K. Danner. 1974. Persistent infections caused by Borna virus. *Infection* **2:**64–69.

Metzler, A., Ehrensperger, F., and R. Wyler. 1978. Natürliche Bornavirus-Infektion bei Kaninchen. *Zentbl. Vetmed. Reihe B* **25:**161–164.

Metzler, A., U. Frei, and K. Danner. 1976. Virologically confirmed outbreak of Borna's disease in a Swiss herd of sheep. *Schweiz. Arch. Tierheilkd.* **118:**483–492.

Metzler, A., H.-P. Minder, X. Wegmann, and W. Zindel. 1979. Die Borna'sche Krankheit, ein veterinärmedizinisches Problem von regionaler Bedeutung. *Schweiz. Arch. Tierheilkd.* **121**:207–213.

Möhlmann, H., and A. Maas. 1960. Wertigkeitsprüfung des Borna-Trockenimpfstoffes "Dessau" bei Pferden unter den Verhältnissen der Praxis. *Arch. Exp. Vet. Med.* **14**:1267–1280.

Monken, C. E., B. Wu, and A. Srinivasan. 1995. High resolution analysis of HIV-1 quasispecies in the brain. *AIDS* **9**:345–349.

Morales, J. A., S. Herzog, C. Kompter, K. Frese, and R. Rott. 1998. Axonal transport of Borna disease virus along olfactory pathways in spontaneously and experimentally infected rats. *Med. Microbiol. Immunol.* **177**:51–68.

Müller, L. F., and R. Fritzsch. 1955. Die Augenveränderungen bei der Bornaschen Krankheit. *Wien. Tieraerztl. Monschr.* **42**:866–871.

Nakamura, Y., S. Asahi, T. Nakaya, M. K. Bahmani, S. Saito, K. Yasui, H. Mayama, K. Hagiwara, C. Ishihara, and K. Ikuta. 1996. Demonstration of Borna disease virus RNA in peripheral blood mononuclear cells derived from domestic cats in Japan. *J. Clin. Microbiol.* **34**:188–191.

Nakamura, Y., M. Kishi, T. Nakaya, S. Asahi, S. Tanaka, H. Sentsui, K. Ikeda, and K. Ikuta. 1995. Demonstration of Borna disease virus RNA in peripheral blood mononuclear cells from healthy horses in Japan. *Vaccine* **13**:1076–1079.

Nakamura, Y., M. Watanabe, W. Kamitani, H. Taniyama, T. Nakaya, Y. Nishimura, H. Tsujimoto, S. Machida, and K. Ikuta. 1999. High prevalence of Borna disease virus in domestic cats with neurological disorders in Japan. *Vet. Microbiol.* **70**:153–169.

Narayan, O., S. Herzog, K. Frese, H. Scheefers, and R. Rott. 1983. Pathogenesis of Borna disease in rats: immune-mediated viral ophthalmoencephalopathy causing blindness and behavioral abnormalities. *J. Infect. Dis.* **148**:305–315.

Nicolau, S., and I. A. Galloway. 1928. Borna disease and enzootic encephalomyelitis of sheep and cattle. *Spec. Rep. Ser. Med. Res. Council* **121**:7–90.

Nishino, Y., M. Funaba, R. Fukushima, T. Mizutani, T. Kimura, R. Iizuka, H. Hirami, and M. Hara. 1999. Borna disease virus infection in domestic cats: evaluation by RNA and antibody detection. *J. Vet. Med. Sci.* **61**:1167–1170.

Nöske, K., T. Bilzer, O. Planz, and L. Stitz. 1998. Virus-specific CD4$^+$ T cells eliminate Borna disease virus from the brain via induction of cytotoxic CD8$^+$ T cells. *J. Virol.* **72**:4387–4395.

Nowotny, N., and J. Kolodziejek. 2000. Human bornaviruses and laboratory strains. *Lancet* **355**:1462–1463.

Nowotny, N., J. Kolodziejek, C. O., Jehle, A. Suchy, P. Staeheli, and M. Schwemmie. 2000. Isolation and characterization of a new subtype of Borna disease virus. *J. Virol.* **74**:5655–5658.

Nowotny, N., and H. Welssenböck. 1995. Description of feline nonsuppurative meningoencephalomyelitis ("staggering disease") and studies of its etiology. *J. Clin. Microbiol.* **33**:1668–1669.

Okamoto, M., H. Furuoka, K. Hagiwara, W. Kamitani, R. Kirisawa, K. Ikuta, and H. Taniyama. 2002a. Borna disease in a heifer in Japan. *Vet. Rec.* **150**:16–18.

Okamoto, M., Y. Kagawa, W. Kamitani, K. Hagiwara, R. Kirisawa, H. Iwai, K. Ikuta, and H. Taniyama. 2002b. Borna disease in a dog in Japan. *J. Comp. Pathol.* **126**:312–317.

Planz, O., and L. Stitz. 1999. Borna disease virus nucleoprotein (N) is a major target for CD8$^+$-T-cell-mediated immune response. *J. Virol.* **73**:1715–1718.

Reeves, N. A., C. R. Helps, D. A. Gunn-Moore, C. Blundell, P. L. Finnermore, G. R. Pearson, and D. A. Harbour. 1998. Natural Borna disease virus infection in cats in the United Kingdom. *Vet. Rec.* **143**:523–526.

Richt, J. A., A. Grabner, and S. Herzog. 2000. Borna disease in horses. *Vet. Clin. N. Am. Equine Pract.* **16**:579–595.

Richt, J. A., S. Herzog, K. Haberzetl, and R. Rott. 1993. Demonstration of Borna disease virus-specific RNA in secretions of naturally infected horses by the polymerase chain reaction. *Med. Microbiol. Immunol.* **182**:293–304.

Richt, J. A., S. Herzog, A. Schmeel, K. Frese, and R. Rott. 1994. Current knowledge about Borna disease, p. 55–60. *In* H. Nakajima and W. Plowright (ed.), *Equine Infectious Diseases*, vol. VII. R & W Publications, Newmarket, United Kingdom.

Richt, J. A., I. Pfeuffer, M. Christ, K. Frese, K. Bechter, and S. Herzog. 1997. Borna disease virus infection in animals and humans. *Emerg. Infect. Dis.* **3**:343–352.

Richt, J. A., and R. Rott. 2001. Borna disease virus: a mystery as an emerging zoonotic pathogen. *Vet. J.* **161**:24–40.

Rott, R., and H. Becht. 1995. Natural and experimental Borna disease in animals. Borna disease. *Curr. Top. Microbiol. Immunol.* **190**:17–30.

Schmidt, J. 1912. Untersuchungen über das klinische Verhalten der seuchenhaften Gehirn-Rückenmarksentzündung (Bornaschen Krankheit) des Pferdes nebst Angaben über diesbezügliche therapeutische Versuche. *Berl. Muench. Tieraerztl. Wochenschr.* **28**:581–603.

Schmidt, J. 1952. Die Bornakrankheit des Pferdes. 55 Jahre Forschung und Lehre. *Arch. Exp. Vet. Med.* **6**:177–187.

Schneider, P. A., T. Briese, W. Zimmermann, H. Ludwig, and W. I. Lipkin. 1994. Sequence conservation in field and experimental isolates of Borna disease virus. *J. Virol.* **68**:63–68.

Schüppel, K.-F., J. Kinne, and M. Reinacher. 1994. Bornavirus-Antigennachweis bei Alpakas (Lama pacos) sowie bei einen Faultier (Choloepus didactylus) und einem Zwergflusspferd (Choeropsis liberiensis), p. 189–194. *In* R. R. Hofmann and R. Ippen (ed.), *Verhandlungsbericht XXXVI Internationales Symposium über Erkrankungen von Zootieren.*

Schüppel, K.-F., M. Reinacher, J. Lebelt, and D. Kulka. 1995. Bornasche Krankheit bei Primaten, p. 115–120. *In* R. R. Hofmann and R. Ippen (ed.), *Verhandlungsbericht XXXVII Internationales Symposium über Erkrankungen von Zootieren.*

Sierra-Honigmann, A. M., S. A. Rubin, M. G. Estefanous, R. H. Yolken, and K. M. Carbone. 1993. Borna disease virus in peripheral blood mononuclear and bone marrow cells of neonatally and chronically infected rats. *J. Neuroimmunol.* **45**:31–36.

Staeheli, P., C. Sauder, J. Hausmann, F. Ehrensperger, and M. Schwemmle. 2000. Epidemiology of Borna disease virus. *J. Gen. Virol.* **81**:2123–2135.

Stitz, L., T. Bilzer, J. A. Richt, and R. Rott. 1993. Pathogenesis of Borna disease. *Arch. Virol.* **7**(Suppl.):135–151.

Stitz, L., B. Dietzschold, and K. M. Carbone. 1995. Immunopathogenesis of Borna disease. *Curr. Top. Microbiol. Immunol.* **190**:75–92.

Ström, B., B. Andrén, and A.-L. Lundgren. 1992. Idiopathic non-suppurative meningoencephalomyelitis (staggering disease) in the Swedish cat: a study of 33 cases. *Eur. J. Companion Anim. Pract.* **3**:9–13.

Suchy, A., H. Weissenböck, P. Caplazi, S. Herzog, and N. Nowotny. 2000. Equine Borna disease in Austria: evidence for a new endemic area of the natural disease. *Equine Pract.* **22**:26–27.

Suchy, A., H. Weissenböck, R. Waller, P. Schmidt, and N. Nowotny. 1997. Nachweis der Bornaschen Krankheit bei einem Pferd in Österreich. *Wien. Tieraerztl. Monschr.* **84**:317–321.

Takahashi, H., T. Nakaya, Y. Nakamura, S. Asahi, Y. Onishi, K. Ikebuchi, T. A. Takahashi, T. Katoh, S. Sekiguchi, M. Takazawa, H. Tanaka, and K. Ikuta. 1997. Higher prevalence of Borna disease virus infection in blood donors living near thoroughbred horse farms. *J. Med. Virol.* **52**:330–335.

Taniyama, H., M. Okamoto, K. Hirayama, K. Hagiwara, K. Kirisawa, W. Kamitani, and K. Ikuta. 2001. Equine Borna disease in Japan. *Vet. Rec.* **148:**480–482.

Theil, D., R. Fatzer, I. Schiller, P. Caplazi, A. Zurbriggen, and M. Vandevelde. 1998. Neuropathological and aetiological studies of sporadic non-suppurative meningoencephalomyelitis of cattle. *Vet. Rec.* **143:**244–249.

Tsujimura, K., T. Mizutani, H. Kariwa, K. Yoshimatsu, M. Ogino, Y. Morii, H. Inagaki, J. Arikawa, and I. Takashima. 1999. A serosurvey of Borna disease virus infection in wild rats by a capture ELISA. *J. Vet. Med. Sci.* **61:**113–117.

Vahlenkamp, T. W., H. K. Enbergs, and H. Müller. 2000. Experimental and natural borna disease virus infections: presence of viral RNA in cells of the peripheral blood. *Vet. Microbiol.* **76:**229–244.

Vandervelde, M., and K. G. Braund. 1979. Polioencephalomyelitis in cats. *Vet. Pathol.* **16:**420–427.

von Sind, J. B. 1767 and 1781. *Der im Feld und auf der Reise geschwind heilende Pferdearzt, welcher einen gründlichen Unterricht von den gewöhnlichsten Krankheiten der Pferde im Feld und auf der Reise wie auch einen auserlesenen Vorrath der nützlichsten und durch die Erfahrung bewährtesten Heilungsmitteln eröffnet,* 2nd and 3rd ed. Frankfurt, Germany.

Waelchli, R. O., F. Ehrensperger, A. Metzler, and C. Winder. 1985. Borna disease in a sheep. *Vet. Rec.* **117:**499–500.

Weissenböck, H., N. Nowotny, P. Caplazi, J. Kolodziejek, and F. Ehrensperger. 1998a. Borna disease in a dog with lethal meningoencephalitis. *J. Clin. Microbiol.* **36:**2127–2130.

Weissenböck, H., N. Nowotny, and J. Zöher. 1994. Feline meningoencephalomyelitis ("staggering disease") in Österreich. *Wien. Tieraerztl. Monschr.* **81:**195–201.

Weissenböck, H., A. Suchy, P. Caplazi, S. Herzog, and N. Nowotny. 1998b. Borna disease in Austrian horses. *Vet. Rec.* **143:**21–22.

Wörz, J. J. 1858. *Die halb-acute Gehirn-Entzündung oder Kopf-Krankheit der Pferde.* Ebner & Seubert, Stuttgart, Germany.

Yamaguchi, K., T. Sawada, T. Naraki, R. Igata-Yi, H. Shiraki, Y. Horii, T. Ishii, K. Ikeda, N. Asou, H. Okabe, M. Mochizuki, K. Takahashi, S. Yamada, K. Kubo, S. Yashiki, R. W. Waltrip II, and K. M. Carbone. 1999. Detection of Borna disease virus-reactive antibodies from patients with psychiatric disorders and from horses by electrochemiluminescence immunoassay. *Clin. Diagn. Lab. Immunol.* **6:**696–700.

Zimmermann, W., R. Dürrwald, and H. Ludwig. 1994. Detection of Borna disease virus RNA in naturally infected animals by a nested polymerase chain reaction. *J. Virol. Methods* **46:**133–143.

Zwick, W. 1939. Bornasche Krankheit und Enzephalomyelitis der Tiere, p. 254–354. *In* E. Gildenmeister, E. Haagen, and O. Waldmann (ed.), *Handbuch der Viruskrankheiten,* vol. 2. Fischer, Jena, Germany.

Zwick, W., O. Seifried, and J. Witte. 1927. Experimentelle Untersuchungen über die seuchenhafte Gehim-und Rückenmarksentzündung der Pferde (Bornasche Krankheit). *Z. Infektkrankh. Parasitare Krankh. Hyg. Haustiere* **30:**42–136.

Zwick, W., and J. Witte. 1932. Zur Frage der Schutzimpfung und der Inkubationfrist bei der Bornaschen Krankheit. *Schweiz. Arch. Tierheilkd.* **64:**116–124.

Borna Disease Virus and Its Role in Neurobehavioral Disease
Edited by K. M. Carbone
© 2002 ASM Press, Washington, D.C.

Chapter 5

Experimental Infection: Pathogenesis of Neurobehavioral Disease

Mikhail V. Pletnikov, Daniel Gonzalez-Dunia, and Lothar Stitz

EXPERIMENTAL MODELS OF BDV INFECTION

The first descriptions of a disease characterized by central nervous system (CNS) symptoms in horses can be found in the veterinary literature at the end of the 18th century. More sophisticated reports on a "feverish disease of the head" (*hitzige Kopfkrankheit*), brain fever, subacute meningitis, or hypersomnia of horses appeared at the beginning of the 19th century (Autenrieth, 1813). The disease drew full attention in 1895, when almost all horses of a cavalry regiment in the town of Borna in Saxony near Leipzig succumbed to an epidemic with severe CNS symptoms. After this event, the term Borna disease (BD) was introduced. Although BD caused by the BD virus (BDV) had been studied since the 1920s, the nature of this virus remained obscure until the 1990s.

The viral etiology of BD was proven in 1924, when Zwick and Selfried demonstrated its transmissibility and fulfilled Koch's postulates by transmitting the disease from horses to rabbits and back to horses (Zwick et al., 1924). However, more intensive investigations of BD were initiated in the 1980s, largely due to the interest of renowned virologist Rudolf

Mikhail V. Pletnikov • Department of Psychiatry and Behavioral Sciences, The Johns Hopkins University School of Medicine, Ross 618, 720 Rutland Ave., Baltimore, MD 21205. **Daniel Gonzalez-Dunia** • Unité des virus lents, CNRS URA 1930, Institut Pasteur, 28 rue du Dr Roux, 75724 Paris Cedex 15, France. **Lothar Stitz** • Institut für Immunologie, Bundesforschungsanstalt für Viruskrankheiten der Tiere, Paul Ehrlich Str. 28, 72076 Tübingen, Germany.

Rott. Although BD was initially studied for almost 80 years because of its relevance to veterinary science, we now know that BD represents a valuable model for studying the immunopathological mechanisms of virus-induced CNS disease. In general, experimental BDV infection of adult immunocompetent hosts produces severe immune-mediated meningoencephalitis, similar to the syndrome observed in naturally infected animals.

Natural BD has been observed in a variety of animal species, including cats, dogs, cattle, sheep, and horses (see chapter 4). An interesting finding was the presence of infectious virus or viral antigen in the salivary glands of horses (Zwick et al., 1926; 1927) and primates (Nicolau and Galloway, 1927) and lachrymal glands of primates (Stitz et al., 1980). These findings seem to support the hypothesis that natural infection occurs via excretions and the olfactory route (Morales et al., 1988; Richt et al., 1993; Bilzer et al., 1995). However, oral infection via the recurrent pharyngeal nerve cannot be excluded (Bilzer et al., 1995). The direct access of virus to the CNS via nerve endings, e.g., olfactory receptor neurons (Johnson, 1982; Ochs, 1982), has been demonstrated for other viruses, including neurotropic influenza virus (Reinacher et al., 1983), herpes simplex virus (Tomlinson and Esiri, 1983), and Semliki Forest virus (Kaluza et al., 1986).

The host spectrum in experimental infections is remarkably broad. Rats (Narayan et al., 1983; Hirano, 1983), mice (Kao et al., 1984; Rubin et al., 1993; Hallensleben et al., 1998), hamsters (Anzil et al., 1973), Mongolian gerbils (Watanabe et al., 2001), rabbits (Zwick, 1939; Krey et al., 1979), guinea pigs (Zwick, 1939), tree shrews (Sprankel et al., 1978), rhesus monkeys (Stitz et al., 1980), and chickens (Zwick, 1939) are all susceptible to BDV infection. Nevertheless, the course of BDV infection, the incubation period, the mortality, and the severity of clinical manifestations vary significantly among species, and even among strains within a species. For example, while BDV infection causes severe neurological abnormalities and high mortality in rabbits (Krey et al., 1979), BDV-infected tree shrews predominantly exhibit alterations in social behavior (Sprankel et al., 1978). Despite high virus titers in the brain of BDV-infected mice, the mouse was originally thought to be resistant to BD (Kao et al., 1984). Subsequent investigations, however, demonstrated that certain strains of mice are susceptible to BDV-induced disease (Rubin et al., 1993; Hallensleben et al., 1998), consistent with the data obtained on BD susceptibility of different strains of rats (Herzog et al., 1991). Even though findings obtained from experimental BDV infection of other species gave many insights into species-specific pathogenic processes, BDV infection of the rat is the most common model for studying the pathogenesis of BD.

PATHOGENESIS OF BD

BDV Replication and Dissemination in the CNS of Adult-Infected, Immunocompetent Rats

After experimental infection of adult rats by various routes, including intracerebral (i.c.), intraocular, intranasal (i.n.) and intramuscular injections, infectious virus and virus-specific antigens can be detected in high concentrations in the cerebrospinal fluid, brain, retina, peripheral nerves, and adrenal gland (Narayan et al., 1983; Carbone et al., 1987; Morales et al., 1988; Deschl et al., 1990).

After experimental i.n. infection, virus-specific antigens can first be identified in the neuroreceptors of the olfactory epithelium and, subsequently, in the brain. Immunohistological demonstration of viral antigen in neuroreceptor cells is possible as early as 6 days postinfection (p.i.) (Morales et al., 1988). Thereafter, the virus replicates rather rapidly in cells of the CNS similar to i.c. infection, although the development of clinical signs of BD following i.n. inoculation requires a period longer than that of disease latency after i.c. inoculation. At days 4 to 6 p.i., virus-specific proteins can be detected by Western blot analysis, and BDV-specific proteins are detectable by immunohistochemistry (IHC) in single ependymal cells of the lateral ventricles. These cells show a distinct granular staining in the nucleus and, sometimes, cytoplasmic staining. Six days p.i., a few neurons in the hippocampus (layers CA3 and CA4) and frontal cortex contain virus specific proteins. Eight days p.i., the number of neurons containing BDV-antigen increases significantly, e.g., in the CA3 region, diencephalon, and amygdala. At this time point, a fine granular staining of the cellular extensions of neurons can be observed in addition to the strong staining of the nucleus and pericaryon. By day 10 p.i., BDV antigens can be demonstrated in cells located in all cortical and brainstem areas. The intensity of the staining reaction increases until day 22 p.i., particularly in the neuropil of the stratum oriens and stratum radiatum of the CA3 and CA4 regions of the hippocampus. Thereafter, the intensity of the staining reaction decreases, and beyond day 70 p.i., BDV is essentially found in the hilus area of the hippocampus, the septal nuclei, and periventricular regions only. During the later stages of the infection, the cytoplasmic staining decreases and the intranuclear reaction predominates again in almost all cells. The types of cells containing BDV-specific proteins include neurons, ependymal cells, astrocytes, and oligodendrocytes, but not endothelial cells of brain blood vessels (Narayan et al., 1983; Gosztonyi and Ludwig, 1984; Deschl et al., 1990; Carbone et al., 1989; Carbone et al., 1993; Stitz et al., 1998).

The determinants for BDV tropism in the CNS are not fully under-stood but are likely to be multiple. During early infection, the kinetics and topography of viral antigen appearance in the CNS neurons are strongly suggestive of a transneuronal spread of the virus. It has been suggested that BDV spreads within the CNS in the form of ribonucleoproteins (RNPs) rather than fully enveloped particles (Cubitt et al., 1994; Gosztonyi et al., 1993). This hypothesis has been further strengthened by the demon-stration that BDV RNPs are infectious (Cubitt et al., 1994). Although the cellular receptor for BDV is unknown, since the stratified (or laminated) distribution of viral antigens in the hippocampus coincides with that of ex-citatory amino acid receptors, in particular glutamate receptors, a hypoth-esis was proposed that BDV virions or RNPs may use such receptors for their transneuronal transfer (Gosztonyi and Ludwig, 1995). In adult-infected, immunocompetent rats that survive the acute infection and de-velop chronic disease, virus antigen and/or nucleic acid can be found in cells of the peripheral nervous system, such as Schwann cells, and within peripheral nerve axons (Carbone et al., 1989), stressing the importance of the spread of the virus via axonal transport (Krey et al., 1979; Carbone et al., 1987; Morales et al., 1988). Furthermore, virus-specific antigen and ge-nomic RNA were detected in the Auerbach's plexus and the plexus mesentericus in the intestines (Carbone et al., 1987). Another clue to the reasons for BDV's neurotropism was deduced from the finding that BDV phosphoprotein, an important cofactor for BDV replication, is phosphory-lated primarily by the epsilon isotype of protein kinase C (Schwemmle et al., 1997). The regional distribution of the epsilon isotype in limbic cir-cuitry coincides with that of BDV (Salto et al., 1993), and thus may con-tribute to the preferential replication of BDV in the limbic system (Hornig et al., 2001).

Although highly neurotropic, the virus can be located by culture and/or reverse transcription-PCR in extraneural tissues (Bilzer et al., 1995; Shankar et al., 1992), including thymus and peripheral blood mononuclear cells under specific circumstances (Sierra-Honigmann et al., 1993). In the late chronic stage of disease, BDV RNA has been demonstrated in blood in fibroblastic stromal cells of the bone marrow and the thymus (Rubin et al., 1995). Other studies have been unable to identify BDV in nonneural tis-sues (Herzog et al., 1985; Stitz et al., 1998). When identified, the spread of BDV outside the nervous system was associated with specific host charac-teristics, demonstrating that some of the BDV neurotropism lies with host specific factors. For example, when BDV was detected in peripheral nerves of rats infected as immunocompetent adults, the virus was not found in or-gan-specific cells and was strictly restricted to the nervous tissue. In con-trast, rats infected with BDV as immunoincompetent neonates or adults immunosuppressed by cyclosporine have the virus in nonneuronal tissues as well (Stitz et al., 1991; Stitz et al., 1998) (see below).

Neuropathology of BDV Infection in the Central Nervous System of Adult-Infected Immunocompetent Rats

Using classical methods, Zwick and coworkers (between 1926 and 1933), Nicolau and Galloway (between 1927 and 1929), Seifried and Spatz (1930), and Pette and Környey (1935) were among the first to describe many BDV-induced pathological changes. The pathology of BDV in different animal species has been described elsewhere (Gosztonyi and Ludwig, 1995; Bilzer et al., 1995; Caplazi and Ehrensperger, 1998). Pathological lesions are found predominantly in the gray matter of the CNS in a variety of animal species, including natural hosts. Since the type of pathological alterations between naturally infected horses and experimentally infected rats differ only with respect to the degree of the inflammatory response, we will summarize the immunohistological and pathological findings from studies of rats. However, where they exist, certain peculiarities of other animal species or strains will also be discussed.

Pathology of the CNS

The clinical onset of acute BD is paralleled by the development of a mononuclear inflammatory reaction in the CNS and peripheral nervous system with severe perivascular cuffing of T cells and macrophages very early after infection (Color Plate 3 [see color insert]) (Deschl et al., 1990; Richt et al., 1990). Encephalitic inflammatory lesions are also found in brain parenchyma. In general, the inflammation is initially centered in the limbic system but spreads to other areas of the brain during infection (Narayan et al., 1983a, 1983b; Deschl et al., 1990; Carbone et al., 1987). Numerous B cells are found, peaking later than all other cells participating in the inflammatory reaction. The development of neurological symptoms is directly correlated with the appearance of inflammatory cells (Narayan et al., 1983a, 1983b; Hirano et al. 1983; Bilzer and Stitz, 1994). Late after infection, i.e., more than 2 to 3 months p.i., the inflammatory reaction starts to decrease and, finally, disappears almost completely despite continuing virus replication. A dramatic loss of neural tissue and a severe hydrocephalus ex vacuo can be observed (Fig. 1) (Narayan et al., 1983a, 1983b; Planz et al., 1993; Bilzer and Stitz, 1993; Bilzer and Stitz, 1994).

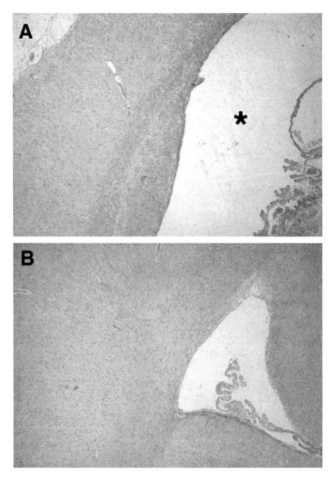

Figure 1. Cortical brain atrophy as a consequence of BDV infection in rats. Note the profound atrophy of the brain parenchyma and hydrocephalus ex vacuo (*) in the BDV-infected rat (A) compared to the intact brain parenchyma in the sham-inoculated rat (B). Original magnification, ×30 (present magnification, ×20). Hematoxylin-and-eosin staining was used. Courtesy of Thomas Bilzer.

Time course analysis

In general, two patterns of pathological changes can be observed during the early phase of experimental infection in adult rats, depending mostly on the route of infection. After intranasal infection of rats, likely comparable to the findings in naturally infected horses, an edema of the olfactory bulb and the rhinencephalon can be found before and during the development of the inflammatory reaction in the brain. In contrast, after intracerebral infection of a wide variety of animal species, a meningoencephalomyelitis develops without edema.

Infectious virus and viral proteins can be found as early as 4 days p.i., but histopathological lesions are found beginning at 8 days p.i. (Narayan et al., 1983a, 1983b; Deschl et al., 1990; Bilzer and Stitz, 1994). At this time point, a focal accumulation of monohistiocytic cells is observed in the leptomeninges. Thereafter, slight perivascular and parenchymal infiltrates are seen in the frontoparietal and entorhinal cortex, amygdala, septal nuclei, and hippocampus.

The accumulation of inflammatory cells increases during the course of the disease, resulting in severe perivascular and parenchymal infiltration. Alterations have been described in one of the major cortical neurotransmitters, acetylcholine, with progressive deterioration of forebrain cholinergic systems paralleling the progression of BDV encephalitis (Gies et al., 1998; Gies et al., 2001). The encephalitis peaks around day 21 p.i., and beyond day 30 p.i., the perivascular inflammatory reaction starts to decrease. By about day 70 p.i., the cellular reaction is composed of one or two mononuclear cell layers in a rare perivascular cuff, and in many cases, there is a total absence of inflammatory cells ("burned-out" encephalitis).

The local immune reaction in the brain results in a progressive loss of neurons, mainly in the neocortex and hippocampus, with the peak cell loss between days 60 and 70 p.i. (Bilzer and Stitz, 1994). Beginning at day 30 p.i., a successive dilatation of the lateral ventricles is noted, and a macroscopically visible hydrocephalus ex vacuo ensues (Fig. 1) (Narayan et al., 1983a, 1983b; Hirano et al., 1983). The hydrocephalus in BDV-infected rats is not based on aqueductal stenosis or obstruction, because all ventricular cavities and the central canal are open (Irigoin et al., 1990). Since no signs of vascular damage are found in the brains of BDV-infected rats, it is unlikely that the hydrocephalus results from hypoxia (Bilzer and Stitz, 1994).

Pathology in peripheral nerves and organs

Pathognomonic Joest-Degen inclusion bodies have been detected in the nuclei of ganglion cells (Nicolau, 1928; Nicolau and Galloway, 1928b; Nicolau and Stoian, 1928). Histological alterations (Zwick and Seifried, 1924; Bemmann, 1926; Nicolau, 1928; Nicolau and Galloway, 1928a, 1928b; Nicolau et al., 1929a; Zwick et al., 1929) and evidence of virus infection in peripheral nerves and in the autonomic nervous system (Carbone et al., 1987) have been described. However, the contribution of BDV infection in peripheral nerves to clinical symptoms, e.g., paresis and paralysis, was believed to be minor because of the relatively rare incidence of the neuritis with perivascular or interstitial infiltration in peripheral nerves. Wallerian degeneration, e.g., swelling of axons early after infection and a degeneration of axons and myelin sheets in ventral and dorsal nerve root fibers and in the sciatic nerve, is seen but is not necessarily associated with signs of the inflammatory reaction (Carbone et al., 1989; Carbone et al., 1991a). There is a progressive loss of myelinated fibers of the sciatic nerve without indications of regeneration, suggesting cell damage not associated with the immunopathological primary degeneration of Schwann cells or the myelin sheet (Carbone et al., 1989; Carbone et al., 1991a). Thus, BDV-induced peripheral neuropathy is an axonal degeneration and secondary degeneration of the myelin sheets by means of a "dying forward" mechanism.

Immunology of BD in Immunocompetent Rats

Humoral immune response

A vigorous humoral immune response can be seen in BDV-infected rats, but the presence of virus-specific antibodies is not related to the presence of clinical signs. The detection of anti-BDV antibodies has been used to diagnose BDV infection (Lange et al., 1987). In animals with positive BDV serology but without signs of disease, the presence of antibodies may reflect subclinical infection or the presence of the virus in the latent stage, i.e., during the variably long incubation period before clinical symptoms can be seen.

In the serum of experimentally infected rats, antibodies directed against the nucleoprotein (N) and the phosphoprotein (P) predominate, although detection of antibodies against the P can sometimes be difficult. BDV-specific antibodies can be detected in the serum of infected rats by 6 to 8 days p.i. In the cerebrospinal fluid of infected animals, virus-specific antibodies are readily detected, representing an oligoclonal immunoglobulin response (Ludwig et al., 1977). In the rat, abundant local immunoglobulin G production with isotype variations has been demonstrated in the brain without damage of the blood-brain barrier (Hatalski et al., 1998a).

The presence of neutralizing antibodies in BDV-infected hosts is highly controversial. Some investigators reported virus neutralizing activity in serum and cerebrospinal fluid (Danner et al., 1978; Hirano et al., 1983; Ludwig et al., 1993; Kliche et al., 1994; Hatalski et al., 1995; Stitz et al., 1998), whereas others found no evidence of neutralizing antibodies at any stage of the disease (Narayan et al., 1983a, 1983b; Herzog et al., 1985; Carbone et al., 1987). However, monoclonal antibodies (MAbs) that reacted with the major viral glycoprotein (G) were generated, and these antibodies inhibited infection both in vitro and in vivo (Furrer et al., 2001). Interestingly, it appears that neutralizing antibodies are only synthesized in vivo after the virus is present in the blood, which occurs late after infection in the chronic phase of the disease, thus providing an explanation for the delayed presence of neutralizing antibodies. How virus-specific antibodies are involved in the restriction of the virus to the CNS is currently not well defined.

Cellular immune response

In the rat, the encephalitic reaction and the perivascular infiltrates have been characterized by immunohistological methods using MAbs against several surface markers of T lymphocytes, B lymphocytes, and macrophages (Deschl et al., 1990; Richt et al., 1990; Bilzer and Stitz, 1994). Large cells with ovoid to kidney-shaped cytoplasm reacting with ED1 MAb (a macrophage marker) represent the majority of inflammatory cells in perivascular and parenchymal infiltrates.

A common T-lymphocyte marker (Ox 52) recognized cells representing about 50% of all cells present in perivascular infiltrates from day 12 p.i. through days 22 and 30 p.i., and then decreasing slightly, reaching a value of 30% at day 70 p.i. This population of T lymphocytes was further divided into helper and cytotoxic or suppressor phenotypes. The T lymphocyte helper-specific cell marker W3/25 stained a few cells outside the perivascular cuffs in the neuropil as well as the most frequent type of T cells in the perivascular encephalitic lesions. On day 12 p.i., W3/25-positive cells comprised 15% of all cells in perivascular cuffs, increasing thereafter to about 29% at day 22 p.i. Beyond day 30, cells with the helper phenotype declined to a level of 13% by day 70 p.i. Cytotoxic or suppressor T cells, stained by MAb Ox 8 were also found in perivascular cuffs but predominated in the brain parenchyma where they comprised about 10 to 20% of all inflammatory cells (Deschl et al., 1990; Stitz et al., 1991b). This phenotype represented the smallest subpopulation of T cells (by percentage).

Immunopathology of BD

The first suggestion of the importance of the immune reaction for the pathogenesis of BD came from experiments using rhesus monkeys (Stitz et al., 1980). Rhesus monkeys developed a severe disease, with neurological symptoms including paralysis, paresis, and, in the late phase of the disease, increasing apathy. It was observed that monkeys that had undergone splenectomy prior to BDV infection showed a less serious clinical and histopathological picture. Narayan et al. (1983) provided the first detailed description of the histological alterations in the brain with associated clinical signs of disease that sparked further investigations on the immunopathogenesis of this virus-induced encephalopathy.

Subsequently, athymic or immunocompromised (e.g., cyclophosphamide- or cyclosporine-treated or newborn) rats infected with BDV were shown to express no signs of BD or the acute inflammatory reaction (Narayan et al., 1983a, 1983b; Herzog et al., 1984; Herzog et al., 1985; Stitz et al., 1989; Stitz et al., 1991a; Stitz et al., 1991b). Notably, virus-specific nucleic acid and infectious virus, in addition to virus-specific antigen, were found in immunocompromised animals in amounts comparable to those in fully immunocompetent rats (Narayan et al., 1983a, 1983b; Carbone et al., 1987; Herzog et al., 1985; Stitz et al., 1991a; Stitz et al., 1991b) and adoptive transfer of lymphocytes from BDV-immune rats into immunoincompetent animals resulted in full-blown BD (Narayan et al., 1983a, 1983b; Stitz et al., 1989).

B cells

Over a decade of research has provided significant insight into the specific immune mediators of the immunopathological basis of BD. Although numerous B cells are present, encephalitic lesions in the later stages of the acute disease and although antiviral antibodies, including neutralizing antibodies, can be found in the serum of infected rats (Narayan et al., 1983a, 1983b; Hirano et al., 1983; Hatalski et al., 1995), several lines of evidence indicate that antiviral antibodies do not play a significant role in the immunopathogenesis of BD (Narayan et al., 1983a, 1983b; Herzog et al., 1985; Stitz et al., 1989). For example, treatment of BDV-infected rats with subtherapeutic doses of cyclosporine results in the development of an encephalitis and BD even in the absence of an anti-BDV antibody response. Additionally, while BDV-infected cyclosporine-immunosuppressed rats do not develop BD, there is a clear BDV-specific B-cell response with production of anti-BDV antibody (Stitz et al., 1989).

MHC

Major histocompatibility complex (MHC) restriction elements are very important in T-cell-mediated immune phenomena. Soon after BDV infection in rats, MHC class I expression is distributed throughout the brain tissue, whereas MHC class II is restricted to perivascular locations. These self-antigens are detected on perivascular cells but are also seen on cells in the parenchyma, e.g., oligodendrocytes and microglial and ependymal cells (Carbone et al., 1993; Deschl et al., 1990; Richt et al., 1990; Stitz et al., 1991a; Stitz et al. 1991b). MHC class II antigens are also detected in areas without blood-borne inflammatory infiltrates, arguing for a widespread induction and expression of MHC class II in the brain of BDV-infected rats. However, MHC class II antigen has not been detected on neurons in BDV-infected rats (Bilzer and Stitz, 1994). MHC class I antigen was also demonstrated on neurons and astrocytes in vivo and in vitro following BDV infection (Carbone et al., 1993; Bilzer and Stitz, 1993, 1994).

T cells

Virus-specific CD4$^+$ T cells act as helpers and contribute to the immune reaction on the T- and B-cell level. Both Th1 and Th2 cells have been shown to provide help to cytotoxic T lymphocytes and trigger production of gamma interferon (IFN-γ) by cytotoxic T cells (Stuhler and Walden, 1993). Dependent on the virus studied, in vivo experiments have revealed a mandatory role for Th cells in the induction of a cytotoxic T-cell response in some viral infections (Ashman and Müllbacher, 1979; Bennink and Doherty, 1978; Kast et al., 1986; Leist et al., 1989; Zinkernagel et al., 1978; Zinkernagel et al., 1989). Coexpression of MHC class I antigen in association with virus-specific proteins renders cells targets for cytotoxic CD8$^+$ T lymphocytes (Zinkernagel and Doherty, 1979).

Antiviral activity of classical MHC class I-restricted virus-specific T cells has been found for many virus infections (Byrne and Oldstone, 1984; Baenziger et al., 1986; Müller et al., 1989; Kägi et al., 1994; Zinkernagel and Doherty, 1979; Luckacher et al., 1985; Sethi et al., 1988). In infections in which MHC class II-restricted cytotoxic T-cell activity was elicited in vitro, there has been no direct evidence for in vivo antiviral effector cell lysis (Jacobson et al., 1984; Wong et al., 1984; Browning et al., 1990a; Browning et al., 1990b; Kaplan et al., 1984; Yasukawa and Zarling, 1984). Thus, it was interesting that initial reports suggested that CD4$^+$ cells played the major role in the immunopathogenesis of BDV. Subsequently, however, a body of data has accumulated that provides strong evidence for a central importance of CD8$^+$ T cells in induction of BD. CD8$^+$ T cells are now believed to play the major role in the immunopathogenesis of BD, triggering the local CD4$^+$-T-cell-mediated delayed-type hypersensitivity reaction in the brain after BDV infection (Stitz et al., 1992).

Although antibodies directed against CD4$^+$ T cells ameliorate BD to some extent, the antibodies have to be given at high doses and for a prolonged time. However, treatment with MAbs specific for CD8$^+$ cells or specific for a pan-T-cell marker given early after infection of thymectomized rats was able to decrease or even prevent the local inflammatory reaction, encephalitis (Stitz et al., 1992). When anti-CD8 antibody treatment is started after BDV infection, there is some delay of the inflammatory reaction and BD, but the ultimate severity of encephalitis or disease is not affected. The limited effect of MAbs given after BDV infection suggests a rapid activation of T cells in the periphery of BDV-infected rats at the time of infection (i.e., before detection of significant immune response in the brain) that is not blocked by postinfection administration of anti-T-cell antibodies (Stitz et al., 1989). This might be due to the fact that after i.c. inoculation, considerable amounts of the virus gain immediate access to immune tissues outside the CNS via the blood (Mims, 1960).

Transforming growth factor β2 (TGF-β2) acts as a multifunctional cytokine with potent inhibitory activity on growth, differentiation, and effector functions of activated T and B lymphocytes and macrophages (reviewed by Wahl et al. [1989] and Palladino et al. [1990]). Treatment of BDV-infected rats with TGF-β2 revealed a transient reduction in the severity of clinical symptoms that was paralleled by a significant reduction of the inflammatory reaction in the brain (Fontana et al., 1989; Stitz et al., 1991a, 1991b). Although IHC revealed slightly reduced CD4$^+$-T-cell numbers and no changes in macrophage counts in the encephalitic lesions of TGF-treated rats, CD8$^+$ T cells were virtually absent from the perivascular inflammatory reaction at early time points after infection and TGF-β2 treatment. The reappearance of CD8$^+$ T cells in TGF-treated rats late in the course of infection was directly correlated with the onset and degree of severity of clinical symptoms. In addition, in the brain of TGF-treated BDV-infected rats, the expression of MHC class II antigen was significantly reduced, whereas MHC class I expression was not. Since CD8$^+$ T cells are potent producers of immune interferon, and since IFN-γ also regulates MHC class I and class II expression (Fierz et al., 1985; G. H. Wong et al., 1984; G. H. W. Wong et al., 1984), the absence of CD8$^+$ T cells in the brains of TGF-treated rats was associated with the observed reduction of MHC class II antigen expression (Stitz et al., 1991). BDV-infected astrocytes produce IFN-α/β in vitro (Planz et al., 1993), a soluble immune mediator that was previously described as astrocyte IFN (Tedeschi et al., 1986). Type I interferons and, in particular, astrocyte IFN up-regulate MHC class I but not class II expression (Tedeschi et al., 1986; Halloran et al., 1989), providing a good explanation for the IFN-γ-independent presence of MHC class I in TGF-treated rats. In summary, experiments with TGF-treated rats demonstrated that initial inhibition of the encephalitic reaction and clinical symptoms correlated with the absence of CD8$^+$ T cells and reduced expression of self-restriction elements for cell-mediated immune responses, even in the presence of CD4$^+$ T cells.

Lymphocytes obtained from regional lymph nodes of rats that had been immunized with a purified virus-specific antigen, BDV N, were cultured and restimulated in vitro by a protocol for the cultivation of CD4$^+$ T cells (Richt et al., 1990; Richt et al., 1989). Analysis of this cell line (NM-1) revealed specificity for BDV, MHC class II restriction and the phenotypical markers of CD4$^+$ helper and inflammatory cells (Richt et al., 1989). Passive transfer of NM-1 cells into BDV-infected cyclophosphamide-immunosuppressed, healthy recipients resulted in severe disease and death as early as 5 days after transfer (Richt et al., 1989, 1990). In contrast, passive transfer into uninfected rats did not result in encephalitis or disease, demonstrating that NM-1 was a BDV-specific T-cell line that, by itself, was not encephalitogenic. These results, together with the immunohistological characterization of inflammatory cells in the brain of BDV-infected rats and data obtained with other T-cell lines (Planz et al., 1995), strongly suggested that BD is caused by a delayed-type hypersensitivity reaction.

The in vivo significance of cytotoxic CD4$^+$ T cells suggested by the NM-1 studies was put in question by the finding that MHC class II-restricted cytotoxicity is difficult to demonstrate in lymphocyte preparations isolated directly from the brain (Bilzer and Stitz, 1994; Planz et al., 1993). In addition, adoptive transfer experiments with lymphocyte preparations that were isolated from the brain and that showed high MHC class I-restricted cytotoxic activity, but not MHC class II restriction, revealed an early onset of severe neurological symptoms, a massive disseminated infiltration of the brain parenchyma with CD8$^+$ T cells, and severe neurodegeneration (Sobbe et al., 1997). One explanation for the unique cytotoxic properties of the NM-1 cell line is that CD4$^+$ T cells may have acquired cytotoxic activity upon in vitro cultivation (Fleischer, 1984; Cash et al., 1994).

Although CD4$^+$-T-cell clones can induce inflammatory reactions in the absence of CD8$^+$ T cells, in vivo disease outcomes have been shown to be dependent on CD8$^+$ T cells (Thivolet et al., 1991; Fowell and Mason, 1993; Ando et al., 1993). Other CD4$^+$ T cells characterized by their cytokine patterns, such as the Th1 or T-helper intermediate type with specificity for either N or P, were shown to lack cytotoxic activity in vitro (Planz et al., 1995). Adoptive transfer of BDV-specific helper T-cell lines into cyclophosphamide-immunosuppressed BDV-infected recipients resulted in an increase of anti-BDV antibody titers and severe encephalitis associated with BD-specific neurological symptoms within 2 to 3 weeks after transfer. Since in vivo adoptive transfer of these noncytotoxic CD4$^+$-T-cell lines resulted in neurological disease that was comparable to BD (Planz et al., 1995), cytotoxic CD4$^+$ T cells are clearly not needed to induce the disease. Interestingly, IHC analysis of the brains of rats with BD uniformly revealed the presence of CD8$^+$ T cells in encephalitic lesions, but CD4$^+$ cells were found in the brains of recipients of the virus-specific CD4$^+$-T-cell line irrespective of whether neurological symptoms developed. Recipient rats treated with antibodies against CD8$^+$ T cells develop neither serious encephalitis nor disease symptoms (Planz et al., 1995), and the inflammatory cells seen in these nondiseased rats are comprised of exclusively CD4$^+$ T cells and macrophages but no CD8$^+$ T cells (Bilzer and Stitz, 1994; Stitz et al., 1992). Therefore, while CD4$^+$ T cells appear to accumulate in the brain and cause perivascular inflammatory lesions, CD8$^+$ T cells are the effector cells causing immunopathogenic BD.

CD4$^+$-T-cell lines specific for the unglycosylated P antigen were shown to carry the α/β T-cell receptor and the β4 integrin (VLA-4) (Planz et al., 1995). The latter has been shown to be the crucial molecule in allowing entry of activated cells into the brain after binding to vascular cell adhesion molecule 1 on endothelial cells (Hickey et al., 1991; Baron et al., 1993; Wekerle et al., 1986). The concept has been proven valid also for BDV infection when anti-α4 integrin blocked the interaction of T cells with the blood-brain barrier endothelium, resulting in an inhibition of the disease process (Rubin et al., 1998).

Since astrocytes are target cells of BDV infection in the rat brain (Ludwig et al., 1988; Carbone et al., 1989; Deschl et al., 1990; Bilzer et al., 1993) and are potent antigen-presenting cells in the CNS (Fierz et al., 1985; Fontana et al., 1984), it was of interest to investigate T-cell–astrocyte interactions in BDV-infected rats. The expression of MHC class II on BDV-infected astrocytes is a prerequisite for these cells to serve as targets for in vitro cytotoxicity by the CD4$^+$-T-cell line NM-1 (Richt and Stitz, 1992). NM-1 was able to lyse syngeneic, IFN-γ-treated, persistently infected astrocytes, and antibodies directed against MHC class II antigens significantly reduced lysis. Interestingly, elevation of astrocyte expression of MHC class II by IFN-γ was required for astrocytes to serve as BDV antigen-presenting cells to the BDV-specific CD4$^+$-T-cell line in vitro (Richt et al., 1990), as BDV infection alone was incapable of inducing the expression of MHC class II in astrocytic cultures in vitro (Stitz et al., 1991a; Stitz et al., 1999b; Richt et al., 1992; Planz et al., 1993). This finding is in contrast to coronavirus infection in rats (Massa et al., 1986; Suzumura et al., 1986). Since BDV-infected astrocytes are able to present BDV-specific antigens, BDV infection does not appear to interfere with vital cell functions (Richt and Stitz, 1992).

The involvement of natural killer (NK) cells in the local inflammatory reaction in the brain is still unclear; although present in the brain (Deschl et al., 1989; Hatalski et al., 1998b), no NK cell activity has ever been demonstrated in brain lymphocyte preparations. Nevertheless, NK cells might participate in immunopathogenesis by virtue of their producing cytokines in the peripheral blood after BDV infection (Planz et al., 1993).

Recently, determining the viral target molecule and specific peptide epitopes has further substantiated the role of CD8[+] T cells in the immune response. The immunodominant viral protein for the CD8[+]-T-cell-mediated cytotoxic response was determined, using a recombinant vaccinia virus that expressed the viral matrix protein (M), P, N, or G. It was shown that the N protein represents the major epitope for cytotoxic T cells, and when rats that had been immunized with recombinant vaccinia virus expressing N were challenged with BDV, they were found to harbor reduced viral loads (Lewis et al., 1999).

There was also a weak indication for a subdominant epitope on G (Planz and Stitz, 1999). This finding was verified in the mouse model (Hausmann et al., 1999). Finally, the relevant naturally processed target peptide within the nucleoprotein was identified: the peptide ASYAQMTTY. Moreover, this peptide represents the first naturally processed viral target structure for rat CD8[+] T cells (Planz et al., 2001).

Despite the vigorous immune response in the brain, including the activity of cytotoxic T cells, BDV persists in the brain. A similar situation has been reported for lymphocytic choriomeningitis virus infection in mice, in which virus clearance is not accomplished despite the presence of cytotoxic T-cell activity (Allan and Doherty, 1985). An example of the apparent protection from BD in rats has been reported by preinfection inoculation of a BDV-specific CD4[+]-T-cell line (Richt et al., 1993). However, it has not been clarified whether antiviral antibodies, antibodies, or clonotypic T cells directed against the T-cell receptors or whether the possible induction of CD8[+] T cells by cytokines produced by these CD4[+] T cells was responsible for the antiviral effect. In addition, in BDV-infected rats, immunopathology and disease were prevented after transfer of CD4[+] T cells due to the function of cytotoxic CD8[+] T cells, which also led to elimination of the virus from the brain (Nöske et al., 1998).

BDV is not directly cell cytotoxic, although BDV-infected cells show disturbances in cell cycle progression and display changes in their morphology (Planz and Stitz, unpublished data) and the serious and often fatal forms of BD are believed to be immunopathogenic. Treatment of BDV-infected rats with anti-CD8 MAbs not only reduces or inhibits inflammation as described but also prevents neuronal degeneration and overt loss of brain substance (Bilzer and Stitz, 1993, 1994). Therefore, CD8[+] T cells are also involved in brain tissue destruction after BDV infection, resulting in organ atrophy and clinically in chronic debility and dementia (Bilzer and Stitz, 1993, 1994; Planz et al., 1993). In contrast, in vivo treatment with MAbs directed against CD4[+] T cells does not prevent significant loss of brain tissue (Planz et al., 1993). By which mechanisms CD8[+] T cells cause tissue destruction is still unsolved. CD8[+] T cells are potent producers of cytokines (Paliard et al., 1988; Street and Mosmann, 1991) that activate macrophages and induce a delayed-type hypersensitivity reaction, including the activation of nonspecific host inflammatory cells that finally results in tissue injury. To what extent other deleterious cytokines and radicals are involved in the tissue destruction is not yet clear. Alternatively, virus-specific CD8$^+$ T cells might kill their target cells after activation of their cytolytic mechanism, including the action of perforin and other effector molecules (Müller et al., 1989; Kägi et al., 1994; Henkart, 1985; Clark, 1994). In this respect, it is of interest and importance that upregulation of perforin mRNA in the brains of BDV-infected rats has been detected in parallel with the first signs of tissue destruction and the presence of CD8$^+$ T cells (Sobbe et al., 1998). However, it has been recently shown that perforin-mediated lysis apparently does not play a major role in immunopathogenesis in the mouse model of BDV infection.

In conclusion, BD in rats appears to be a CD4$^+$-T-cell-dependent immunopathological disease in which CD8$^+$ T cells and/or CD8$^+$-T-cell-mediated cytodestructive mechanisms are operative, leading to tissue destruction and organ atrophy and clinically to organ dysfunction and disease.

Molecular Mechanisms of Immune Response in BD

Leukocyte populations can generate cytokines, chemokines (Quagliarello et al., 1991), neurotoxins, or reactive oxygen intermediates (Nathan, 1992). These soluble factors not only play a central role in modulating immune responses and inflammatory reactions but also can have direct cytotoxic effects (Selmaj, 1992; Quagliarello et al., 1991).

In rats inoculated as adults, BDV infection is associated with a surge in expression of mRNAs encoding proinflammatory cytokines interleukin 1α (IL-1α), IL-2, IL-6, TNF-α, and IFN-γ (Shankar et al., 1992; Hatalski et al., 1998b). After reaching the peak of expression at 5 weeks p.i. (i.e., the acute phase of BD), expression of these mRNAs declines over the following 10 weeks (i.e., the chronic phase of BD). In contrast, expressions of mRNAs for TGF-β and IL-4 begin to increase later, 4 to 5 weeks p.i., and continue to increase to 15 weeks p.i. (Hatalski et al., 1998b). The pattern of IL-4 mRNA expression indicates a switch from a Th1 cellular immune response (i.e., the acute phase of BD) to a Th2 humoral immune response (i.e., the chronic phase of BD) (Hatalski et al., 1998b). In addition to cytokines, BDV infection in immunocompetent rats induces an upregulation of mRNAs for chemokines, IP-10 and RANTES (Sauder et al., 2000), and COX-2 and CGRP (Rohrenbeck et al., 1999). Similarly, levels of mRNA for inducible nitric oxide synthase (iNOS) and superoxide dismutase, as an indicator of free oxygen radicals, are significantly upregulated by BDV (Koprowski et al., 1993; Bilzer and Stitz, unpublished data). BDV-induced elevation of iNOS mRNA correlated with the degree of CNS inflammation and levels of TNF-α, IL-1, and IL-6 mRNAs (Selmaj, 1992), suggesting that TNF-α and IL-1 may stimulate infiltrating macrophages to generate NO (Nathan, 1992). Future studies are needed to gain better insights into molecular and cellular effects of cytokine during BD.

Behavioral Disease in Experimentally Infected Rats

Behavioral alterations in BDV-infected immunocompetent animals have been commonly evaluated in the Lewis rat model. An early report showed that rats became disoriented after infection (Nitzschke, 1963). Narayan et al. and Hirano et al. were the first to provide more-detailed descriptions of behavioral deficits induced by BDV infection in the rat (Narayan et al., 1983a, 1983b; Hirano et al., 1983). Similar to the course of natural BD in horses, the behavioral disease in adult-infected rats is characterized by an initial frenzied phase followed by a chronic passive state. Depending upon dose and route of inoculation (Carbone et al., 1987) abnormalities are usually first observed approximately 20 days p.i., when rats are very alert. During the next few days, rats become frenzied and exhibit exaggerated motor responses to minor stimuli. They appear disoriented and lack coordination without signs of paralysis. Some rats can be aggressive and attack their cage mates. Infected rats frequently develop ravenous appetites, approaching their food and water in the same frenzied manner. Approximately 30 to 40 days p.i., animals start exhibiting an extrapyramidal syndrome and stereotypy, including head bobbing with retrocollis; dystonias and flexed postures; and sniffing, chewing, scratching, and grooming. Masturbation, hoarding, and inges-tive disturbances (hyperphagia and polydipsia) along with self-mutila-tion (chewing the digits or tail) can be also observed. Constant erection (priapism) is often noted in infected males. The state of frenzy and hy-peractivity lasts for 30 to 40 days and then disappears (Narayan et al., 1983b).

By day 60 after inoculation, when inflammation subsides, rats become much calmer and spend most of their time resting or sleeping. They do not groom themselves. When picked up suddenly, they can be startled and bite at everything within reach, including cage mates. This reaction may be associated with blindness. Interestingly, at this stage of infection, hy-peractivity is no longer seen, and rats appear docile. Heightened sexual ac-tivity observed at the previous stage subsides, even when a normal female is introduced into the cage (Narayan et al., 1983a, 1983b). A small portion of animals (5 to 10%) becomes obese, achieving body weights as much as 300% of normal (Fig. 2). By 180 days p.i., rats usually show premature senescence, decreased activity, and cachexia.

The early phase of restless locomotion and excitation is rather common in encephalitic afflictions such as rabies and picornavirus infections (Johnston, 1998). Similarly, much of the behavioral disease in BDV-infected immunocompetent rats is most likely to be due to the inflammatory response in the brain parenchyma, since there is a temporal correlation between the hyperactive-aggressive phase in BD and the peak of inflammation between 30 and 40 days p.i. (Narayan et al., 1983a, 1983b). Then, a decline of encephalitis parallels the quiescent phase of BD, although infectious virus titers continue to be high in the rat's brain. A leading role of inflammation in the production of behavioral abnormalities in BDV-infected rats was further demonstrated in the experiments using hamsters and black-hooded rats. In those animals, the lack of the inflammatory response was accompanied by no apparent gross behavioral and neurological signs of disease, despite the high viral load of the CNS (Anzil et al., 1973; Herzog et al., 1991).

Inflammation-associated hyperactivity may be explained both by direct effects of proinflammatory molecules (e.g., cytokines and/or chemokines) on neuron functioning (e.g., release of neurotransmitter) and by indirect cytokine-mediated neuronal damage leading to cell loss (Bruce-Keller, 1999; Becher et al., 2000). For example, proinflammatory molecules have been shown to produce behavioral deficits (Campbell,

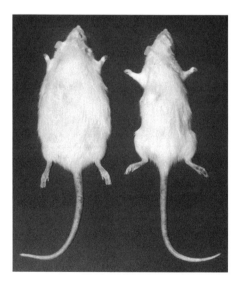

Figure 2. Obese (left) and nonobese (right) rats infected with BDV as adults.

1991; Rothwell et al., 1995) by affecting chemical neurotransmission (Galoyan, 2000). The correlation of cytokine levels in BDV-infected rat brains with the degree of inflammatory response and severity of neurological symptoms supports the hypothesis that cytokine-mediated cell damage and/or loss may also be responsible for behavioral deficits. This may be the case especially for BDV-associated damage to the hippocampus. Experimental lesions to the hippocampus have been consistently shown to induce hyperactivity in rats and mice (Panksep, 1999). Given that the hippocampus harbors a high viral load, this brain structure may be a primary target for virus-induced specific inflammatory responses and cytokine-mediated cell loss (Gonzalez-Dunia et al., 1999) that could lead to hyperactivity and frenzied behavior observed in infected rats. Thus, the predominant damage of the limbic system by the inflammatory infiltrates and/or direct effects of virus and cytokines or chemokines on relevant neural pathways could explain the hyperactivity and stereotypic behaviors in BDV-infected rats.

A series of investigations has been performed to explore a pathogenic role of BDV-altered chemical neurotransmission in the production of locomotor hyperactivity and stereotypic behaviors. Lipkin et al. published data showing a BDV-associated decrease in brain levels for mRNAs coding for cholecystokinin, glutamic acid decarboxylase, and somatostatin in acutely infected rats and a BDV-associated increase in chronically infected rats (Lipkin et al., 1988). Of note, actin levels were not altered in either acutely or chronically infected rats, suggesting that the effects of BDV were not generalized but were instead restricted to specific genes. Fluctuating BDV-associated alterations in mRNA levels during acute and chronic phases were suggested to reflect the presence and recession of inflammation. It is possible that reported alterations in levels for mRNAs for cholecystokinin, glutamic acid decarboxylase, and somatostatin might account for some aspects of abnormal locomotor activity during BD. It remains unclear whether this dissociation between different neurochemical alterations and similar behavioral outcomes in adult and neonatal BDV infections is due to differential pathogenic mechanisms.

Further studies into the mechanisms of locomotor hyperactivity and stereotypic behavior revealed selective neurochemical alterations in the dopamine brain system, suggesting a syndrome of dopamine (DA) hypersensitivity (Solbrig et al., 1994; Solbrig et al., 1996b). Pharmacological challenges showed that the central DA system of adult-infected rats is more sensitive to DA agents than that of sham-inoculated animals. For example, BD rats showed increased sensitivity to the indirect DA agonist D-amphetamine, manifested by increased amphetamine-induced locomotion and stereotypy (Solbrig et al., 1994). The atypical neuroleptic clozapine, which has D1 and D2 antagonist activity, and the selective D1 antagonist SCH23390 reduced activity in BD rats but not in control rats. In contrast, the D2-selective antagonist raclopiride had no effects on loco-motor responses in BDV-infected rats. Although elevated locomotion and behavior stereotypic to cocaine administration were seen 45 days after infection in both BDV-infected and control rats, only BDV-infected animals responded to cocaine with generalized and atonic seizures. Enhanced sensitivity to seizure-induced actions of cocaine was suggested to also indicate BDV-increased DA neurotransmission (Solbrig et al., 1998).

Putative neurochemical mechanisms of heightened responses to DA compounds were further evaluated by high-performance liquid chro-matography and receptor autoradiography techniques. It was shown that BDV infection resulted in depletion of DA by 47.3% in the caudate-puta-men, 29.4% in the nucleus accumbens, and 30.4% in the olfactory tubercle (Solbrig et al., 1995). In prefrontal cortex, BDV infection produced a sig-nificant (630%) increase in DA metabolite, 3,4-dihydroxyphenol acetic acid (DOPAC), without changing DA tissue content. As a result, the DOPAC/DA ratio, an index of DA turnover, was increased in BDV-infected animals. Changes in levels of DA and DOPAC in tissue were as-sociated with BDV-induced reduction of DA neurons in substantia nigra, pars compacia, and noradrenergic cells in locus coeruleus (Solbrig et al., 1994).

BDV-associated changes in density of DA receptors were examined by quantitative receptor autoradiography. Adult BDV infection produced regional and selective alterations in the density of DA receptors. In the caudate-putamen, a significant BDV-associated decrease in density of DA_2 receptors and DA reuptake sites but not DA_1 receptors was reported (Sol-brig et al., 1994, 1998). Similarly, in the core of the nucleus accumbens, BDV infection reduced the density of DA uptake sites and DA_2 and DA_3 receptors (Solbrig et al., 1996b). In contrast, in the prefrontal cortex, the density of DA_2 and DA_1 receptors remained unaltered by BDV infection (Solbrig et al., 1996a). Selective vulnerability of different subtypes of DA receptors has been attributed to the competition for splicing machinery be-tween the virus and spliced messages for DA_2 and DA_3 receptors but not unspliced messages for DA_1 receptors (Briese et al., 1999).

Solbrig et al. further explored a role of neurotrophic factors in BDV-associated alterations of DA neurotransmission (Solbrig et al., 2000). They reported a significant BDV-induced increase in levels of mRNAs for all tested members of growth factors (β-NGF, BDNF, NT-3, and NT-4), a sig-nificant increase in CNTF, and a significant decrease in GDNF mRNA lev-els in striatum of adult BDV-infected rats (Solbrig et al., 2000). BDV-induced changes in neurotrophin expression might lead to an increased tyrosine hydroxylase activity and enhanced amphetamine sensitivity. Thus, BDV-induced alterations in the mesocorticolimbic dopaminergic system may underlie the hyperactivity syndrome in infected rats.

A pathogenic role of cholinergic system alternations in BD was also addressed (Gies et al., 1998; Gies et al., 2001). A decrease in the number of choline acetyltransferase-positive fibers was observed to begin as early as day 6 p.i. and to progress to a nearly complete loss of cholinergic fibers in the hippocampus and neocortex by day 15 p.i. (Gies et al., 1998; Gies et al., 2001). Effects of adult BDV infection on serotonin and norepinephrine brain systems have not yet been thoroughly studied.

One of the most striking clinical manifestations of BD is the obesity syndrome that usually develops in a small number of rats that survived adult infection (Fig. 2) (Ludwig et al., 1988). The pathogenic mechanisms of obesity in BDV-infected rats are poorly understood. The recent findings have suggested that a putative "obesity" substrain of the virus may cause the obesity syndrome (Herden et al., 2000). Intracerebral injections of the obesity-inducing virus isolate (BDV-ob) produced a significant increase in the body weight of the infected animals as early as 14 days p.i. Interestingly, compared to rats infected with regular strains of BDV, obese BDV-infected rats exhibited minimal, if any, neurological signs, indicating selectivity in BDV-induced damage to the brain. Compared to the infection with a conventional strain of BDV, in BDV-ob infection, inflammatory lesions and BDV antigen localization were restricted to certain brain areas (e.g., the septum and ventromedian hypothalamus) (Herden et al., 2000). BDV-ob produced low infectivity that was undetectable at late time points, indicating that infection with this strain may cause only a transient low-level virus replication confined to certain brain regions, perhaps due to neutralization of virus infectivity by the immune system. Since electrolytic or chemical lesions to the ventromedian hypothalamus induce obesity in rats (Bray and York, 1979), inflammation-induced cell damage in the hypothalamus may be also responsible for the causation of the obesity syndrome in BDV-infected rats.

Behavioral Disease after Experimental Infection in Other Species

Investigations of experimental adult BDV infection in other species replicated findings from the rat model and extended our understanding of the pathogenesis of BD. Those studies revealed common and host-specific features of BDV-associated neurobehavioral disease.

Although BDV-infected rabbits show early and progressive decreases in body weight, they do not show signs of disease until 15 and 20 days after i.c. inoculation (Nicolau and Galloway, 1928; Zwick, 1939; Krey et al., 1979; Ludwig et al., 1988). In contrast to BDV-infected rats, infected rabbits' movements become slow and they appear depressed, and the rabbits do not exhibit excitement or hyperactivity (Ludwig et al., 1988). When the rabbit is placed on its side it makes efforts to recover its balance, beating the air with its hind legs before eventually recovering the normal position. While the depression referred to above suggests modifications in the meninges and cerebrum, the symptoms described later point to changes in the spinal cord. The animal assumes a characteristic attitude in the cage with the head in the angle formed by two walls; it appears somnolent, and the somnolence lasts until the end of the disease. The symptoms of the CNS disease (e.g., amaurosis) gradually intensify. Paresis of ears and trismus are seen. The muscles of the back become soft and flaccid. Paresis begins with hind limbs and spreads to front limbs. The animal ceases to feed, either from loss of appetite or difficulty in deglutition, further contributing to the weight loss.

The symptoms of the disease in rhesus monkeys begin with signs of apathy and loss of threatening behavior. Subsequently, infected animals become anorexic and refuse water. Infected rhesus monkeys exhibit a number of neurological symptoms consistent with those described for horses, sheep, and rabbits (Stitz et al., 1980).

BDV infection in tree shrews (*Tupaia glis*), which exhibit a complex social organization and behavioral repertoire, provided the first example of detailed BDV-induced behavioral abnormalities in the absence of inflammation and generalized, life-threatening neurological disease (Sprankel et al., 1978). The clinical manifestation of the behavioral disease in tree shrews was largely dependent on the housing conditions, i.e., socially isolated and group-housed animals demonstrated different disease outcomes. Socially isolated BDV-infected females exhibited exaggerated spontaneous locomotor activity and associated increase in feeding behavior that did not lead to weight gain, reminiscent of the phase of hyperactivity observed in BDV-infected rats (Narayan et al., 1983a). The hyperactivity phase was followed by the phase of clinical neurological symptoms, spatial and temporal disorientation, and alterations in comfort behavior. Following a slow recovery, the animals remained unusually docile and were much less timid than before infection (Sprankel et al., 1978).

Unlike socially isolated tree shrews, none of the BDV-infected tree shrews kept in pairs showed signs of hyperactivity or neurological symptoms. Instead, BDV infection produced a significant increase in all components of social behavior. There was a remarkable change in the sexual behavior in infected pairs, i.e., a reverse of social roles in the initiation of sexual interaction. Although males usually initiated sexual interaction among control tree shrews, BDV-infected females significantly increased the initiation of sexual behavior. In contrast, the sexual activity of infected male tree shrews declined. This was the first and remains the only documentation of gender effects on BDV-associated behavioral abnormalities (Sprankel et al., 1983).

Another interesting outcome of BDV infection in female tree shrews was the failure to nurse or to provide maternal care (Sprankel et al., 1978). Whether poor nursing was due to the social stress or BDV-associated hormonal disturbances is unclear. It also remains unknown why clinical manifestations of BD were not observed in all infected animals despite the comparable viral load and similar levels of antibodies detected in serum in all infected tree shrews. The pathogenic mechanisms of abnormal social activity in infected tree shrews remain obscure. Besides characteristic perivascular lymphocyte infiltrations and intranuclear Joest-Degen inclusion bodies in the brain, no other pathologic alterations were noted. The syndrome of disinhibition towards the environmental stimuli observed in infected animals has been suggested to be due to BDV-induced damage to the limbic system that has been implicated in the regulation of social interaction (Sprankel et al., 1978).

The importance of host factors in modulating BD outcome has been further demonstrated in experimentally BDV-infected mice. Slowed growth rates and minimal encephalitis along with the lack of neurobehavioral disease had been initially reported in infected mice (Nicolau and Galloway, 1927; Kao et al., 1984). Rubin and colleagues showed that a lower susceptibility to BD in mice might be explained by mouse strain-specific differences (Rubin et al., 1993). They found that while by day 55 p.i., MRL/*lpr*, MRL/+, and BALB/c mice had mononuclear cell encephalitis, the degree of intensity of encephalitis ranged from mild (BALB/c) to severe (MRL/+), with comparable BDV replication. Interestingly, although BDV infection induced encephalitis to a similar degree in MRL/+ and MRL/*lpr* mice, only MRL/+ mice exhibited locomotor hyperactivity (Rubin et al., 1993). In addition to revealing mouse strain differences, this study demonstrated another important feature of BDV infection in mice, i.e., the dissociation between inflammatory response and behavioral deficits, indicating that the onset of BD in different mouse strains might reflect variations in the composition and immunological properties of the cellular infiltrates (Rubin et al., 1993). Alternatively, host factors could also modulate the vulnerability of brain cells to the inflammatory reaction (Gonzalez-Dunia et al., 1998).

Taken together, the results of experimental BDV infection in adult immunocompetent animals have provided us with a variety of BD outcomes and extended our knowledge of the pathogenesis of BD.

PATHOGENESIS OF BDV-INDUCED NEURODEVELOPMENTAL DAMAGE

Virus Infection in Neonatally BDV-Infected Rats

Initially described in the early 1980s and extensively characterized by Carbone and coworkers (Narayan et al., 1983a, 1983b; Hirano et al., 1983; Carbone et al., 1991a; Carbone et al., 1991b), interest in the novel features of neonatal BDV infection of rats has recently spread to many groups studying BDV. It is now generally recognized that this model may help to understand the pathogenesis of human neuropsychiatric disorders such as autism and schizophrenia, where prenatal or perinatal injury to the developing CNS appears to play a role (Ciaranello and Ciaranello, 1995; Carbone and Pletnikov, 2000). Moreover, neonatal BDV infection occurs with minimal signs of inflammatory reaction in the CNS and offers the possibility to investigate direct effects of BDV infection on brain function in the absence of confounding global brain damage caused by the inflammation (Carbone et al., 1991a; Carbone et al., 1991b). This may be particularly important since there is evidence suggesting a higher prevalence of natural BDV infections without overt clinical manifestations than previously thought (Nakamura et al., 1995).

The first neurobehavioral studies of neonatal BDV infection of rats were performed in Wistar rats (Hirano et al., 1983; Dittrich et al., 1989), but most of the recent studies have focused on the Lewis strain. In Wistar newborn rats, it was shown that the virus could persist in the CNS and cause learning deficiencies, but there are only limited data on virus tropism and neuropathology. Hence, here we will concentrate on results obtained with the Lewis rat strain.

Infection of neonates is generally performed within 24 h of birth, by i.c. inoculation. A few days after infection, markers of viral infection (viral antigens and RNA) can be found in neurons of discrete CNS areas, most notably the olfactory bulb, hippocampus (CA3 and CA4 areas), the frontal cortex, and the deep cerebellar nuclei. Subsequently, viral antigen spreads rapidly to connecting neurons. By 6 to 10 days p.i., BDV markers label intensely the cell bodies of neurons, in particular in the hippocampus, cortex, and cerebellum (Bautista et al., 1995; Gonzalez-Dunia et al., 2000; Gosztonyi and Ludwig, 1995; Hornig et al., 1999; Sauder et al., 1999). Of interest, Purkinje cells (PCs) are the predominant, if not only, cells infected in the cerebellar cortex (Fig. 3) (Bautista et al., 1995; Eisenman et al., 1999). At about 3 weeks p.i., viral antigen is detected in virtually all areas of the CNS in neurons. The distinct viral antigen staining of neuronal cell bodies is accompanied by a progressively more diffuse staining of the neuropil. Secondarily to the infection of neurons, viral antigen is also found in CNS glial cells, in particular astrocytes but also oligodendrocytes, ependymal cells, as well as Schwann cells in the peripheral nervous system. Astrocytes appear to be infected at later time points than in the immunocompetent infected adult (Carbone et al., 1989; Carbone et al., 1991a), possibly because infection of astrocytes occurs only after BDV release by neurons. In agreement with this hypothesis is the situation in the cerebellum, where cerebellar astrocytes become infected well after the early infection of PCs. Finally, no infection has been demonstrated at any time in microglia in the CNS of BDV-infected neonates, consistent with the demonstration that macrophage cell lines are apparently resistant to BDV infection (Carbone et al., 1989; Weissenbock et al., 2000).

As early as 1963, Nitzschke had already described the presence of infectious virus in various organs, including the spleen, liver, and kidney, and even in the blood of rats infected as neonates. Subsequent studies have shown that, in the late stages of infection, BDV diffuses centrifugally from the CNS of neonatally infected rats, probably by using an anterograde axonal transport. Viral markers can be detected in peripheral nerves of all tissues and organs. Consequently, any ectodermal or epithelial tissue that receives central, peripheral, or autonomic innervation can become in-

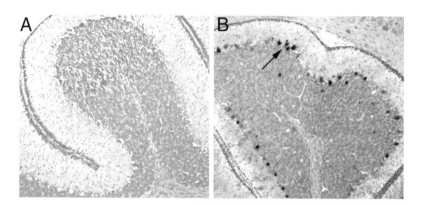

Figure 3. BDV antigen expression in PCs of the cerebellum at day 10 p.i. immunostaining of BDV nucleoprotein in sham-inoculated (A) and neonatally BDV-infected (B) Lewis rats. Note the expression of BDV antigen in many PCs in a BDV-infected rat (arrow). Original magnification, ×100 (present magnification, ×70). Courtesy of Aymeric Hans, Unité des virus lents, Institut Pasteur, Paris, France.

fected with BDV, including organs such as the liver, heart, or gut (Gosztonyi and Ludwig, 1995; Herzog et al., 1984; Stitz et al., 1998). This delayed invasion of BDV in extraneural tissues may be due to the absence of neutralizing antibodies in neonatally BDV-infected rats, antibodies which have been shown to play an important role in controlling BDV infection outside the CNS (Stitz et al., 1998).

It has been also demonstrated that neonatally BDV-infected rats excrete the virus in tears, saliva, and urine and can infect intact rats housed together in the same cage (Nitzschke 1963; Morales et al., 1988; Sierra-Honigmann et al., 1993; Stitz et al., 1998). Since there have been few descriptions of natural neonatal BDV infection and there is no convincing evidence that naturally BDV-infected animals excrete the virus outside the body, it remains to be established whether excretion of the virus by an infected animal is a mechanism of virus dissemination. Nevertheless, given the evidence for the presence of viral antigens in the olfactory system of diseased naturally infected horses, it is conceivable that natural BDV infection may occur via the olfactory route (Morales et al., 1988; Richt et al., 1993; Bilzer et al., 1995) or the recurrent pharangeal nerve (Bilzer et al., 1995) if the virus is excreted in saliva of infected animals. This suggestion would be in line with the phenomenon of the direct access of virus to the CNS via nervous endings, e.g., olfactory receptor neurons (Johnson, 1982; Ochs, 1982), as it has been demonstrated for infections with other viruses such as neurotropic influenza virus (Reinacher et al., 1983), herpes simplex virus (Tomlinson and Esiri, 1983), and Semliki Forest virus (Kaluza et al., 1986).

Developmental Damage to the Brain

Viral infections of the CNS are a significant cause of congenital disease in newborns. Moreover, many neuropsychiatric disorders of children, such as autism, may result from early brain injury during critical periods of pre- or postnatal brain development (Ciaranello and Claranello, 1995). Even though there is compelling evidence that BDV has a noncytolytic strategy of replication (Herzog and Rott, 1980), BDV persistence in neonates is associated with discrete brain damage, limited to specific neuronal populations. In this context, the features of neurodevelopmental damage after neonatal infection of Lewis rats with BDV are amenable to the study of the pathogenesis of behavioral abnormalities associated with perinatal virus infection (see below).

Following neonatal infection, BDV will preferentially damage the CNS areas that experience an extensive postnatal maturation (Carbone et al., 1991a; Carbone et al., 1991b; Rubin et al., 1999a). As a result, the dentate gyrus (DG) in the hippocampus undergoes progressive degeneration. There is also developmental injury to the cerebellum. Less salient, but nonetheless important, is virus-induced damage to the neocortex, as well as alterations in synaptic density and plasticity (Gonzalez-Dunia et al., 2000). This brain pathology might lead to a number of behavioral deficits, including locomotor hyperactivity and poor learning and memory, as well as abnormal social behavior. In addition, neonatal BDV infection produces a remarkable inhibition of weight gain (Bautista et al., 1994). The basis for runting is not clear since levels of glucose, growth hormone, and insulin-like growth factor 1 are normal following perinatal BDV infection (Bautista et al., 1994).

Damage to the hippocampus

The hippocampal formation, especially neurons of the CA3 and CA4 areas, is one of the first targets of neonatal BDV infection. An early infection of the DG has been reported, although not consistently (Gonzalez-Dunia et al., 1996; Gonzalez-Dunia et al., 2000; Sauder et al., 1999). As the infection progresses, the hippocampus consistently harbors the highest viral load (Gosztonyi and Ludwig, 1995). Despite this high replication of BDV, there is no overt damage to the neurons in the CA region. In contrast, there is a progressive involution of the DG that ultimately leads to its complete destruction by about 6 weeks p.i. (Fig. 4) (Carbone et al., 1991a; Carbone et al., 1991b). Since the vast majority (>85%) of granule neurons of DG are generated after birth (Gould and McEwen, 1993), the proliferating capacity of these neurons may be one of the explanations for their selective vulnerability to neonatal infection with BDV. Several studies employing techniques for the evaluation of neuronal pyknosis and density, or using terminal deoxynucleotidyl nick end labeling (TUNEL), have consistently shown that DG neurons die by an apoptosis-related mechanism, which peaks at about 4 weeks p.i. (Color Plate 4 [see color insert]) (Hornig et al., 1999; Rubin et al., 1999b; Sauder et al., 2000; Weissenbock et al., 2000). Apoptosis is accompanied by concordant modifications in the gene expression pattern of apoptosis-related genes, most notably an increased expression of caspase 1 and Fas and a decreased expression of *bcl-x* (Hornig et al., 1999). Nevertheless, the upstream mechanisms of BDV-induced DG degeneration are still not understood.

One can hypothesize that a greater vulnerability of DG granule cells may be linked to viral interference with pathways essential for DG granule cell maturation. DG damage may also be due to neuroendocrine disturbances. Adrenalectomy is a classical example of a stress resulting in apoptosis of DG granule cells (Sloviter et al., 1989; Vaher et al., 1994), where the resulting high levels of glucocorticoid receptor expression by DG neurons underscore the key role of glucocorticoids in promoting DG neurogenesis and survival. However, whether or not BDV-altered levels

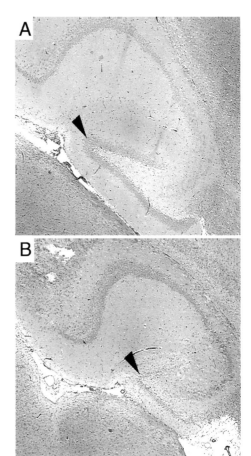

Figure 4. Degeneration of the DG of the hippocampus in neonatally BDV-infected rats at day 30 p.i. (A) Sham-inoculated rat; (B) BDV-infected rat. Note the disappearance of DG in the BDV-infected rat (arrowhead) compared to control DG. Hematoxylin and eosin staining was used. Original magnification, ×100 (present magnification, ×80).

of glucocorticoids might account for the DG degeneration remains unclear since there is no evidence for BDV infection of the adrenal glands and/or BDV-associated changes in glucocorticoid levels per se. A possible hypothesis involving resident glial cells and released soluble factors will be addressed further later in this chapter.

Damage to the cerebellum

Cerebellar hypoplasia is one of the most salient morphological features of BDV-induced neurodevelopmental damage (Fig. 5). Damage to the cerebellum has also been observed in other perinatal virus infections, including lymphocytic choriomeningitis virus, rubella, mumps, rat par-

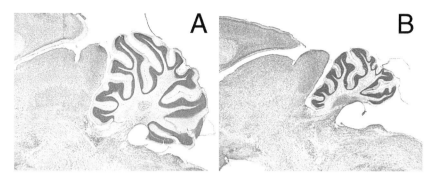

Figure 5. Hypoplasia of the cerebellum following neonatal BDV infection at day 30 p.i. Shown are representative sagittal sections of the cerebellum of a sham-inoculated rat (A) and a BDV-infected rat (B). Hematoxylin and eosin staining was used. Original magnification, ×12.5 (present magnification, ×8).

vovirus, or reovirus type III (Monjan et al., 1971; Oster-Granite and Herndon, 1985; Raine and Fields, 1973; Takano et al., 1994; Waxham and Wolinsky, 1984). In most cases, the cerebellum developmental arrest was attributed to either an immune-mediated or a virus-induced lysis of the dividing immature cerebellar granule cells. However, it is clear that BDV-induced damage to the cerebellum in neonates follows a different pattern.

During the early postnatal period, the cerebellum undergoes a dramatic (>20-fold) increase in size and acquires its foliage and laminar organization. This is accompanied by an intense proliferation and radial migration of cerebellar granule neurons, from the external granular layer towards the internal granule layer. Although PCs are all generated between embryonic days 13 and 15, a significant maturation of PC continues after birth (Goldowitz and Hamre, 1998).

In contrast to the other viral systems mentioned above, BDV does not appear to infect cerebellar granule cells following neonatal inoculation (Bautista et al., 1995). Although the cerebellum of neonatally BDV-infected rats is reduced in size, there is a normal foliation and laminar organization, even though a premature loss of the external granular layer and thinning of the internal granular layer were reported (Bautista et al., 1995). This finding was, however, not always clearly shown in all studies so far (Eisenman et al., 1999). Since PCs are the first cerebellar cells infected by BDV, it is surprising that the profound effects of neonatal BDV infection on PC survival were published only recently (Eisenman et al., 1999; Hornig et al., 1999; Zocher et al., 2000). It has now been clearly shown that neonatal BDV infection induces a prominent loss of PCs, reaching up to 75% of cell loss by 7 months p.i., although this loss may be nonuniform throughout the cerebellar cortex (K. M. Carbone and D. Gonzalez-Dunia, unpublished data). The exact timing of the onset of PC loss is still unclear, although one study estimated that it started somewhere between days 27 and 33 p.i. (Zocher et al., 2000). However, another report demonstrated that BDV-associated cerebellar damage, and presumably PC death, was not observed when rats were infected at postnatal day 15. This may indicate that the selective vulnerability of PCs to BDV infection is dependent in part on the developmental stage of the brain at the time of infection (Rubin et al., 1999a). It is clear that a more rigorous quantitative analysis of PC numbers is needed to precisely evaluate the timing of PC dropout.

Hence, BDV-induced developmental injury to the cerebellum is likely due to the prominent loss of PCs, together with a more discrete, and probably secondary, loss of granule cells, the presynaptic partners of PCs. Moreover, evidence indicates that PCs play a main role in supporting multiplication, maturation, and migration of granular cells. It is therefore conceivable that the loss of such a support following neonatal infection with BDV may negatively impact cerebellar granule cell survival (Bautista et al., 1995; Smeyne et al., 1995).

The precise mechanism for PC death is not known. Apoptosis in the cerebellum can be identified in only a few apoptotic granule cells, and PCs did not seem to be labeled by TUNEL or at least were labeled at levels well below the reported 75% loss of this cell population (Weissenbock et al., 2000; Zocher et al., 2000). Also, given a key role of astrocytes in the postnatal cerebellar development (e.g., secreting trophic factors and providing the physical tract upon which the granule cells migrate), it is possible that BDV-associated prominent astrocytosis in the cerebellum observed as early as at 3 days p.i. may affect the cerebellar cell survival (Bautista et al., 1995; Sauder et al., 1999).

Damage to the neocortex

Early after the description of the perinatal infection with BDV, it was demonstrated that BDV induced cortical shrinkage in neonatally infected rats (Bautista et al., 1994). In recent studies, it was confirmed that a significant proportion of cortical neurons is lost following perinatal infection with BDV. Whole-brain mass starts to decrease at about 2 weeks p.i., and apoptotic nuclei are found in the cerebral cortex at 3 weeks p.i. (Hornig et al., 1999; Weissenbock et al., 2000). Moreover, a morphometric analysis established that by 45 days p.i. about 30% of neuronal bodies were lost in the cortical area of neonatally infected rats (Gonzalez-Dunia et al., 2000). The selective decrease in cells with a diameter over 100 μm and with positive immunostaining for parvalbumin suggested that both pyramidal and gamma-aminobutyric acid-ergic cortical neurons exhibited vulnerability to neonatal BDV infection. It remains unclear whether neuronal death in the cortex is directly due to infection with BDV or is a consequence of astrocytosis and microgliosis leading to release of neurotoxic soluble factors.

Synaptic pathology

BDV-induced neuronal damage may also be attributed to disturbances in specialized functions of neurons. In particular, synaptic density and neuronal plasticity are likely to play important roles in neural functions during neural development and in processes of learning and memory. A recent study has examined the expression of the growth-associated protein 43 (GAP-43) and synaptophysin (SYN), two well-established markers of neuroplasticity and synaptic density, respectively (Gonzalez-Dunia et al., 2000). GAP-43 is a presynaptic membrane phosphoprotein that accumulates in neuronal growth cones. SYN is a 38-kDa calcium-binding protein present in the membranes of presynaptic vesicles. A semi-quantitative assessment of levels of immunoreactivity (IR) for these markers at different times after neonatal BDV infection revealed a progressive decrease in IR for GAP-43 and SYN in the neocortex and hippocampus (Gonzalez-Dunia et al., 2000). These disturbances did not appear to correlate directly with viral load or astrocytosis, suggesting differential vulnerability among various neuronal populations. Additionally, since SYN was sometimes found in cell bodies or in axonal spheroids, axonal transport in some BDV-infected neurons may have been also affected. This finding is reminiscent of those obtained in the adult immunocompetent rat model for BDV infection, which demonstrated axonal flow damage in the cortical cholinergic innervation prior to encephalitis (Gies et al., 1998). Thus, BDV-induced synaptic and axonal flow damage may have serious consequences in the supply and trafficking of growth factors required for proper neuronal function (Gonzalez-Dunia et al., 2000).

Immune Responses in Neonatally BDV-Infected Rats

In contrast to infection of immunocompetent adult rats, neonatal BDV infection is characterized by the absence of widespread encephalitis. The exact causes for the lack of significant immune infiltrates in this model are not completely elucidated. It has been postulated that perinatal infection leads to an early infection of the thymus during immune system maturation, resulting in the negative selection of BDV-reactive T-cell clones and BDV-specific "immune" or "split" tolerance (Rubin et al., 1995). However, direct proof of this hypothesis is still lacking (Carbone et al., 1991a; Carbone et al., 1991b). Nevertheless, mild and transient immune T-cell infiltrates were actually found in the CNS of neonatally BDV-infected rats between days 22 and 33 p.i. (Sauder et al., 1999; Hornig et al., 1999; Weissenbock et al., 2000). It has been argued that these immune infiltrates did not play a role in BDV-induced neurodevelopmental damage because they were not localized in sites of neuronal damage (Weissenbock et al., 2000) and were resolved at later time points p.i.

Astrocytosis and microgliosis

Despite the lack of cell-mediated immune response in the CNS of BDV-infected rats, BDV-induced activation of resident immune cells, i.e., astrocytes and microglia, is likely to play a major role in virus infection-associated neurodevelopmental damage. Astrocytosis is usually determined by an increase in the number and size of cells expressing an astrocyte-specific marker, the glial fibrillary acidic protein (GFAP). A significant increase in IR of GFAP is already seen as early as 3 days after neonatal BDV infection (Bautista et al., 1995). It steadily increases thereafter, most notably in areas of neuronal damage such as the DG in the hippocampus, the cerebellum and the neocortex (Color Plate 5 [see color insert]) (Bautista et al., 1995; Gonzalez-Dunia et al., 1996; Stitz et al., 1995). Moreover, a strong activation of microglial cells, identified by immunostaining with a specific rat marker such as ED-1, was also demonstrated in the CNS following neonatal BDV infection (Sauder and de la Torre, 1999; Weissenbock et al., 2000).

Proliferation and activation of astrocytes and microglia is a hallmark of neuronal damage, although the events responsible for glial cell activation are not well understood. While BDV replication in astrocytes may contribute to their activation, the events that lead to microglia activation remain obscure because microglial cells do not appear to be infected. One hypothesis is that microglia activation may be induced by soluble factors released by BDV-infected neurons or astrocytes.

Astrocyte functions are essential to neurons, not only in providing a substrate for neuronal migration during development, but also in eliminating neurotoxins and in producing various trophic factors, including cytokines (Eddleston and Mucke, 1993). Activated astrocytes and microglia may have a deleterious impact on neuronal function. For example, high levels of tissue factor (TF) were demonstrated in the CNS of neonatally BDV-infected rats (Gonzalez-Dunia et al., 1996). TF is a membrane-bound protein that belongs to the class II cytokine receptor family and is mainly produced by astrocytes. TF is the primary initiator of the coagulation protease cascade that results in the generation of the protease thrombin. In addition to their role in coagulation, there is increasing evidence that such proteases function in the CNS by regulating brain development and plasticity. Any imbalance in the protease activities may contribute to neuronal damage. Therefore, chronic astrocyte activation leading to a sustained TF up-regulation in neonatally BDV-infected rats may be also implicated in brain damage.

Expression of chemokines and cytokines

Upon stimulation, astrocytes and microglia have the capacity to produce several soluble factors, including cytokines and chemokines that can have diverse effects on neuronal function (Rothwell and Hopkins, 1995). Using sensitive RNase protection analyses, several groups have demonstrated alterations in cytokine gene expression in brains of neonatally BDV-infected rats (Hornig et al., 1999; Plata-Salaman et al., 1999; Sauder et al., 1999). Elevated levels of the proinflammatory cytokines IL-6, TNF-α, IL-1α, and IL-1β were consistently found in the hippocampus and cerebellum as early as 1 week p.i. Elevated levels of TGF-β1 mRNA were also demonstrated (Plata-Salaman et al., 1999). The regional localization of these elevated levels of proinflammatory cytokine mRNAs coincided with sites of major glial cell activation, supporting the hypothesis that astrocytes and microglia appear to be the major source for cytokine production. It is interesting to note that iNOS was detected in few macrophages and only at later time points, suggesting that NO may not be a major factor implicated in neuronal loss following neonatal infection with BDV (Hornig et al., 1999).

Considering the important role of cytokines in regulating neuronal physiology (Rothwell and Hopkins, 1995), the elevated levels of proinflammatory cytokines are likely to contribute to neuronal damage in neonatally BDV-infected rats, in particular in the hippocampus, since the neuronal activity of this brain region can be significantly affected by cytokines. For example, IL-1β or TNF-α can inhibit long-term potentiation in the CA1 and DG areas of the hippocampus (Cunningham et al., 1996), whereas IL-1 can disturb calcium fluxes in hippocampal neurons (Plata-Salaman et al., 1994).

Also, a sustained expression of the chemokines IP-10 and RANTES has been demonstrated in the brains of newborn rats infected with BDV, as early as 2 weeks p.i. (Sauder et al., 2000). Elevated mRNA levels for IP-10 were studied by in situ hybridization and were particularly conspicuous in the cerebellar astrocytes and, most notably, the Bergman glia. Interestingly, the elevated levels of chemokine mRNAs were not linked to leukocyte attraction, indicating a role of chemokines in supporting neuronal function (Asensio and Campbell, 1999). For example, elevated levels of IP-10 mRNA in the Bergman glia have been suggested to contribute to death of PCs or to act as an "astrocyte alarm signal" of PC loss (Asensio and Campbell, 1999).

Profile of Gene Expression in Brains of Neonatally BDV-Infected Rats

In addition to cytokines, chemokines, TF, and apoptosis genes, the expression of other factors potentially implicated in neuronal damage following perinatal infection with BDV has also been investigated. Postnatal brain development is strongly dependent on trophic support by neurotrophins, which play major roles in promoting neuronal proliferation, migration, and survival (Levi-Montalcini et al., 1996). It is therefore highly interesting that levels of mRNAs coding for neurotrophins and neurotrophin receptor genes are significantly altered following neonatal BDV infection (Hornig et al., 1999; Zocher et al., 2000). RNase protection analysis revealed BDV-induced reduction of levels of mRNA for the neurotrophins BDNF, NT-3, and NGF in the hippocampus by 2 weeks p.i. This phenomenon coincided with a decreased expression of mRNAs for the receptors for BDNF and NT-3, namely, TrkB and TrkC. It is tempting to speculate that alterations in neurotrophin secretion and/or susceptibility may contribute to brain dysgenesis following perinatal infection with BDV.

BDV-Induced Developmental Alterations in Monoamine Brain Systems

Recently, developmental alterations in the monoamine system of neonatally BDV-infected rats have been examined in order to evaluate a pathogenic role of disturbed neurochemical transmission in hyperactivity and hyperreactivity exhibited by infected rats.

Effects of neonatal BDV infection on the postnatal development of brain monoamine systems were evaluated in developing and adult Lewis rats neonatally infected with BDV (Pletnikov et al., 2000). Concentrations in tissue of norepinephrine (NE); DA and its metabolite, DOPAC; and serotonin (5-HT) and its metabolite, 5-hydroxyindole-3-acetic acid (5-HIAA), were assayed by means of high-performance liquid chromatography with electrochemical detection in frontal cortex, cerebellum, hippocampus, hypothalamus, and striatum of neonatally BDV-infected and sham-inoculated male Lewis rats 8, 14, 21, 60, and 90 days of age. Both NE and 5-HT concentrations were significantly affected by neonatal BDV infection. The cortical and cerebellar levels of NE and 5-HT were significantly greater in BDV-infected rats than control animals at postnatal day (PND) 60 and 90. The level of NE in hippocampus tissue was unaffected. Neonatally BDV-infected rats had lower 5-HT levels in the hippocampus at PND 8 and significantly elevated levels at PND 21 and onwards. Neither striatal levels of 5-HT nor hypothalamic levels of 5-HT and NE were affected by neonatal BDV infection, suggesting that the monoamine systems in these prenatally maturing brain regions are less sensitive to effects of neonatal viral infection. The 5-HIAA/5-HT ratio was not altered in BDV-infected rats, indicating no changes in the serotonin turnover in the brain regions damaged by the virus. Neither DA nor the DOPAC/DA ratio was affected by neonatal BDV infection in any of the brain regions examined (Pletnikov et al., 2000).

The data demonstrate significant and specific changes in the monoamine systems of neonatally BDV-infected rats. The observed monoamine disturbances may explain some behavioral deficits, including hyperactivity and increased anxiety in infected rats.

Behavioral Deficits

Neonatal BDV infection produces a constellation of behavioral abnormalities in locomotion, fear-related, cognitive and social behaviors.

Neonatal BDV infection-associated sensorimotor deficits

In the rat, cerebellum-controlled behaviors have a discrete, organized pattern of evolution, paralleling the physical development of the cerebellum: e.g., the ability to maintain static quadruped posture precedes the ability to maintain quadruped posture during movement, which is followed by the acquisition of simple motor skills (Altman, 1975).

Neonatal BDV infection produces distinct impairments in motor and postural skills in Lewis rats. Importantly, no evidence of gross ataxia is observed, and the neonatally infected rats have a normal swimming speed (Rubin et al., 1999a). This finding is consistent with previous observations that cerebellar lesions made during the neonatal period do not affect these motor behaviors (LaLonde, 1997). However, neonatally BDV-infected rats do exhibit behavioral deficits that could be explained by developmental damage to the cerebellum. For example, neonatally infected rats demonstrate mild gait ataxia, hind paw spasticity, and a decreased ability to hang from a dowel when tested as adults, i.e., at 12 to 76 weeks of age (Hornig et al., 1999). Recently, a developmental time course of sensorimotor deficits in developing BDV-infected rats (PND 4 to 30) was evaluated using a battery of behavioral tests (Pletnikov et al., 2001). BDV-induced motor deficits and impaired coordination were selective and correlated with the time course of BDV damage to the cerebellum. BDV-induced motor disturbances were not seen until day 14 p.i., when cerebellar developmental abnormalities are detected by histological analysis. By day 21 p.i., BDV-infected rats exhibit deficient negative geotropism and fore- and hindlimb placing and grasping. The ability to hold on to a bar and to cross a suspended bar is also impaired in BDV-infected rats. Decreased responsiveness to the acoustic startle stimuli (day 30 p.i.) and attenuated habituation of the acoustic startle response (day 23 p.i.) are also noted (Pletnikov et al., 2001). Interestingly, despite BDV-associated low startle responsiveness, prepulse inhibition of the acoustic startle remains unaffected (day 30 and 120 p.i.) or even abnormally high (day 18 and 30 p.i.) in BDV-infected rats.

Thus, BDV-induced abnormal development of the cerebellum is associated with selective deficits in sensorimotor and postural skills in Lewis rats.

Neonatal BDV infection-associated emotional disturbances

Experimental lesions to the hippocampus and to the medial part of the cerebellum have been shown to lead to emotional disturbances in rats (Pankseep, 1999). In the first formal experimental study of behavioral abnormalities in neonatally BDV-infected rats, Dittrich et al. reported that compared to uninfected animals, BDV-infected Wistar rats exhibited hyperactivity in the open field and a greater number of transitions in the white-black box paradigm, suggesting a decreased level of anxiety (Dittrich et al., 1989). Emotional abnormalities due to neonatal BDV infection were further evaluated in Lewis rats tested as adults (Pletnikov et al., 1999a; Pletnikov et al., 1999b). Compared to healthy animals, and in contrast with the report of Dittrich et al., Pletnikov et al. found that BDV-infected rats exhibit signs of significant fear responses, e.g., locomotor hyperactivity and elevated defecation, in a highly aversive, brightly lit open field. In a less aversive, dimly lit open field, signs of reduced stress were apparent, as uninfected rats exhibited more ambulation, while infected rats significantly decreased their locomotor hyperactivity and defecation response. BDV-infected rats also demonstrated increased sensitization of the startle response by preceding foot shocks, suggesting a tendency toward elevated escape behavior. Prolonged novelty-induced behavioral inhibition observed in 1-month-old BDV-infected rats was another indicator of possible disturbances in emotionality in neonatally BDV-infected rats (Hornig et al., 1999).

The neurobiological basis of emotional alterations in BDV-infected rats is obscure. Cerebellar damage, degeneration of the DG of the hippocampus, and cortical injury could all contribute to disturbed emotionality in infected rats. In addition, putative chronic anxiety in BDV-infected rats may be associated with functional damage to amygdala neurons that are infected by BDV.

Neonatal BDV infection-associated cognitive abnormalities

The limbic system and, in particular, the hippocampus have been long implicated in the neuronal pathways underlying learning and memory processes in animals (Rolls, 2000). Given the consistent reports on BDV-induced hippocampal damage, evaluating putative cognitive abnormalities in neonatally BDV-infected rats has been a focus of many investigations.

One of the first behavioral studies of neonatal BDV infection-associated cognitive deficits was to examine spatial discrimination learning based on performance in the Y-maze and the hole board (Dittrich et al., 1989). In the Y-maze, the neonatally BDV-infected Wistar rats were trained to discriminate between two symmetrical arms of a Y-maze where food was placed only at the end of the right arm. Compared to uninfected animals, the infected rats made a significantly greater number of incorrect choices (Dittrich et al., 1989). Similarly, in the hole board paradigm designed to reflect an ability to process and remember spatial information, the rats were trained to search for food pellets placed diagonally in different holes. The mean number of errors in BDV-infected rats was higher than those in uninfected control animals, and it took a significantly longer time for BDV-infected rats to locate all baited holes (Dittrich et al., 1989).

Both the hippocampus and cerebellum play a major role in the acquisition of spatial navigation tasks, and lesions to these brain regions have been shown to affect acquisition and/or retention of a hidden platform location in the Morris water maze (MWM) (Lalonde, 1997; Petrosini et al., 1998). The MWM is a classic test for studying spatial learning and memory via navigation based on visual cues (Eichenbaum et al., 1990). An advantage of the MWM is the use of a swimming paradigm, rather than a running one, since, unlike running, swimming is minimally affected by cerebellar damage (Petrosini et al., 1998). This was confirmed in neonatally BDV-infected rats, where the maximum swimming speed between infected and uninfected groups was not different (Rubin et al., 1999a). In the MWM, neonatally BDV infected rats performed significantly worse than control rats (Rubin et al., 1999a). At day 72 p.i., the BDV-infected rats were deficient in their ability to learn the location of the platform over a series of swim trials, as indicated by their failure to significantly reduce the time to find the submerged platform.

Another behavioral task requiring the integrity of the limbic system is contextual fear conditioning (Fanselow, 2000). In this task, rats exhibited species-specific fear responses to the context (e.g., the test chamber) previously paired with aversive stimuli (e.g., electrical foot shock or sudden loud noise). Freezing (i.e., a complete immobility) and defecation response can be used to assess the amount of contextual fear conditioning. In contrast to untrained naive animals, normal trained rats usually exhibit more freezing and/or defecation in the context previously paired with aversive stimulation, indicating that contextual fear conditioning has been successful and, therefore, that the memory about the aversive context has formed (Fanselow, 2000). Compared to control Lewis rats, BDV-infected Lewis rats demonstrate attenuated conditional freezing in the context previously paired with either sudden loud noise or foot shock, suggesting deficits in contextual conditioning. Interestingly, conditioned defecation response to the context was spared in BDV-infected rats, indicating that some components of the brain system mediating fear conditioning appear to be unaffected by the virus infection (Pletnikov et al., 1999a).

Effects of neonatal BDV infection on aversive learning and memory were studied by assessing avoidance of pain (either taste aversion or shock). Compared to uninfected animals, neonatally BDV-infected Wistar rats demonstrated a significantly reduced inhibition of responses to aversive taste and/or shock following the training procedure, indicating deficient learning and/or memory about past aversive experiences (Dittrich, 1989).

Thus, neonatally BDV-infected rats exhibit a number of learning and memory abnormalities that may be due to BDV-induced developmental damage to the hippocampus, cortex, and cerebellum. Additionally, impairment of neuronal functioning due to putative direct (e.g., the virus replication) or indirect (cytokine or chemokine effects) viral toxicity may explain the observed deficits in the cognitive domain (Becher et al., 2000).

Neonatal BDV infection-associated alterations in social behavior

BDV-induced damage to the cerebellum and hippocampus may underlie abnormal social interaction and communication. Pletnikov and colleagues found social behavioral deficits in neonatally BDV-infected Lewis rats when tested at day 30 to 33 p.i. (Pletnikov et al., 1999b). Studies were conducted using the resident/intruder paradigm. A resident rat was isolated for one week in order to increase social motivation (Pankseep et al., 1984), and an unfamiliar rat (intruder) was placed in the resident's cage. This scenario is conducive to social interactions between young rats, often resulting in play behavior (measured as number of "pins," similar to a pin observed in a wrestling match). When play activity of the resident was analyzed, the control rat pairs exhibited significantly more pins than the pairs where either one rat or both rats were infected with BDV. To evaluate whether reduced play activity in the BDV-infected rats was due to a decreased drive to engage their partner in social play, an observational paradigm was used to evaluate specific play-soliciting behaviors (e.g., pouncing, crawling over or under, and darting). These studies showed that the control resident rats have significantly more play solicitations than the BDV-infected resident rats, regardless of the intruder's infection status, indicating normal play readiness on the part of the healthy, but not BDV-infected, rats. The reduced play activity in BDV-infected rats was not due to reduced locomotor activity or deficits in nonplay social behavior

(Pletnikov et al., 1999b). In fact, compared to control animals, nonplay social interaction is elevated in BDV-infected rats, suggesting that the entire
organization of the timely expression of different types of social interaction was significantly disturbed by BDV infection. These data have interesting neurodevelopmental implications, suggesting that play activity and
social nonplay activity are under the control of different neural systems
undergoing unequal maturation during postnatal life.

Thus, neonatal BDV infection produces a number of distinct behavioral abnormalities that can be attributed to regional developmental brain
damage and selective neurochemical and molecular alterations in infected
rats. A possibility of relating brain pathology to behavioral deficits in the
neonatal BDV infection model opens new perspectives in studying the
mechanisms by which environmental factors, including virus infection,
derail the normal brain and behavior development.

FUTURE DIRECTIONS

Molecular Mechanism of Effects of BDV Infection in Neuronal and Glial Cells

The study of the pathogenesis of neurological diseases caused by
BDV infection is a formidable challenge. Among many factors, one must
consider the neurodevelopmental stage at the time of infection, the immune status of the host, and presumably the viral strain used. Moreover,
it may be difficult sometimes to separate effects directly linked to BDV infection per se from the consequences of brain stress or damage, resulting,
for example, in the secondary release of soluble factors.

Reductionistic approaches in organotypic and cell culture systems
can provide new insights into direct effects of BDV infection on the function of neuronal or glial cells. Even if the significance of results obtained in
vitro is dependent on a subsequent validation in vivo, in vitro approaches
are likely to be instrumental in future studies of the molecular pathogenesis of BDV infection.

Until recently, few studies have examined the impact of BDV infection on CNS-derived cells. Most studies have focused on established cell
lines or primary cultures, although organotypic culture systems (e.g.,
brain slices) have not been evaluated yet. Early studies on neuronal and
glial cell lines infected with BDV demonstrated different behavior patterns
of BDV and a possible role of neurotrophic factors, such as NGF, in regulating BDV replication in PC12 and C6 cells (Carbone et al., 1993). More recently, it has been shown that BDV infection of the astrocyte-derived cell
line C6 led to TF upregulation, paralleling the results observed in brains of

neonatally BDV-infected rats (Gonzalez-Dunia et al., 1996). The use of an established cell line for further analysis of the molecular bases for this phenomenon showed that TF up-regulation was due to an increased transcriptional activity of the TF promoter together with a stabilization of TF mRNA (Gonzalez-Dunia et al., 1996). In another series of experiments, a BDV-induced inhibition of glutamate uptake was demonstrated in primary cultures of feline astrocytes, suggesting a pathogenic mechanism of BDV neurotoxicity in vivo (Billaud et al., 2000).

Direct effects of BDV on neuronal cultures largely remain unstudied. A recent report has demonstrated that PC12 cells, a classical model for studying neuronal differentiation, became resistant to NGF-induced neuronal differentiation upon infection with BDV (Hans et al., 2001). This effect was linked to BDV-induced perturbations in the signal transduction cascade triggered by NGF and, most notably, a chronic activation of the mitogen-activated protein kinase ERK1/2. Interestingly, a selective blockade of the ERK1/2 signaling cascade has been found to prevent BDV replication (Planz et al., 2001). These findings supported the hypothesis that BDV-associated neurodevelopmental damage may be caused by or lead to neurotrophin unresponsiveness of BDV-infected neurons. Moreover, BDV-infected PC12 cells displayed an impaired expression of the neuroplasticity-related genes GAP-43 and SYN, a feature also demonstrated in the CNS of neonatally BDV-infected rats (Gonzalez-Dunia et al., 2000).

Hence, it is probable that in vitro approaches using primary or established cell lines as well as organotypic cultures will bring important information on the molecular bases for the CNS disturbances caused by BDV infection. If confirmed in the natural situation, these approaches may be particularly helpful in better understanding the specific mechanisms for the BDV neuropathogenesis.

Role of Genetic Factors in Neurobehavioral Disease

Effects of genetic factors on BDV-induced neurobehavioral abnormalities are not new to BDV research. For example, Herzog and colleagues reported differential outcomes of BDV infection in adult animals from different rat strains, pointing out a likely role of host genetic factors in determining the inflammatory response and the severity of the disease (Herzog et al., 1991). In addition, the specific conditions of a particular host might be able to influence disease outcome by causing the species or strain-specific selection of unique virus mutants, thereby creating more virulent or attenuated substrains. For example, recent investigations by Nishino and her coworkers suggested that serial passage of BDV through mouse brain appeared to cause a small number of mutations in the BDV genome, resulting in a more virulent substrain of the BDV (Nishino et al., 2002).

Studies on different mouse strains after BDV infection revealed effects of genetic background on the type and degree of clinical manifestations of BD in infected mice, demonstrating that, after infection as adults, mice of the MRL strain, but not BALB/c or SJL strain, showed evidence of behavioral disease (Rubin et al., 1993). Further, Staeheli and his collaborators showed differences in BD outcomes among newborn mice of different strains (Hallensleben et al., 1998). Virus infection of newborn mice resulted in severe neurological disease, but the percentage of animals showing neurological signs differed widely among inbred strains. Mice of the MRL strain were most susceptible to BD, while only a small percentage of mice of C3H and CBA strains developed BD, although the neurological signs of BD were similarly strong in all three strains. In contrast, mice of BALB/c and C57BL/6 strains exhibited much more attenuated, if any, symptoms of BD.

Newborn and adult-infected mice show signs of significant inflammation in the brain. While there was dissociation between inflammatory encephalitis and signs of disease in adult-infected mice (Rubin et al., 1993), in newborn-infected mice there was a correlation between the severity of the inflammatory response in the brain and the degree of clinical manifestation of BD for each mouse strain (Hallensleben et al., 1998). The strain-specific histopathological features of neonatal BDV infection in diseased mice included weak astrocytosis, an inverse correlation between lymphocytic infiltrations and presence of BDV-infected neurons, and an inverse correlation between high levels of viral RNA and signs of neurological disease. The findings may indicate that virus replication in brain cells did not cause BD, but instead, BD is induced by the antiviral activity of the immune system that eliminates virus-infected cells. The later hypothesis was supported in a series of experiments on mice with a targeted disruption of the β2-microglobulin gene (Hallensleben et al., 1998). These mice do not express MHC class I antigen and, as a result, lack CD8$^+$ T cells. It has been shown that neither β2-microglobulin-deficient infected C57BL/6 nor β2-microglobulin-deficient infected MRL mice developed signs of neurological disease, despite comparable levels of the virus in the β2-microglobulin-deficient and wild-type mice. In general, the proposed immune tolerance explanation for the inflammation-free outcome of neonatally BDV-infected rats is not seen in neonatally BDV-infected mice (Hallensleben et al., 1998). Future investigations will elucidate the different kinetics of BDV spread between rats and mice to explain the failure of the mechanisms of immune tolerance in neonatally infected mice. Now that BDV infection in mice has been demonstrated to be a feasible investigative model, advancements in gene targeting and the availability of a great number of mice with transgenic and knockout mutations will further facilitate genetic analysis of the BD pathogenesis.

Further demonstrating dissociation between inflammatory response and severity of signs of BD, BDV infection in newborn gerbils leads to severe neurological disease and death of infected animals without significant signs of CNS inflammation or neuronal damage (Watanabe et al., 2001). Importantly, during the asymptomatic phase of the disease, the virus replication was predominantly detected in the cerebral cortex and hippocampus. In contrast, the appearance of neurological signs coincided with a high level of expression in the lower brain stem and cerebellum. These observations suggested that replication of the virus and its neurotoxic effects on certain neuronal populations of the brain were critical for the development of neurological disorders in neonatally BDV-infected gerbils. The unique pattern of BDV dissemination in the brains of diseased gerbils may be related to the selective tropism of BDV for brain stem neurons (Watanabe et al., 2001). Thus, future experiments will focus on exploring what specific features of neuronal metabolism in gerbils may lead to the severe neurological disorder and accelerated death.

Furthermore, there may be differences in BD outcomes within a species, as indicated by strain-related virus-associated abnormalities in different strains of rats. Our preliminary studies have demonstrated strain-specific brain pathology, neurochemical alterations, and behavioral deficits in BDV-infected Lewis and Fisher 344 rats (Pletnikov et al., 2001). Although neonatal BDV infection has been mostly studied in Lewis rats, comparisons to BDV-induced neurodevelopmental damage in other strains of rats may be instrumental in delineating genetic factors that influence brain pathology and clinical symptoms in genetically different rats. As it has been shown with numerous compounds, no matter how well pathogenic mechanisms of a disease have been studied or how well responses to a drug have been characterized, there is always a possibility of a limited application of knowledge obtained with a single rodent strain (Festing, 2001). Thus, comparing inbred rat strains allows for studying general and unique pathogenic processes of abnormal brain development and may stimulate a more successful search for pharmacological treatments for behavioral disorders.

Effects of Sex on BDV-Induced Neurodevelopmental Damage

Another aspect of genetic background effects on BDV-induced developmental damage that has not been well delineated is putative differences in BD expression in female and male rats. Current knowledge is limited to the neurological and behavioral abnormalities observed in BDV-infected tree shrews that were clearly sex related and, therefore, were suggestive of a role of sex hormones in modulating neurobehavioral deficits (Sprankel et al., 1978). Pilot studies indicated that female rats appeared to be more severely damaged than male rats by the neonatal BDV infection (Pletnikov, unpublished results). Thus, the mechanisms of participation of sexual hormones in shaping BDV-associated damage also deserve future investigations.

Animal Models of Neuropsychiatric Diseases

For decades, BDV infection of the rat brain has been a valuable animal model for exploring the mechanisms of virus injury to the brain. This work has significantly advanced the understanding of the immunopathogenesis mechanisms of BD in adult-infected rats and the mechanisms of abnormal brain and behavior development in neonatally BDV-infected rodents. Furthermore, the results of BDV research have had widespread application as scientists in the area continue to develop new animal models that may be able to mirror selective human neurobehavioral disorders and/or pathogenic processes. Preliminary steps toward development of a BDV rat model of obesity can be a case in point (Herden et al., 2000). The BDV animal model of obesity is based on the use of a putative, obesity-inducing substrain of BDV. If this putative strain is isolated, a new animal model of obesity may be developed, and distinctive pathogenic features of BDV-ob infection will not only be of a great interest to the BDV community but may also have far-reaching implications for studies of environmental factors in the causation of obesity in humans.

New models of BDV infection in other species can be developed to explore the mechanisms of viral toxicity without obvious histopathological changes. For example, in a series of elegant behavioral tests, Sauder and colleagues have used C57BL/10J mice that lack $CD8^+$ T cells and show asymptomatic, persistent BDV infection. In particular, the authors examined performance of infected mice in the MWM, and correlated the MWM performance with the levels of expression of some chemokines. These studies showed that BDV infection can disturb the function of the mammalian CNS without causing overt neuronal loss and that selective BDV-induced disturbances in chemokine production might be responsible for selective behavioral alterations (Sauder et al., 2001).

New information from BDV animal model studies is particularly relevant to the long-lasting debates about possible BDV infection in humans, for which neither overt inflammation nor visible brain damage has been documented (Ludwig et al., 2001). In this context, animal models with virus-induced functional rather than structural alterations (e.g., selective neurochemical or neuroimmune pathways) may serve better to recapitulate possible BDV-associated disease syndromes in patients in whom the existence of BDV infection seemed to be demonstrated but whose clinical picture of virus infection was not consistent with the conventional experimental BDV models (Ludwig et al., 2001). Thus, new animal models of BDV infection with subtle ultrastructural or functional alterations may be able to better reflect the human conditions of virus infections and associated neurobehavioral disorders.

This chapter is dedicated to Rudolf Rott, the founder of modern BDV research.

REFERENCES

Allan, J. E., and P. C. Doherty. 1985. Immune T cells can protect or induce fatal neurological disease in murine lymphocytic choriomeningitis. *Cell. Immunol.* **90:**401–407.

Altman, J., and K. Sudarshan. 1975. Postnatal development of locomotion in the laboratory rat. *Anim. Behav.* **23:**896–920.

Ando, K., T. Moriyama, L. G. Guidott, S. Wirth, R. D. Schreiber, and H. J. Schlicht. 1993. Mechanisms of class I restricted immunopathology. A transgenic mouse model of fulminant hepatitis. *J. Exp. Med.* **178:**1541–1554.

Anzil, A., K. Blinzinger, K. and A. Mayr. 1973. Persistent Borna virus infection in adult hamsters. *Arch. Gesamt. Virusforsch.* **40:**52–57.

Asensio, V. C., and I. L. Campbell. 1999. Chemokines in the CNS: plurifunctional mediators in diverse states. *Trends Neurosci.* **22:**504–512.

Ashman, R. B., and A. A. Müllbacher. 1979. T helper cell for anti-viral cytotoxic T cell responses. *J. Exp. Med.* **150:**1277–1282.

Autenrieth, C. F. 1823. *Ueber die hitzige Kopf-Krankheit der Pferde.* Auf Verlangen des Münsinger Vereins zur Beförderung der Pferdezucht auf der Alb und zunächst fuer diese Gegend. Bey Heinrich Laupp, Tübingen, Germany.

Baenziger, J., H. Hengartner, R. M. Zinkernagel, and G. A. Cole. 1986. Induction or prevention of immunopathological disease by cloned cytotoxic T cell lines specific for lymphocytic choriomeningitis virus. *Eur. J. Immunol.* **16:**387–393.

Bautista, J. R., S. A. Rubin, T. H. Moran, G. J. Schwartz, and K. M. Carbone. 1995. Developmental injury to the cerebellum following perinatal Borna disease virus infection. *Dev. Brain Res.* **90:**45–53.

Bautista, J. R., G. J. Schwartz, J. C. de la Torre, T. H. Moran, and K. M. Carbone. 1994. Early and persistent abnormalities in rats with neonatally acquired Borna disease virus infection. *Brain Res. Bull.* **34:**31–36.

Becher, B., A. Prat and J. P. Antel. 2000. Brain-immune connection: immuno-regulatory properties of CNS-resident Cells. *Glia* **29:**293–304.

Bennink, J. R., and P. C. Doherty. 1978. Different rules govern help for cytotoxic T cells and B cells. *Nature* **276:**829–831.

Billaud, J. N., C. Ly, T. R. Phillips, and J. C. de La Torre. 2000. Borna disease virus persistence causes inhibition of glutamate uptake by feline primary cortical astrocytes. *J. Virol.* **74:**10438–10446.

Bilzer, T., O. Planz, W. I. Lipkin, L. Stitz. 1995. Presence of CD4+ and CD8+ T cells and expression of MHC class I and MHC class II antigen in horses with Borna disease virus-induced encephalitis. *Brain Pathol.* **5:**223–230.

Bilzer, T., and L. Stitz. 1993. Brain cell lesions in Borna disease are mediated by T cells. *Arch. Virol. Suppl.* **7:**153–158.

Bilzer, T., and L. Stitz. 1994. Immune-mediated brain atrophy. CD8+ T cells contribute to tissue destruction during borna disease. *J. Immunol.* **153:**818–823.

Bray, G. A., and D. A. York. 1979. Hypothalamic and genetic obesity in experimental animals. *Physiol. Rev.* **59:**719–803.

Briese, T., M. Hornig, and W. I. Lipkin. 1999. Bornavirus immunopathogenesis in rodents: models for human neurological diseases. *J. Neurovirol.* **5:**604–612.

Browning, M., C. S. Reiss, and A. S. Huang. 1990a. The soluble viral glycoprotein of vesicular stomatitis virus efficiently sensitizes target cells for lysis by CD4+ T lymphocytes. *J. Virol.* **64:**3810–3816.

Browning, M. J., A. S. Huang, and C. S. Reiss. 1990b. Cytolytic T lymphocytes from the BALB/c-H-2dm2 mouse recognize the vesicular stomatitis virus glycoprotein and are restricted by class II MHC antigens. *J. Immunol.* **145:**985–994.

Bruce-Keller, A. 1999. Microglial-neuronal Interactions in synaptic damage and recovery. *J. Neurosci. Res.* **58:**191–201.

Byrne, J. A., and M. B. Oldstone. 1984. Biology of cloned cytotoxic T lymphocytes specific for lymphocytic choriomeningitis virus: clearance of virus in vivo. *J. Virol.* **51:**682–686.

Cambell, I. L. 1991. Cytokines in viral diseases. *Curr. Opin. Immunol.* **3:**486–491.

Caplazi, P., A. Waldvogel, L. Stitz, U. Braun, and F. Ehrensperger. 1994. Borna disease in naturally infected cattle. *J. Comp. Pathol.* **111:**65–72.

Carbone, K., and M. Pletnikov. 2000. Borna again, starting from the beginning. *Mol. Psychiatry* **5:**577.

Carbone, K. M., C. S. Duchala, J. W. Griffin, A. L. Kincaid, and O. Narayan. 1987. Pathogenesis of Borna disease in rats: evidence that intra-axonal spread is the major route for virus dissemination and the determinant for disease incubation. *J. Virol.* **61:**3431–3440.

Carbone, K. M., T. R. Moench, and W. I. Lipkin. 1991a. Borna disease virus replicates in astrocytes, Schwann cells and ependymal cells in persistently infected rats: location of viral genomic and messenger RNAs by in situ hybridization. *J. Neuropathol. Exp. Neurol.* **50:**205–214.

Carbone, K. M., S. W. Park, S. A. Rubin, R. W. Waltrip II, and G. B. Vogelsang. 1991b. Borna disease: association with a maturation defect in the cellular immune response. *J. Virol.* **65:**6154–6164.

Carbone, K. M., S. A. Rubin, Y. Nishino, and M. Pletnikov. 2001. Borna disease: virus induced neurobehavioral disease pathogenesis. *Curr. Opin. Microbiol. Rev.* **4:**467–475.

Carbone, K. M., S. A. Rubin, A. M. Sierra-Honigmann, and H. M. Lederman. 1993. Characterization of a glial cell line persistently infected with Borna disease virus (BDV): influence of neurotrophic factors on BDV protein and RNA expression. *J. Virol.* **67:**1453–1460.

Carbone, K. M., B. D. Trapp, J. W. Griffin, C. S. Duchala, and O. Narayan. 1989. Astrocytes and Schwann cells are virus-host cells in the nervous system of rats with Borna disease. *J. Neuropathol. Exp. Neurol.* **48:**631–644.

Cash, E., A. Minty, P. Ferrara, D. Caput, D. Fradelizi, and O. Rott. 1994. Macrophage-inactivating IL-13 suppresses experimental autoimmune encephalomyelitis in rats. *J. Immunol.* **153:**4258–4267.

Ciaranello, A. L., and R. D. Ciaranello. 1995. The neurobiology of infantile autism. *Annu. Rev. Neurosci.* **18:**101–28.

Clark, D. A. 1994. The whole truth about perforin. *Nature* **369:**16–18.

Cubitt, B., and J. C. de la Torre. 1994. Borna disease virus (BDV), a nonsegmented RNA virus, replicates in the nuclei of infected cells where infectious BDV ribonucleoproteins are present. *J. Virol.* **68:**1371–1381.

Danner, K., D. Heubeck, and A. Mayr. 1978. *In vitro* studies on Borna disease. I. The use of cell cultures for the demonstration, titration and production of Borna virus. *Arch. Virol.* **57:**63–75.

Deschl, U., L. Stitz, S. Herzog, K. Frese, and R. Rott. 1990. Determination of immune cells and expression of major histocompatibility complex class II antigen in encephalitic lesions of experimental Borna disease. *Acta Neuropathol.* (Berlin) **81:**41–50.

Ding, A. H., C. F. Nathan, and D. J. Stuehr. 1988. Release of reactive nitrogen intermediates and reactive oxygen intermediates from mouse peritoneal macrophages. Comparison of activating cytokines and evidence for independent production. *J. Immunol.* **141:**2407–2412.

Dittrich, W., L. Bode, H. Ludwig, M. Kao, and K. Scheider. 1989. Learning deficiencies in Borna disease virus-infected but clinically healthy rats. *Biol. Psychiatry* **20:**818–828.

Eddleston, M., and L. Mucke. 1993. Molecular profile of reactive astrocytes—implications for their role in neurologic disease. *Neuroscience* **54:**15–36.

Eichenbaum, H., C. Stewart, and R. G. Morris. 1990. Hippocampal representation in place learning. *J. Neurosci.* **10:**3531–3542.

Eisenman, L. M., R. Brothers, M. H. Tran, R. B. Kean, G. M. Dickson, B. Dietzschold, and D. C. Hooper. 1999. Neonatal Borna disease virus infection in the rat causes a loss of Purkinje cells in the cerebellum. *J. Neurovirol.* **5:**181–189.

Fanselow, M. S. 2000. Contextual fear, gestalt memories, and the hippocampus. *Behav. Brain Res.* **110:**73–81.

Festing, M. F. 2001. Experimental approaches to the determination of genetic variability. *Toxicol. Lett.* **120:**293–300.

Fierz, W., B. Endler, K. Reske, H. Wekerle, and A. Fontana. 1985. Astrocytes as antigen-presenting cells. I. Induction of Ia antigen expression on astrocytes by T cells via immune interferon and its effect on antigen presentation. *J. Immunol.* **134:**3785–3793.

Fleischer, B. 1984. Acquisition of specific cytotoxic activity by human T4+ T lymphocytes in culture. *Nature* **308:**365–367.

Fontana, A., W. Fierz, and H. Wekerle. 1984. Astrocytes present myelin basic protein to encephalitogenic T-cell lines. *Nature* **307:**273–276.

Fontana, A., K. Frei, S. Bodmer, E. Hofer, M. H. Schreier, M. A. Palladino, Jr. 1989. Transforming growth factor-beta inhibits the generation of cytotoxic T cells in virus-infected mice. *J. Immunol.* **143:**3230–3234.

Fowell, D., and D. Mason. 1993. Evidence that the T cell repertoire of normal rats contains cells with the potential to cause diabetes. Characterization of the CD4+ T cell subset that inhibits this autoimmune potential. *J. Exp. Med.* **177:**627–636.

Furrer, E., T. Bilzer, L. Stitz, and O. Planz. 2001. Neutralizing antibodies in persistent Borna disease virus infection: prophylactic effect of gp94-specific monoclonal antibodies in preventing encephalitis. *J. Virol.* **75:**943–951.

Galoyan, A. 2000. Neurochemistry of brain neuroendocrine immune system: signal molecules. *Neurochem. Res.* **25:**1343–1355.

Gies, U., T. Bilzer, L. Stitz, and J. F. Staiger. 1998. Disturbance of the cortical cholinergic innervation in Borna disease prior to encephalitis. *Brain Pathol.* **8:**39–48.

Gies, U., T. J. Gorsc, J. Mulder, O. Planz, L. Stitz, T. Bilzer, P. G. Luiten, and T. Harkany. 2001. Cortical cholinergic decline parallels the progression of Borna disease virus encephalitis. *Neuroreport* **12:**3767–3772.

Goldowitz, D., and K. Hamre. 1998. The cells and molecules that make a cerebellum. *Trends Neurosci.* **21:**375–382.

Gonzalez-Dunia, D., M. Eddleston, N. Mackman, K. M. Carbone, and J. C. de la Torre. 1996. Expression of tissue factor is increased in astrocytes within the central nervous system during persistent infection with Borna disease virus. *J. Virol.* **70:**5812–5820.

Gonzalez-Dunia, D., C. Sauder, and J. C. de la Torre. 1997. Borna disease virus and the brain. *Brain Res. Bull.* **44:**647–664.

Gonzalez-Dunia, D., M. Watanabe, S. Syan, M. Mallory, E. Masliah, and J. C. de la Torre. 2000. Synaptic pathology in Borna disease virus persistent infection. *J. Virol.* **74:**3441–3448.

Gosztonyi, G., and H. Ludwig. 1984. Borna disease of horses. An immunohistological and virological study of naturally infected animals. *Acta Neuropathol.* (Berlin) **64:**213–221.

Gosztonyi, G., and H. Ludwig. 1995. Borna disease—neuropathology and pathogenesis. *Curr. Top. Microbiol. Immunol.* **190:**39–73.

Gosztonyi, G., B. Dietzschold, M. Kao, C. E. Rupprecht, H. Ludwig, and H. Koprowski. 1993. Rabies and Borna disease. A comparative pathogenetic study of two neurovirulent agents. *Lab. Investig.* **68:**285–295.

Gould, E., and B. S. McEwen. 1993. Neuronal birth and death. *Curr. Opin. Neurobiol.* **3:**676–682.

Haliensleben, W., M. Schwemmie, J. Hausmann, L. Stitz, B. Volk, A. Pagenstecher, and P. Staeheli. 1998. Borna disease virus-induced neurological disorder in mice: infection of neonates results in immunopathology. *J. Virol.* **72:**4379–4386.

Halloran, P. F., J. Urmson, P. H. Van der Meide, and P. Autenried P. 1989. Regulation of MHC expression in vivo. II. IFN-α/β inducers and recombinant IFN-α modulate MHC antigen expression in mouse tissues. *J. Immunol.* **142:**4241–4247.

Hans, A., S. Syan, C. Crosio, P. Sassone-Corsi, M. Brahic, and D. Gonzalez-Dunia. 2001. Borna disease virus persistent infection activates mitogen-activated protein kinase and blocks neuronal differentiation of pc12 cells. *J. Biol. Chem.* **276:**7258–7265.

Hatalski, C. G., S. Kliche, L. Stitz, and W. I. Lipkin. 1995. Neutralizing antibodies in Borna disease virus-infected rats. *J. Virol.* **69:**741–747.

Hatalski, C. G., W. F. Hickey, and W. I. Lipkin. 1998. Evolution of the immune response in the central nervous system following infection with Borna disease virus. *J. Neuroimmunol.* **90:**137–142.

Hatalski, C. G., W. F. Hickey, and W. I. Lipkin. 1998. Humoral immunity in the central nervous system of Lewis rats infected with Borna disease virus. *J. Neuroimmunol.* **90:**128–136.

Hausmann, J., W. Hallensleben, J. C. de la Torre, A. Pagenstecher, C. Zimmermann, and H. Pircher. 1999. T cell ignorance in mice to Borna disease virus can be overcome by peripheral expression of the viral nucleoprotein. *Proc. Natl. Acad. Sci. USA* **96:**9769–9774.

Henkart, P. A. 1985. Mechanism of lymphocyte-mediated cytotoxicity. *Annu. Rev. Immunol.* **3:**31–58.

Herden, C. S., Herzog, J. A. Richt, A. Nesseler, M. Christ, K. Failing, and K. Frese. 2000. Distribution of Borna disease virus in the brain of rats infected with an obesity-inducing virus strain. *Brain Pathol.* **10:**39–48.

Herzog, S., K. Frese, and R. Rott. 1991. Studies on the genetic control of resitsance of black hooded rats to Borna disease. *J. Gen. Virol.* **72:**535–540.

Herzog, S., C. Kompter, K. Frese, and R. Rott. 1984. Replication of Borna disease virus in rats: age-dependent differences in tissue distribution. *Med. Microbiol. Immunol.* (Berlin) **173:**171–177.

Herzog, S., and R. Rott. 1980. Replication of Borna disease virus in cell culture. *Med. Microbiol. Immunol.* **168:**153–158.

Herzog, S., K. Wonigeit, K. Frese, H. J. Hedrich, and R. Rott. 1985. Effect of Borna disease virus infection on athymic rats. *J. Gen. Virol.* **66:**503–508.

Hickey, W. F., B. L. Hsu, and H. Kimura. 1991. T-lymphocyte entry into the central nervous system. *J. Neurosci. Res.* **28:**254–260.

Hirano, N., M. Kao, and H. Ludwig. 1983. Persistent, tolerant or subacute infection in Borna disease virus-infected rats. *J. Gen. Virol.* **64:**1521–1530.

Hornig, M., M. Solbrig, N. Horscroft, H. Weissenbock, and W. I. Lipkin. 2001. Borna disease virus infection of adult and neonatal rats: models for neuropsychiatric disease. *Curr. Top. Microbiol. Immunol.* **253:**157–177.

Hornig, M., H. Weissenbock, N. Horscroft, and W. I. Lipkin. 1999. An infection-based model of neurodevelopmental damage. *Proc. Nat. Acad. Sci. USA* **96:**12102–12107.

Irigoin, C., E. M., Rodriguez, M. Heinrichs, K. Frese, S. Herzog, and A. Oksche. 1990. Immunocytochemical study of the subcommissural organ of rats with induced postnatal hydrocephalus. *Exp. Brain Res.* **82:**384–392.

Jacobson, S., J. R. Richert, W. E. Biddison, A. Satinsky, R. J. Hartzman, and H. F. McFarland. 1984. Measles virus-specific T4$^+$ human cytotoxic T cell clones are restricted by class II HLA antigens *J. Immunol.* **133:**754–757.

Johnson, R. T. 1982. Selective vulnerability of neural cells to viral infections. *Adv. Neurol.* **36:**331–337.

Johnson, R. T. 1998. *Viral Infections of the Nervous System.* Lippincott-Raven, Philadelphia, Pa.

Kägi, D., B. Ledermann, and K. Bürki. 1994. Cytotoxicity mediated by T cells and natural killer cells is greatly impaired in perform-deficient mice. *Nature* **369:**31–37.

Kaluza, G., G. Lell, M. Reinacher, L. Stitz, and W. R. Willems. 1987. Neurogenic spread of Semliki Forest virus in mice. *Arch. Virol.* **93:**97–110.

Kao, M., H. Ludwig, and G. Gosztonyi. 1984. Adaptation of Borna disease virus to the mouse. *J. Gen. Virol.* **65:**1845–1849.

Kaplan, D. R., R. Griffith, V. L. Braciale, and T. J. Braciale. 1984. Influenza virus-specific human cytotoxic T cell clones: heterogeneity in antigen specificity and restriction by class II MHC products. *Cell. Immunol.* **88:**193–199.

Kast, W. M., A. M. Bronkhorst, L. P. DeWaal, and C. J. M. Melief. 1986. Cooperation between cytotoxic and helper T lymphocytes in protection against lethal Sendai virus infection: protection by T cells is MHC-restricted and MHC-regulated: a model for MHC-disease associations. *J. Exp. Med.* **164:**723–738.

Kliche, S., T. Briese, A. H. Henschen, L. Stitz, and W. I. Lipkin. 1994. Characterization of a Borna disease virus glycoprotein, gp18. *J. Virol.* **68:**6918–6923.

Koprowski, H., Y. M. Zheng, E. Heber-Katz, N. Fraser, L. Rorke, and Z. F. Fu. 1993. In vivo expression of inducible nitric oxide synthase in experimentally induced neurologic diseases. *Proc. Natl. Acad. Sci. USA* **90:**3024–3027. (Erratum, **90:**5378.)

Krey, H., H. Ludwig, and R. Rott. 1979. Spread of infectious virus along the optic nerve into the retina in Borna disease virus-infected rabbits. *Arch. Virol.* **61:**283–288.

Krey, H., L. Stitz, and H. Ludwig. 1982. Virus-induced pigment epithelitis in rhesus monkeys. Clinical and histological findings. *Ophthalmologica* **185:**205–213.

Lalonde, R. 1997. Visuospatial abilities. *Int. Rev. Neurobiol.* **41:**191–215.

Leist, T. P., M. Kohler, and R. M. Zinkernagel. 1989. Impaired generation of antiviral cytotoxicity against lymphocytic choriomeningitis and vaccinia virus in mice treated with CD4-specific monoclonal antibody. *Scand. J. Immunol.* **30:**679–686.

Levi-Montalcini, R., S. D. Skaper, R. Dal Toso, L. Petrelli, and A. Leon. 1996. Nerve growth factor: from neurotrophin to neurokine. *Trends Neurosci.* **19:**514–520.

Lewis, A. J., J. L. Whitton, C. G. Hatalski, H. Weissenbock, and W. I. Lipkin. 1999. Effect of immune priming on Borna disease. *J. Virol.* **73:**2541–2546.

Lipkin, W. I., K. M. Carbone, M. C. Wilson, C. S. Duchala, O. Narayan, and M. B. Oldstone. 1988. Neurotransmitter abnormalities in Borna disease. *Brain Res.* **475:**366–370.

Luckacher, A. E., L. A. Morrison, V. L. Braciale, B. Malissen, and T. J. Braciale. 1985. Expression of specific cytolytic activity by H-2 I region-restricted, influenza virus-specific T lymphocyte clones. *J. Exp. Med.* **162:**171–187.

Ludwig, H., H. Becht, and L. Groh. 1973. Borna disease, a slow virus infection: biological properties of the virus. *Med. Microbiol. Immunol.* (Berlin) **158:**275–289.

Ludwig, H., and L. Bode. 2001. Borna disease virus: new aspects on infection, disease, diagnosis and epidemiology. *Rev. Sci. Tech.* **19:**259–288.

Ludwig, H., L. Bode, and G. Gosztonyi. 1988. Borna disease: a persistent virus infection of the central nervous system. *Prog. Med. Virol.* **35:**107–151.

Ludwig, H., K. Furuya, L. Bode, N. Klein, R. Durrwald, and D. S. Lee. 1993. Biology and neurobiology of Borna disease viruses (BDV), defined by antibodies, neutralizability and their pathogenic potential. *Arch. Virol. Suppl.* **7:**111–133.

Ludwig, H., and P. Thein. 1977. Demonstration of specific antibodies in the central nervous system of horses naturally infected with Borna disease virus. *Med. Microbiol. Immunol.* **163:**215–226.

Massa, P. T., R. Dörries, and V. Ter Meulen. 1986. Viral particles induce antigen expression on astrocytes. *Nature* **320:**543–546.

Mims, C. A. 1960. Intracerebral injections and the growth of viruses in the mouse brain. *Br. J. Exp. Pathol.* **41:**52–59.

Monjan, A. A., D. H. Gilden, G. A. Cole, and N. Nathanson. 1971. Cerebellar hypoplasia in neonatal rats caused by lymphocytic choriomeningitis virus. *Science* **171:**194–196.

Morales, J. A., S. Herzog, C. Kompter, K. Frese, and R. Rott. 1988. Axonal transport of Borna disease virus along olfactory pathways in spontaneously and experimentally infected rats. *Med. Microbiol. Immunol.* (Berlin) **177:**51–68.

Müller, C., D. Kägi, and T. Aebischer. 1989. Detection of perforin and granzyme A mRNAs in infiltrating cells during LCMV infection of mice. *Eur. J. Immunol.* **19:**1253–1259.

Nakamura, Y., M. Kishi, T. Nakaya, S. Asahi, H. Tanaka, H. Sentsui, K. Ikeda, and K. Ikuta. 1995. Demonstration of Borna disease virus RNA in peripheral blood mononuclear cells from healthy horses in Japan. *Vaccine* **13:**1076–1079.

Narayan, O., S. Herzog, K. Frese, H. Scheefers, and R. Rott. 1983a. Behavioral disease in rats caused by immunopathological responses to persistent borna virus in the brain. *Science* **220:**1401–1403.

Narayan, O., S. Herzog, K. Frese, H. Scheefers, and R. Rott. 1983b. Pathogenesis of Borna disease in rats: immune-mediated viral ophthalmoencephalopathy causing blindness and behavioral abnormalities. *J. Infect. Dis.* **148:**305–315.

Nathan, C. 1992. Nitric oxide as a secretory product of mammalian cells. *FASEB J.* **6:**3051–3064.

Nicolau, S. 1928. Les modifications histo-pathologiques des capsules surrénales et des glandes salivaires des lapins morts d'encéphalomeyélite enzootique expérimentale (maladie de Borna). *C. R. Acad. Sci.* **186:**655–657.

Nicolau, S., and I. A. Galloway. 1927. Preliminary note on the experimental study of enzootic encephalo-myelitis (Borna disease). *Br. J. Exp. Pathol.* **8:**336–341.

Nicolau, S., and I. A. Galloway. 1928. Étude sur les inclusions intranucléaires caractérisant la maladie de Borna. *C. R. Soc. Biol. Fil.* **99:**1455–1457.

Nicolau, S., and N. Stroian. 1928. Altérations du système nerveux de l'estomac et de l'intestin des lapins morts d'encéphalo-myélite enzootique expérimentale (maladie de Borna). *C. R. Soc. Biol. Fil.* **99:**1102–1106.

Nishino, Y., D. Kobasa, S. A. Rubin, M. V. Pletnikov, and K. M. Carbone. 2002. Enhanced neurovirulence of Borna disease virus variants associated with nucleotide changes in the glycoprotein and L polymerase genes. *J. Virol.* **76:**8650–8658.

Nitzschke, E. 1963. Untersuchungen ueber die experimentelle Bornavirus-Infektion bei der Ratte. *Zentbl. Vetmed. Reihe B* **10:**470–527.

Noske, K., T. Bilzer, O. Planz, and L. Stitz. 1998. Virus-specific CD4$^+$ T cells eliminate Borna disease virus from the brain via induction of cytotoxic CD8$^+$ T cells. *J. Virol.* **72:**4387–4395.

Oster-Granite, M. L., and R. M. Herndon. 1985. The pathogenesis of parvovirus-induced cerebellar hypoplasia in the Syrian hamster *Mesocricetus auratus*. Fluorescent antibody, foliation, cytoarchitectonic, golgi and electron microscopic studies. *J. Comp. Neurol.* **169:**481–522.

Paliard, X., R. W. Malefijt, J. E. de Vries, and H. Spits. 1988. Interleukin-4 mediates CD8 induction on human CD4+ T-cell clones. *Nature* **335:**642–644.

Palladino, M. A., R. E. Morris, H. F. Starnes, and A. D. Levinson. 1990. The transforming growth factor-β. A new family of immunoregulatory molecules. *Ann. N. Y. Acad. Sci.* **593:**181–187.

Pankseep, J. 1990. The psychoneurology of fear: evolutionary perspective and the role of animal models in understanding human anxiety, p. 3–58. *In* G. D. Burrows, M. Roth, and R. Noyes (ed.), *Handbook of Anxiety,* vol. 3. *The Neurobiobiology of Anxiety.* Elsevier, Amsterdam, The Netherlands.

Pankseep, J., S. Siviy, and L. Normansell. 1984. The psychobiology of play: theoretical and methodological perspectives. *Neurosci. Biobehav. Rev.* **8:**465–492.

Petrosini, L., M. Leggio, and M. Molinari. 1998. The cerebellum in the spatial problem solving: a co-star or a guest star? *Prog. Neurobiol.* **56:**191–210.

Pette, H., and S. Környey. 1935. Über die Pathogenese und die Histologie der Bornaschen Krankheit im Tierexperiment. *Dtsch. Z. Nervenheilkd.* **136:**20–65.

Planz, O., T. Bilzer, M. Sobbe, and L. Stitz. 1993. Lysis of major histocompatibility complex class I-bearing cells in Borna disease virus-induced degenerative encephalopathy. *J. Exp. Med.* **178:**163–174.

Planz, O., T. Bilzer, and L. Stitz. 1995. Immunopathogenic role of T-cell subsets in Borna disease virus-induced progressive encephalitis. *J. Virol.* **69:**896–903.

Planz, O., T. Dumrese, S. Hulpusch, M. Schirle, S. Stevanovic, and L. Stitz. 2001. A naturally processed rat major histocompatibility complex class I-associated viral peptide as target structure of Borna disease virus-specific CD8+ T cells. *J. Biol. Chem.* **276:** 13689–13694.

Planz, O., S. Pleschka, and S. Ludwig. 2001. MEK-specific inhibitor U0126 blocks spread of Borna disease virus in cultured cells. *J. Virol.* **75:**4871–4877.

Planz, O., and L. Stitz. 1999. Borna disease virus nucleoprotein (p40) is a major target for CD8$^+$-T-cell-mediated immune response. *J. Virol.* **73:**1715–1718.

Plata-Salaman, C. R., S. E. Ilyin, D. Gayle, A. Romanovitch, and K. M. Carbone. 1999. Regional cytokine, cytokine receptor and neuropeptide mRNA changes associated with behavioral and neuroanatomical abnormalities in persistent, noninflammatory virus infection of neonatal rats. *Ann. N. Y. Acad. Sci.* **890:**469.

Pletnikov, M., S. Rubin, K. Carbone, T. Moran, and G. J. Schwartz. 2001. Neonatal Borna disease virus infection (BDV)-induced damage to the cerebellum is associated with sensorimotor deficits in developing Lewis rats. *Dev. Brain Res.* **126:**1–12.

Pletnikov, M., S. Rubin, G. Schwartz, K. Carbone, and T. H. Moran. 2000. Effects of neonatal rat Borna disease virus (BDV) infection on the postnatal development of brain monoaminergic systems. *Dev. Brain Res.* **119:**179–185.

Pletnikov, M., S. Rubin, G. Schwartz, T. Moran, T. Sobotka, and K. M. Carbone. 1999a. Persistent neonatal Borna disease virus (BDV) infection of the brain causes chronic emotional abnormalities in adult rats. *Physiol. Behav.* **66:**823–831.

Pletnikov, M., S. Rubin, K. Vasudevan, T. Moran, and K. M. Carbone. 1999b. Developmental brain injury associated with abnormal play behavior in neonatally Borna disease virus-infected Lewis rats: a model of autism. *Behav. Brain Res.* **100:**43–50.

Pletnikov, M. V., M. L. Jones, S. A. Rubin, T. H. Moran, and K. M. Carbone. 2001. Rat model of autism spectrum disorders. Genetic background effects on Borna disease virus-induced developmental brain damage. *Ann. N. Y. Acad. Sci.* **939:**318–319.

Powell, M. B., D. Mitchell, J. Lederman, J. Buckmeier, S. S. Zamvil, and M. Graham. 1990. Lymphotoxin and tumor necrosis factor-alpha production by myelin basic protein-specific T cell clones correlates with encephalitogenicity. *Int. Immunol.* **2:**539–544.

Quagliarello, V. J., B. Wispelwey, W. J. Long, Jr., and W. M. Scheld. 1991. Recombinant human interleukin-1 induces meningitis and blood-brain barrier injury in the rat. Characterization and comparison with tumor necrosis factor. *J. Clin. Investig.* **87:**1360–1366.

Raine, C. S., and B. N. Fields. 1973. Reovirus type III encephalitis: a virologic and ultra-structural study. *J. Neuropathol. Exp. Neurol.* **32:**19–33.

Reinacher, M., J. Bonin, O. Narayan, and C. Scholtissek. 1983. Pathogenesis of neurovirulent influenza A virus infection in mice. Route of entry of virus into brain determines infection of different populations of cells. *Lab. Investig.* **49:**686–692.

Richt, J., L. Stitz, U. Deschi, K. Frese, and R. Rott. 1990. Borna disease virus-induced meningo-encephalomyelitis caused by a virus-specific CD4+ T cell-mediated immune reaction. *J. Gen. Virol.* **71:**2565–2573.

Richt, J. A., S. Herzog, K. Haberzettl, and R. Rott. 1993. Demonstration of Borna disease virus-specific RNA in secretions of naturally infected horses by the polymerase chain reaction. *Med. Microbiol. Immunol.* (Berlin) **182:**293–304.

Richt, J. A., and L. Stitz. 1992. Borna disease virus-infected astrocytes function in vitro as antigen-presenting and target cells for virus-specific CD4-bearing lymphocytes. *Arch. Virol.* **124:**95–109.

Richt, J. A., L. Stitz, H. Wekerle, and R. Rott. 1989. Borna disease, a progressive meningoencephalo-myelitis as a model for CD4+ T cell-mediated immunopathology in the brain. *J. Exp. Med.* **170:**1045–1050.

Rohrenbeck, A. M., M. Bette, D. C. Hooper, F. Nyberg, L. E. Eiden, and B. Dietzschold. 1999. Upregulation of COX-2 and CGRP expression in resident cells of the Borna disease virus-infected brain is dependent upon inflammation. *Neurobiol. Dis.* **6:**15–34.

Rolls, E. 2000. Memory systems in the brain. *Annu. Rev. Psychol.* **51:**599–630.

Rothwell, N. J., and S. J. Hopkins. 1995. Cytokines and the nervous system. II. Actions and mechanisms of action. *Trends Neurosci.* **18:**130–136.

Rubin, S. A., J. R. Bautista, T. H. Moran, G. J. Schwartz, and K. M. Carbone. 1999a. Viral terato-genesis: brain developmental damage associated with maturation state at time of infection. *Dev. Brain Res.* **112:**237–244.

Rubin, S. A., A. M. Sierra-Honigmann, H. M. Lederman, R. W. Waltrip II, J. J. Eiden, and K. M. Carbone. 1995. Hematologic consequences of Borna disease virus infection of rat bone marrow and thymus stromal cells. *Blood* **85:**2762–2769.

Rubin, S. A., P. Sylves, M. W. Vogel, M., Pletnikov, T. H. Moran, G. J. Schwartz, and K. M. Carbone. 1999b. Borna disease virus-induced hippocampal dentate gyrus damage is associated with spatial learning and memory deficits. *Brain Res. Bull.* **48:**23–30.

Rubin, S. A., R. W. Waltrip II, J. R. Bautista, and K. M. Carbone. 1993. Borna disease virus in mice: host-specific differences in disease expression. *J. Virol.* **67:**548–552.

Rubin, S. A., T. A. Yednock, and K. M. Carbone. 1998. In vivo treatment with anti-α4 integrin suppresses clinical and pathological evidence of Borna disease virus infection. *J. Neuroimmunol.* **84:**158–163.

Ruddle, N. H., C. M. Bergman, K. M. McGrath, E. G. Lingenheld, M. L. Grunnet, and S. J. Padula. 1990. An antibody to lymphotoxin and tumor necrosis factor prevents transfer of experimental allergic encephalomyelitis. *J. Exp. Med.* **172:**1193–1200.

Ruddle, N. H., and D. S. Schmid. 1987. The role of lymphotoxin in T-cell-mediated cytotoxicity. *Ann. Inst. Pasteur Immunol.* **138**:314–320.

Saito, N., A. Itouji, Y. Totani, I. Osawa, H. Koide, N. Fujisawa, K. Ogita, and C. Tanaka. 1993. Cellular and intracellular localization of epsilon-subspecies of protein kinase C in the rat brain presynaptic localization of the epsilon-subspecies. *Brain Res.* **607**:241–248.

Sauder, C., and J. C. de la Torre. 1999. Cytokine expression in the rat central nervous system following perinatal Borna disease virus infection. *J. Neuroimmunol.* **96**:29–45.

Sauder, C., W. Hallensleben, A. Pagenstecher, S. Schneckenburger, L. Biro, D. Pertlik, J. Hausmann, M. Suter, and P. Staeheli. 2000. Chemokine gene expression in astrocytes of Borna disease virus-infected rats and mice in the absence of inflammation. *J. Virol.* **74**:9267–9280.

Schwemmle, M., B. De, L. C. Shi, A. Banerjee, and W. I. Lipkin. 1997. Borna disease virus P-protein is phosphorylated by protein kinase c-epsilon and casein kinase II. *J. Biol. Chem.* **272**:21818–21823.

Seifried, O., and H. Spatz. 1930. Die Ausbreitung der enzephalitischen Reaktion bei der Bornaschen Krankheit der Pferde und deren Beziehung zu der Enzephalitis epidemica, der Heine-Medinschen Krankheit und der Lyssa des Menschen. Eine vergleichend-pathologische Studie. *Z. Ges. Neurol. Psychiat.* **124**:317–383.

Selmaj, K. W. 1992. The role of cytokines in inflammatory conditions of the central nervous system. *Semin. Neurosci.* **4**:221–229.

Sethi, K. K., H. Naher, and I. Stroehmann. 1988. Phenotypic heterogeneity of cerebrospinal fluid-derived HIV-specific and HLA-restricted cytotoxic T-cell clones. *Nature* **335**:178–181.

Shankar, V., M. Kao, A. N. Hamir, H. Sheng, H. Koprowski, and B. Dietzschold. 1992. Kinetics of virus spread and changes in levels of several cytokine mRNAs in the brain after intranasal infection of rats with Borna disease virus. *J. Virol.* **66**:992–998.

Sierra-Honigmann, A. M., S. A. Rubin, M. G. Estafanous, R. H. Yolken, and K. M. Carbone. 1993. Borna disease virus in peripheral blood mononuclear and bone marrow cells of neonatally and chronically infected rats. *J. Neuroimmunol.* **45**:31–36.

Simmons, R. D., and D. O. Willenborg. 1990. Direct injection of cytokines into the spinal cord causes autoimmune encephalomyelitis-like inflammation. *J. Neurol. Sci.* **100**:37–42.

Sloviter, R. S., G. Valiquette, G. M. Abrams, E. C. Ronk, A. L. Sollas, L. A. Paul, and S. S. Neubort. 1989. Selective loss of hippocampal granule cells in the mature rat brain after adrenalectomy. *Science* **243**:535–538.

Smeyne, R. J., T. Chu, A. Lewin, F. S. Bian, S. Crisman, C. Kunsch, S. A. Lira, and J. Oberdick. 1995. Local control of granule cell generation by cerebellar Purkinje cells. *Mol. Cell. Neurosci.* **6**:230–251.

Sobbe, M., T. Bilzer, S. Gommel, K. Noske, O. Planz, and L. Stitz. 1997. Induction of degenerative brain lesions after adoptive transfer of brain lymphocytes from Borna disease virus-infected rats: presence of CD8[+] T cells and perforin mRNA. *J. Virol.* **71**:2400–2407.

Solbrig, M. V., J. H. Fallon, and W. I. Lipkin. 1995. Behavioral disturbances and pharmacology of Borna disease. *Curr. Top. Microbiol. Immunol.* **190**:93–101.

Solbrig, M. V., G. F. Koob, J. H. Fallon, and W. I. Lipkin. 1994. Tardive dyskinetic syndrome in rats infected with Borna disease virus. *Neurobiol. Dis.* **1**:111–119.

Solbrig, M. V., G. F. Koob, J. H. Fallon, S. Reid, and W. I. Lipkin. 1996a. Prefrontal cortex dysfunction in Borna disease virus (BDV)-infected rats. *Biol. Psychiatry* **40**:629–636.

Solbrig, M. V., G. F. Koob, J. N. Joyce, and W. I. Lipkin. 1996b. A neural substrate of hyperactivity in Borna disease: changes in brain dopamine receptors. *Virology* **222**:332–338.

Solbrig, M. V., G. F. Koob, and W. I. Lipkin. 1998. Cocaine sensitivity in Borna disease virus-infected rats. *Pharmacol. Biochem. Behav.* **59**:1047–1052.

Solbrig, M. V., G. F. Koob, L. H. Parsons, T. Kadota, N. Horscroft, T. Briese, and W. I. Lipkin. 2000. Neurotrophic factor expression after CNS viral injury produces enhanced sensitivity to psychostimulants: potential mechanism for addiction vulnerability. *J Neurosci.* **20:**RC104.

Sprankel, H., K. Richarz, H. Ludwig, and R. Rott. 1978. Behavior alterations in tree shrews (*Tupaia glis*) induced by Borna disease virus. *Med. Microbiol. Immunol.* (Berlin) **165:**1–18.

Stitz, L., B. Dietzschold, and K. M. Carbone. 1995. Immunopathogenesis of Borna disease, p. 75–92. *In* H. Koprowski and I. Lipkin (ed.), *Borna Disease.* Springer-Verlag KG, Berlin, Germany.

Stitz, L., H. Krey, and H. Ludwig. 1980. Borna disease in rhesus monkeys as a model for uveo-cerebral symptoms. *J. Med. Virol.* **6:**333–340.

Stitz, L., K. Noske, O. Planz, E. Furrer, W. I. Lipkin, and T. Bilzer. 1998. A functional role for neutralizing antibodies in Borna disease: influence on virus tropism outside the central nervous system. *J. Virol.* **72:**8884–8892.

Stitz, L., O. Planz, T. Bilzer, K. Frei, and A. Fontana. 1991a. Transforming growth factor-beta modulates T cell-mediated encephalitis caused by Borna disease virus. Pathogenic importance of CD8+ cells and suppression of antibody formation. *J. Immunol.* **147:**3581–3586.

Stitz, L., D. Schilken, and K. Frese. 1991b. Atypical dissemination of the highly neurotropic Borna disease virus during persistent infection in cyclosporine A-treated, immunosuppressed rats. *J. Virol.* **65:**457–460.

Stitz, L., M. Sobbe, and T. Bilzer. 1992. Preventive effects of early anti-CD4 or anti-CD8 treatment on Borna disease in rats. *J. Virol.* **66:**3316–3323.

Stitz, L., D. Soeder, U. Deschl, K. Frese, and R. Roff. 1989. Inhibition of immune-mediated meningo-encephalitis in persistently Borna disease virus-infected rats by cyclosporine A. *J. Immunol.* **143:**4250–4256.

Street, N. E., and T. R. Mosmann. 1991. Functional diversity of T lymphocytes due to secretion of different cytokine patterns. *FASEB J.* **5:**171–177.

Stuhler, G., and P. Walden. 1993. Collaboration of helper and cytotoxic T lymphocytes *Eur. J. Immunol.* **23:**2279–2286.

Suzumura, A., E. Lavi, S. R. Weiss, and D. H. Silberberg. 1986. Coronavirus infection induces H-2 antigen expression on oligodendrocytes and astrocytes. *Science* **232:**991–993.

Takano, T., M. Uno, T. Yamano, and M. Shimada. 1994. Pathogenesis of cerebellar deformity in experimental Chiari type I malformation caused by mumps virus. *Acta Neuropathol.* **87:**168–173.

Tedeschi, B., J. N. Barrett, and R. W. Keane. 1986. Astrocytes produce interferon that enhances the expression of H-2 antigens on a subpopulation of brain cells. *J. Cell Biol.* **102:**2244–2253.

Thivolet, C., A. Bendelac, P. Bedossa, J. F. Bach, and C. Carnaud. 1991. CD8+ T cell homing to the pancreas in the nonobese diabetic mouse is CD4+ T cell-dependent. *J. Immunol.* **146:**85–88.

Tomlinson, A. H., and M. M. Esiri. 1983. Herpes simplex encephalitis. Immunohistological demonstration of spread of virus via olfactory pathways in mice. *J. Neurol. Sci.* **60:** 473–484.

Vaher, P. R., V. N. Luine, E. Gould, and B. S. McEwen. 1994. Effects of adrenalectomy on spatial memory performance and dentate gyrus morphology. *Brain Res.* **656:**71–78.

Wahl, S. M., N. McCartney-Francis, and S. E. Mergenhagen. 1989. Inflammatory and immunomodulatory roles of TGF-beta. *Immunol. Today* **10:**258–261.

Watanabe, M., L. Byeong-Jae, W. Kamitani, T. Kobayashi, H. Taniyama, K. Tomonaga, and K. Ikuta. 2001. Neurological diseases and viral dynamics in the brains of neonatally Borna disease virus-infected gerbils. *Virology* **282:**65–76.

Waxham, M. N., and J. S. Wolinsky. 1984. Rubella virus and its effects on the central nervous system. *Neurol. Clin.* **2**:367–385.

Weissenbock, H., M. Hornig, W. F. Hickey, and W. I. Lipkin. 2000. Microglial activation and neuronal apoptosis in Bornavirus infected neonatal Lewis rats. *Brain Pathol.* **10**:260–272.

Wekerle, H., C. Linington, H. Lassmann, and R. Meyermann. 1986. Cellular immune reactivity within the CNS. *Trends Neurosci.* 271–277.

Wong, G. H., P. F. Bartlett, I. Clark-Lewis, F. Battye, and J. W. Schrader. 1984. Inducible expression of H-2 and Ia antigens on brain cells. *Nature* **310**:688–691.

Wong, G. H. W., I. Clark-Lewis, A. W. Harris, and J. W. Schrader. 1984. Effect of cloned interferon-γ on expression of H-2 and Ia antigens on cell lines of hemopoietic, lymphoid, epithelial, fibroblastic and neuronal origin. *Eur. J. Immunol.* **14**:52–56.

Yasukawa, M., and J. M. Zarling. 1984. Human cytotoxic T cell clones directed against herpes simplex infected cells. I. Lysis restricted by HLA class II MB and DR antigens. *J. Immunol.* **133**:422–427.

Zinkernagel, R. M., G. N. Callahan, A. Althage, S. Cooper, J. W. Streilein, and J. J. Klein. 1978. The lymphoreticular system in triggering virus-plus-self-specific cytotoxic T cells: evidence for T help. *J. Exp. Med.* **147**:897–911.

Zinkernagel, R. M., and P. C. Doherty. 1979. MHC-restricted cytotoxic T cells: studies on the biological role of polymorphic major transplantation antigens determining T-cell restriction-specificity, function, and responsiveness. *Adv. Immunol.* **27**:51–177.

Zinkernagel, R. M., M. Eppler, and H. P. Pircher. 1989. Immune-protection versus immunopathology by antiviral T cell responses, p. 906–913. *In* F. Melchers (ed.), *Progress in Immunology*, 7th ed. Springer-Verlag, Berlin, Germany.

Zocher, M., S. Czub, J. Schulte-Monting, J. C. de La Torre, and C. Sauder. 2000. Alterations in neurotrophin and neurotrophin receptor gene expression patterns in the rat central nervous system following perinatal Borna disease virus infection. *J. Neurovirol.* **6**:462–477.

Zwick, W. 1929. Neuere Untersuchungen über die seuchenhafte Gehirn- und Rückenmarksentzündung (Bornasche Krankheit) der Pferde. *Dtsch. Z. Nervenheilkd.* **110**:316–322.

Zwick, W. 1939. Bornasche Krankheit und Enzephalomyelitis der Tiere, p. 254–354. *In* E. Gildenmeister, E. Haagen, and O. Waldmann (ed.), *Handbuch der Viruskrankheiten*, vol. 2. Fischer, Jena, Germany.

Zwick, W., and O. Seifried. 1924. Untersuchungen ueber die in Hessen gehaeuft auftretende seuchenhafte Gehirn- und Rueckenmarksentzuendung (Bornasche Krankheit) bei Pferden. *Berl. Tieraerztl. Wochenschr.* **40**:465–471.

Zwick, W., O. Seifried, and J. Witte. 1927. Experimentelle Untersuchungen uber die seuchenhafte Gehirn- und Rückenmarksentzündung der Pferde (Bornasche Krankheit). *Z. Infektkrankh. Haustiere* **30**:42–136.

Zwick, W., O. Seifried, and J. Witte. 1929. Weitere Beitrage zur Erforschung der Bornaschen Krankheit des Pferdes. *Arch. Tierheilkd.* **59**:511–545.

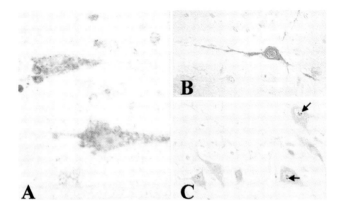

Color Plate 1 (chapter 4). BDV protein expression in brain tissue from horses with Borna disease, shown by IHC. (A) Parietal lobe neurons stained with polyclonal rabbit anti-BDV N antibody, subjected to the avidin-biotin complex technique, and counterstained with Mayer's hematoxylin. Magnification, ×47. (B) Positive immunostaining in neuron in the hippocampus region; stained with monoclonal antibody BO18 and by the avidin-biotin complex technique. Magnification, ×157. (C) Numerous intranuclear Joest-Degen inclusion bodies (arrows), characteristic of BDV infection, in BDV antigen-positive hippocampal neurons. Magnification, ×157. Panels B and C are reprinted from Nowotny et al. (2000).

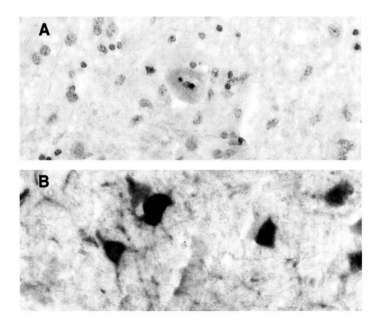

Color Plate 2 (chapter 4). ISH. (A) Demonstration of genomic RNA in horse hippocampus neuron nuclei with sense P (p24) probe. Magnification, ×130. (B) Demonstration of mRNA in cytoplasm with horse hippocampus neuron antisense P probe. Magnification, ×80. Figures kindly provided by H. Weissenböck.

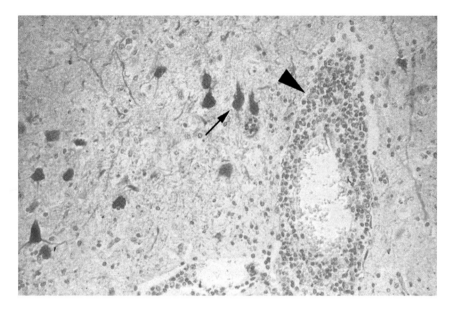

Color Plate 3 (chapter 5). Presence of BDV-specific antigen and perivascular cuffing. Note immunostaining of BDV antigens in neurons (arrow) and mononuclear blood cell infiltrations of brain parenchyma around a blood vessel (arrowhead). Original magnification, ×240 (present magnification, ×220). ABC method staining with MAb 38/17 C1 against nucleoprotein p40 counterstained with hematoxylin. Courtesy of Thomas Bilzer, Insitute for Neuropathology, University of Düsseldorf, Düsseldorf, Germany.

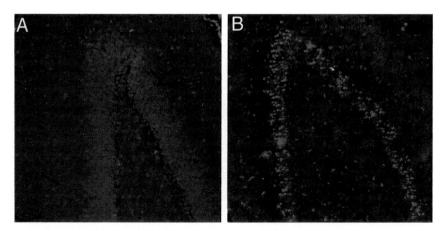

Color Plate 4 (chapter 5). Apoptosis of neurons in the DG of the hippocamus at day 28 p.i. TUNEL staining for apoptotic neurons in sham-inoculated (A) and neonatally BDV-infected (B) rats. Note the massive apoptosis of neurons in the DG of the BDV-infected rat. Original magnification, ×225 (present magnification, ×160). Courtesy of Aymeric Hans.

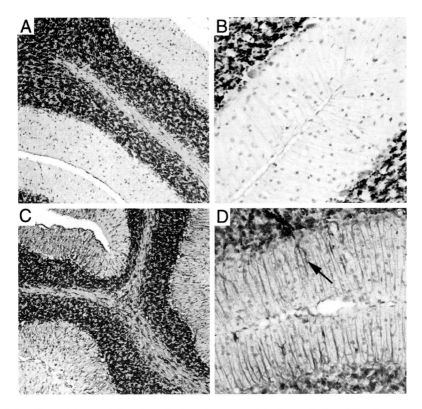

Color Plate 5 (chapter 5). Reactive gliosis and astrocytosis in the cerebellum following neonatal BDV infection at day 45 p.i. Shown are results of immunostaining (diaminobenzidine) for GFAP plus hematoxylin and eosin staining of representative sections of cerebellum of sham-inoculated (A and B) and BDV-infected (C and D) rats. Note the remarkable activation of Bergmann glial cells in cerebellum of BDV-infected rats (arrow). Original magnifications, ×200 (A and C) and ×400 (B and D) (present magnifications, ×130 and ×260, respectively). Courtesy of Aymeric Hans.

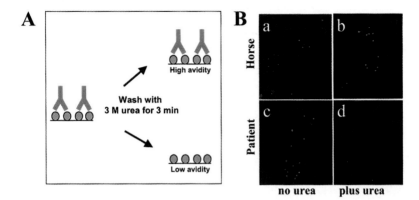

Color Plate 6 (chapter 6). BDV-reactive antibodies from patients with psychiatric diseases may exhibit low avidity in the presence of 3 M urea. (A) To measure the avidity of BDV-reactive antibodies, a short washing step with 3 M urea is introduced in the IFA procedure after the antibodies have bound to antigens. High-avidity antibodies remain bound to the BDV antigen, whereas low-avidity antibodies are washed away and are no longer visible in the IFA. (B) (a) In IFA, antibodies from horses with BD give a typical punctate staining in the nucleus of BDV-infected C6 cells. (b) These antibodies show high avidity since treatment with urea has no effect on the binding efficacy. (c) BDV-reactive antibodies from patients with mental disorders frequently recognize BDV antigens in the nuclei of infected cells. (d) In contrast to sera of horses with BD, the avidity of the human antibodies is low since treatment with urea completely abolishes the specific signals in the IFA.

Chapter 6

Human Borna Disease Virus Infection

Oliver Planz, Karl A. Bechter, and Martin Schwemmle

Finding Borna disease (BD) virus (BDV)-specific serum antibodies in psychiatric patients with major depression but not in healthy controls suggested a possible causal relationship between BDV infection and depressive disorders (Rott et al., 1985; Amsterdam et al., 1985). Subsequent studies supported an increased BDV seroprevalence in patients suffering from various psychiatric syndromes and disorders. However, a considerable number of healthy controls (Bechter et al., 1987) and possibly other human populations (L. Bode, S. Riegel, H. Ludwig, J. D. Amsterdam, W. Lange, and H. Koprowski, Letter, *Lancet* ii:689, 1988) also presented with BDV-serum antibodies. Meanwhile, a number of seroepidemiological studies have corroborating evidence that psychiatric patients present with increased BDV seroprevalence. Nevertheless, interpretation of the available epidemiological data regarding a possible association of BDV infection with human disease has become more difficult rather than easier with increasing information. Because various methods were used to assess BDV infection and because of unknown epidemiological factors in populations investigated, interpretation of the results remains difficult. Here, basic researchers help to evaluate the validity and specificity of laboratory methods applied in various studies while a clinical psychiatrist evaluates clinical studies selected with specific design and end point criteria.

Oliver Planz (Laboratory Evidence of Human BDV Infection) • Institute for Immunology, Federal Research Center for Virus Diseases of Animals, Paul-Ehrlich-Strasse 28, D-72076 Tübingen, Germany. **Karl A. Bechter (Clinical Studies of Human BDV Infection)** • Department of Psychosomatics/Psychotherapy and Department of Psychiatry II, University of Ulm, Ludwig-Heilmeyer-Strasse 2, D-89312 Günzburg, Germany. **Martin Schwemmle (Laboratory Evidence of Human BDV Infection)** • Institute of Medical Virology, University of Zürich, Gloriastrasse 30, CH-8028 Zürich, Switzerland.

LABORATORY EVIDENCE OF HUMAN BDV INFECTION

Serological Evidence

The presence of BDV-reactive antibodies in sera of psychiatric patients was first documented by a conventional indirect immunofluorescence assay (IFA) using BDV-infected Madin-Darby kidney cells (Rott et al., 1985). Since viral replication occurs only in the nucleus of infected cells (Carbone et al., 1991; Briese et al., 1992; Cubitt et al., 1994), the presence of BDV-reactive antibodies is diagnosed by a typical punctate immunostaining of what are most likely aggregated viral ribonucleoprotein (RNP) complexes (Bode et al., 1992) in the nucleoplasm (Color Plate 6 [see color insert]). In initial studies (Amsterdam et al., 1985; Rott et al., 1985; Bechter et al., 1987; Bode et al., letter, 1988; Bode et al., 1992; Rott et al., 1991; Bechter et al., 1992a) with sera from 265 to 5,000 patients, BDV-reactive antibody prevalence in a small but significant fraction of psychiatric patients was 0.6 to 7% versus 0 to 3.5% in healthy controls (Table 1). Similar to the situation in naturally infected horses (Lange et al., 1987; Herzog et al., 1994), the human antibody titers were frequently below 1:40. Thus, anti-BDV antibody may be difficult to detect in the IFA, depending on the BDV-infected cell line used, and this may account for some of the differences in the prevalence rates. Nevertheless, subsequent IFA studies with smaller samples confirmed these data (Table 1), suggesting that the increase in error rates due to reader subjectivity is minimal. Interestingly, high seroprevalence rates (7.1 to 13.99%) were also observed in patients infected with human immunodeficiency virus (HIV), schistosomiasis, and malaria (Bode et al., letter, 1988; Bode et al., 1992; L. Bode, A. L. Komaroff, and H. Ludwig, Letter, *Clin. Infect. Dis.* **15**:1049, 1992), suggesting that opportunistic infection with BDV occurs frequently after immunosuppression (Table 1). This and the observation that BDV-reactive antibodies were also found in sera of chronic fatigue syndrome (CFS) patients and patients with multiple sclerosis (MS) may also indicate that BDV infection is not necessarily linked to psychiatric diseases.

Although double IFA demonstrated colocalization of human and monoclonal antibodies directed against the N or P protein (Bode et al., 1992), it is unclear whether the corresponding human sera do contain indeed BDV-specific or cross-reactive antibodies. The latter antibodies may recognize viral or cellular proteins, especially since relocalization and concentration of cellular proteins to the sites of virus replication often occur after virus infection. In addition, autoantibodies have been detected in many patients with psychiatric disorders (Ganguli et al., 1992; Legros et

Table 1. Seroprevalence of BDV in humans

Assay(s)	Donor origin(s)	Diagnosis or subject group	No. of patients	% Seropositive for BDV	Reference(s)
IFA	United States	Major depressive disorders	265	4.5	Amsterdam et al. (1985)
		Healthy volunteers	105	0	
IFA	Germany	Various psychiatric disturbances	694	0.6	Rott et al. (1985)
		Healthy volunteers	95	0	
IFA	Germany	Various psychiatric disturbances	1,003	6.8	Bechter et al. (1987)
		Surgery patients	133	3.5	
IFA	Germany	HIV infected	460	7.8	Bode et al. (letter, 1988)
		HIV antibody negative	125	1.6	
		HIV-negative drug abusers	106	3.8	
IFA	United States, Germany, Japan	Psychiatric or neurological patients	5,000	4.7	Rott et al. (1991)
		Control hospital patients	1,000	1	
IFA	East Africa	Schistosomiasis and malaria	193	9.8	Bode et al. (1992)
IFA	Germany	Psychiatric patients	2,377	5.9	Bechter et al. (1992a, 1992b)
		Surgery patients	569	3.5	
IFA-IP[a]	Europe	Asymptomatic HIV infection	1,024	7.1	Bode et al. (1992)
		HIV infected	244	13.99	
		HIV-negative blood donors	118	2.5	
IFA-IP	United States	Major depression	550	2.2	Bode et al. (1992)
		Surgery patients	365	2.2	
IFA	Germany	Acute psychiatric patients (follow-up study)	71	19.7	Bode et al. (1993)
IFA	Germany	MS	50	0	Kitze et al (1996)
IFA	Japan	Psychiatric disorders	346	0.9	Kubo et al. (1997)
		Healthy controls	70	0	
IFA	Germany	Major depression	65	3.1	Deuschle et al. (letter)
		Bipolar disorders	8	0	
		Schizophrenic patients	27	0	
		Other psychiatric patients	28	0	
		MS patients	19	0	

Continued on following page

Table 1. *Continued*

Assay(s)	Donor origin(s)	Diagnosis or subject group	No. of patients	% Seropositive for BDV	Reference(s)
		Cerebrospinal diseases	14	7.14	
		Other neurological disease	69	0	
IFA	Switzerland	HIV	16	12.5	Bachmann et al.
		ADC	25	8	(1999)
IFA	Germany	Psychiatric patients	27	14.8	Vahlenkamp et al.
		Healthy controls	13	0	(2000)
IFA	Surinam	Schizophrenia	29	3	Selten et al. (2000)
		Healthy volunteers	26	6	
WBA	USA	Major depression	138	6.5	Fu et al. (1993)
		Healthy controls or nonpsychiatric patients	117	0.85	
WBA	United States	Schizophrenic outpatients	90	14.4	Waltrip et al. (1995)
		Healthy controls	20	0	
WBA	Japan	Psychiatric patients	60	30	Kishi et al. (1995b)
WBA	Germany	Various psychiatric disorders	416	9.6	Sauder et al. (1996)
		Surgery patients	203	1.4	
WBA	Japan	Schizophrenia	67	45.0	Iwahashi et al.
		Medical staff	26	0	(1997)
WBA	Taiwan	Schizophrenia	314	12.1	Chen et al. (1999)
		Asymptomatic family members of schizophrenic patients	132	12.1	
		Blood donors, hospital patients	274	2.9	
		Mental health workers	82	9.8	
WBA	Japan	Psychiatric patients	89	0	Tsuji et al. (2000)
		Healthy volunteers	210	0	
ELISA	Thailand	Asymptomatic HIV infection	60	15	Auwanit et al. (1996)
		AIDS	67	17.9	
		HIV-negative blood donors	103	2.5	
ELISA-WBA	Japan	Blood donors	100	1	Kishi et al. (1995a)
ELISA	Japan	CFS	89	33.7	Kitani et al. (1996)
ELISA	Japan	Blood donors living near horse farms	428	2.6–14.8	Takahashi et al. (1997)
		Blood donors	100	1	

Continued on following page

Table 1. *Continued*

Assay(s)	Donor origin(s)	Diagnosis or subject group	No. of patients	% Seropositive for BDV	Reference(s)
RS-ELISA	Japan	Chronic schizophrenia	70	0	Horimoto et al. (1997)
		Healthy volunteers	40	0	
ECLIA	Japan	Schizophrenia	845	3.08	Yamaguchi et al.
		Mood disorders	251	3.59	(1999)
		Various other psychiatric disorders	366	0.55	
		Neurological diseases	114	0	
		Various ocular diseases	1,393	1.36	
		Multitransfused patients	66	4.55	
		Blood donors	917	1.09	
		HIV infected	85	1.18	
		CFS	75	0	
		Epilepsy	214	1.4	
		Autoimmune diseases	50	0	
		Leprosy	17	0	
ECLIA	Poland	Various psychiatric patients	816	2	Rybakowski et al. (2001)
ELISA-WBA	Sweden	CFS	169	0	Evengard et al.
		Controls	62	0	(1999)
IFA-ECLIA-WBA	Japan	Mood disorder	45	4	Fukuda et al.
		Schizophrenia	45	9	(2001)

[a] IP, immunoprecipitation.

al., 1985; Sirota et al., 1993). Alternative serological techniques, including immunoprecipitation, Western blot assay (WBA), enzyme-linked immunosorbent assay (ELISA) and electrochemiluminescence immunoassay (ECLIA) were developed to confirm and extend the IFA findings. Several studies employing these techniques confirmed to a certain extent the IFA-based findings (Table 1) and revealed prevalence rates between 0 and 45% in psychiatric patients and between 0 and 1.8% in healthy controls. Since most assays used purified viral proteins (Fu et al., 1993; Kishi et al., 1995a; Kishi et al., 1995b; Iwahashi et al., 1997; Chen et al., 1999, Kitani et al., 1996; Takahashi et al., 1997; Yamaguchi et al., 1999; Fukuda et al., 2001; Tsuji et al., 2000; Auwanit et al., 1996), the risk of a cross-reactivity to cellular proteins was substantially reduced. Nevertheless, the critical question of whether BDV-reactive antibodies are caused by an infection with BDV or by related pathogens or immunogens is difficult to exclude, especially if only one viral protein is included in the serological test. The finding of human sera containing antibodies that recognize more than one viral protein in WBA, ELISA, or ECLIA argues against cross-reactive antibodies and in support of specific BDV human seropositivity (Waltrip et al., 1995; Kishi et al., 1995a, 1995b; Horimoto et al., 1997; Auwanit et al., 1996; Kitani et al., 1996).

ECLIA and WBA using recombinant forms of the two major viral proteins, the N and P protein, revealed that the reactivity of human antibodies is predominantly directed against only one of these proteins (Fukuda et al., 2001; Yamaguchi et al., 1999; Rybakowski, 2001; Takahasi et al., 1997; Chen et al., 1999; Iwahashi et al., 1997). It is unclear why, in the majority of cases, antibodies to only one or the other BDV protein can be detected in humans, whereas in naturally infected horses reactivity to both proteins is normally observed.

Due to the high frequency with which sera from patients with schizophrenia and healthy control groups reacted with only one BDV protein in WBA, Waltrip et al. (1995) introduced a more restrictive criterion by assigning seropositivity only if more than one BDV protein is specifically recognized by human sera. Based on this restriction the prevalence rate of seropositive patients with schizophrenia dropped from 32 to 14.4% and that in healthy controls dropped from 20 to 0%, suggesting that detection of antibodies to more than one protein is a useful working criterion for seropositivity. Such restrictive criteria can serve as a helpful tool, as shown in the diagnosis of HIV infection by WBA, where recognition of only one viral protein is not sufficient to indicate a true infection with this virus. Whether similar restrictive criteria should apply for BDV is not clear. Sera of some experimentally infected mice contain, despite high titers in the IFA, no detectable amounts of BDV-reactive antibodies directed against P or N as determined by WBA (C. Billich and M. Schwemmle, unpublished results). Furthermore, screening of Japanese feral horse sera with ECLIA suggested that in the majority of cases BDV-reactive antibodies were directed against the P protein (Yamaguchi et al., 1999). Screening for BDV-reactive human antibodies by three serological test systems including IFA, WBA, and ECLIA revealed that only 1 out of 45 patients with mood disorders was positive for BDV antibodies by all three assays and that the BDV-reactive antibodies were directed against the N protein only (Fukuda et al., 2001). It is tempting to speculate whether BDV infection may eventually lead to different BDV-reactive antibodies in humans: antibodies that recognize predominantly linear epitopes on one particular BDV protein and/or antibodies that recognize conformational epitopes on either single viral proteins or RNP structures. The latter type of antibody is especially difficult to detect with serological test systems using denatured or single viral proteins. In summary, since seropositivity of human sera to only one viral protein cannot be ignored, specific criteria to indicate true BDV positives in tests of human sera remain to be established.

Other studies employing WBA or reverse sandwich-type ELISA (RS-ELISA) as detection methods have completely failed to demonstrate BDV-reactive antibodies in the sera of psychiatric patients with various disorders (Horimoto et al., 1997; Evengard et al., 1999), perhaps through more stringent procedures which reduce the frequency of false positives. Alternatively a lower sensitivity of the serological assays, especially of the RS-ELISA (see also chapter 3), may account for the failure to detect BDV-reactive antibodies in humans. The latter possibility must be seriously entertained, since comparison of the various serological methods (WBA, ELISA, and IFA) in a German multicenter study organized by the Paul Ehrlich Institute indeed revealed great differences between the individual serological assays in their capacity to identify BDV-reactive human sera (Schwemmle, 1999) and concluded that the IFA was the most "valuable" method. Nevertheless, while validation of a suitable screening test is urgently needed, it will be difficult due to the lack of a human reference serum with defined concentrations of BDV-specific antibodies.

Is the serology misleading?

Although there is no "gold standard," it is possible that further improvements and validation of BDV-specific serologically based assays may, in principle, result in a reliable diagnostic tool in the future. However, the recent observation by Allmang et al. (2001) that human BDV antibodies bind their antigens with low avidity might challenge this view and question the diagnostic value of serological tests.

Low-avidity immunoglobulin G (IgG) antibodies appear very early during the course of many primary viral infections (Gutierrez et al., 1996). The maturation of low-avidity IgG towards high-affinity antibodies occurs during the subsequent selection process of B cells. The differences in strength with which low- and high-affinity antibodies recognize their antigens are often used as a diagnostic tool to differentiate between primary infection, reinfection, and reactivation (Gutierrez et al., 1996). Evaluation of antibody avidity is simple and can be carried out with most serological tests, including IFA and WBA, by a brief incubation with denaturing agents such as 6 M urea after antigen binding. Low-avidity antibodies dissociate from their antigen after this procedure, whereas high-avidity antibodies remain bound to the antigen.

Measuring the avidity of 25 samples from psychiatric patients by IFA, Allmang et al. (2001) observed in all cases a pronounced (>5-fold) reduction in the immunofluorescence signal intensities after treatment with only 3 M urea (Color Plate 6) indicating that the BDV-reactive antibodies are of the low-avidity phenotype. In contrast, BDV-specific antibodies from Borna-diseased horses or from experimentally infected monkeys (not shown) were unaffected in their efficacy to bind the antigen. Depletion experiments using recombinant viral proteins revealed that the low-avidity antibodies were predominantly directed against P (Allmang et al., 2001). One interpretation of these results is that all human samples investigated were, by chance, obtained from patients with primary BDV infections. However, longitudinal studies with serum samples from two patients obtained at intervals between 1 and 4 years revealed, at all time points, a similarly high sensitivity to urea despite elevated levels of the BDV-reactive antibodies (Allmang et al., 2001). This suggests that, in humans, there is no or inefficient maturation towards high-affinity antibodies. The simplest interpretation of these results would be that the reactive antibodies were not induced by BDV itself and are therefore of a cross-reactive nature. Cross-reactive antibodies are known to exhibit a low-avidity phenotype (Lehtonen et al., 1986; Schupbach et al., 1988). The existence of cross-reacting antibodies may also explain in part the difficulty and differences between various laboratories to develop a reliable serological test for BDV-specific antibodies in humans. Alternatively, maturation towards high-avidity IgGs might be impaired in BDV-infected humans due to low amounts of viral antigen. Viral persistence at such threshold levels would also explain the difficulties in detecting BDV RNA by nested reverse transcriptase PCR (RT-PCR). Finally, consideration must be given to the effects of using an animal source of BDV antigen when examining human sera, as it is possible that the putative human BDV differs somewhat in antigenic characteristics from the animal isolates.

Due to the small number of sera investigated by Allmang et al. (2001), it is too early to conclude that all previously BDV-positive human sera will react with similar sensitivity to 3 M urea. Because there are cases of human BDV infections identified by nonserological methods it is likely that we may also find BDV-specific antibodies with high avidity. It will be of interest to analyze the avidity of these human antibodies that recognize N or more than one viral protein. However, the frequency of such serologically confirmed cases will certainly be lower, and such cases may no longer be linked to psychiatric diseases. In conclusion, the low avidity of BDV-reactive antibodies questions the diagnostic value of all serological assays. Incorporation of the avidity test into the serological surveys is likely to reveal lower prevalence rates of BDV infection in humans than previously reported.

Independent of the avidity issue, there remains the seroepidemiological evidence that BDV-reactive antibodies are found more frequently in psychiatric patients than in healthy controls. Therefore, it is possible that the identification of the agent responsible for the induction of these antibodies may finally lead to the discovery of a new pathogen or immunogen important in the development of psychiatric diseases. Since all BDV strains show extremely high conservation in their primary protein sequences (Briese et al., 1994; Cubitt et al., 1994; Staeheli et al., 2000; Formella et al., 2000) it is tempting to speculate whether this agent represents a new human BDV variant with only remote similarity to known animal-derived strains. The first important steps to unveil this agent may include the characterization of the corresponding epitopes recognized from the BDV-reactive antibodies.

Antigen Detection and Virus Isolation

BDV antigen was first detected in peripheral blood mononuclear cells (PBMCs) of psychiatric patients by fluorescence-activated cell sorting (FACS) using monoclonal antibodies against P and N (L. Bode, F. Steinbach, and H. Ludwig, Letter, *Lancet* **343:**297–298, 1994), revealing that 15 to 17% of monocytes expressed BDV antigens. Unfortunately, PBMCs of normal control cases were not included in this pilot study. Thus, the link to certain psychiatric diseases based only on this method is unclear. Further, Gonzalez-Dunia et al. reasoned that these findings would suggest that at least 1% of the PBMCs of the patients positive for BDV antigen by FACS are infected with BDV (Gonzales-Dunia et al., 1997), and, in this case, detection of BDV RNA should be possible without the use of the highly sensitive RT-nested PCR. However, as seen with other studies, RT-nested PCR was required for the detection of BDV RNA in some of the PBMC samples positive for BDV RNA by FACS. Thus, the RNA detection data in humans are in concert with findings in neonatally BDV-infected rats, where the number of infected PBMCs is very low and thus the detection of viral RNA generally requires RT-nested PCR (Furrer et al., 2001; Vahlenkamp et al., 2000; Sierra-Honigmann et al., 1993; Sauder et al., 1998). Although caution is warranted when comparing the results of human and animal studies, these data imply that the viral load in human PBMCs is lower than that suggested from the FACS analysis, questioning the reliability of this test. Without further data on the specificity and sensitivity of BDV antigen detection by FACS (e.g., testing PBMCs of BDV-infected rats) the diagnostic value of this tool remains uncertain.

To measure BDV antigen in the cerebrospinal fluid (CSF) and blood, Bode et al. (1998) developed an antigen capture ELISA which uses monoclonal antibodies and polyclonal antiserum to capture and detect the antigen, respectively. With the help of this assay three patients with major depression and two patients with MS were identified as BDV seropositive. Unfortunately, the specificity of this assay remains unclear (see chapter 3).

Only a few groups have succeeded in the isolation of BDV from blood or brain tissue using either a complicated cell culture procedure or infection of newborn gerbils (Table 2). The significance of these findings, however, was brought into question by the observation that the genome sequences of the human isolates were almost identical with the particular laboratory strains used for experiments in the individual laboratories which performed the isolation procedure (M. Schwemmle, C. Jehle, S. Formella, and P. Staeheli, Letter, *Lancet* 354:1973–1974, 1999; Staeheli et al., 2000). Thus, accidental contamination of human samples with laboratory strain viruses cannot be formally excluded. However, Bode et al. (L. Bode, D. E. Dietrich, R. Stoyloff, H. M. Emrich, and H. Ludwig, Letter, *Lancet* 349:178–179, 1997) described differences between some human isolates and laboratory strains in their sensitivity towards amantadine, a compound known to inhibit very efficiently the spread of some influenza virus strains (Davies et al., 1965). Other studies revealed that replication of various BDV laboratory strains remained unaffected in vitro and in vivo (Hallensleben et al., 1997; Stitz et al., 1998; Cubitt et al., 1997). Although it is entirely unclear why only human isolates should exhibit this specific phenotype, it might be a first step in defining a true human BDV strain. Unfortunately, the human isolates in question have not been available for examination by the general scientific community; so this finding remains unconfirmed. Bode et al. (letter, 1997) further reported that treatment of psychiatric patients with amantadine coincided with a decline in the viral load in the PBMCs of these individuals. However, in an open trial of amantadine sulfate treatment in chronically depressed patients, the antidepressant activity of this drug did not correlate with a decline of the vi-

Table 2. Isolation of BDV

Isolation procedure[a]	Tissue used for isolation	Subject specification	No. of patients	No. positive for BDV	Reference
Cell culture	PBMCs	Psychiatric patients	32	3	Bode et al. (1996)
Cell culture	Granulocytes	Psychiatric patient	1	1	Planz et al. (1999)
Gerbils	Brain	Schizophrenic patient	1	1	Nakamura et al. (2000)

[a]Assays used to isolate BDV included human oligodendrocytes (for cell culture of PBMCs), a guinea pig cell line (CRL 1405) (for granulocytes), and newborn Mongolian gerbils (for brain).

ral markers (Ferszt et al., 1999a; Ferszt et al., 1999b). As shown by Lieb et al. (K. Lieb, F. T. Hufert, K. Bechter, J. Bauer, and J. Kornhuber, Letter, *Lancet* **349**:958, 1997) the observed antidepressant effects of amantadine can be easily explained by direct interference of this drug with neurotransmitter systems (Moryl et al., 1993) rather than its putative antiviral effect on BDV.

BDV-Specific Nucleic Acid Detection

Brain

When Mullis first described the new technology of PCR in 1986 it took 6 more years before this method was used for detection of BDV-specific nucleic acid in human brain tissue specimens (Shankar et al., 1992) (Table 3). These authors used RT-PCR to attempt to detect nucleic acid encoding BDV in postmortem human nervous tissue of 16 schizophrenic patients but failed to detect BDV RNA. In addition, no positive PCR signal for BDV was found when the CSF of 48 schizophrenic patients and of nine sets of identical twins discordant for schizophrenia were tested (Sierra-Honigmann et al., 1995). It is possible that false-negative results can be due to primer sequences that correspond to regions of the viral genome that are not evolutionarily conserved in a related human pathogen. The recent discovery of a new BDV subtype, named No/98, which was isolated from a horse with BD (Nowotny et al., 2000) may support this hypothesis. No/98 differs from known BDV genome sequences by more than 15%, and most importantly, this virus escapes detection by the currently used diagnostic RT-PCR protocols (Nowotny et al., 2000).

The first successful demonstration of BDV nucleic acid in human brain tissue was reported in 1996 by de la Torre et al. Using RT-nested PCR and

Table 3. Detection of BDV-specific nucleic acid in brain tissue by RT-PCR

Reference	BDV gene(s) detected
Studies in which BDV-specific nucleic acid was detected	
Nakamura et al., 2000	P, N
Czygan et al., 1999	P, N
Haga et al., 1998	P
Salvatore et al., 1997	P
de la Torre et al., 1996	N
Studies in which BDV-specific nucleic acid was not detected	
Sierra-Honigmann et al., 1995	
Shankar et al., 1992	

in situ hybridization, BDV-specific RNA (N) was detected in autopsy brain samples from four out of five patients with a diagnosis of hippocampus sclerosis and astrocytosis. Specificity of the RT-PCR was demonstrated by Southern blot hybridization using a probe that corresponded to the internal sequence of the BDV N segment (Cubitt et al., 1994). Finally, there was a perfect correlation between the detection of BDV N antigen and RNA in these brains, strongly supporting the hypothesis that BDV is a human pathogen. Nevertheless, sequence analyses of the amplified PCR products were not made available; therefore, PCR contamination of the human samples by laboratory strains of virus cannot be ruled out. Three positive samples from de la Torre and colleagues were evaluated by Czygan and coworkers (Czygan et al., 1999), who detected BDV genes for N, P, and X after first-round RT-PCR, confirming the previous study. However, since sequence analyses revealed that some of these BDV-specific genes were either identical or contained only a few nucleotide changes to the sequence of the laboratory strain He/80, it is also possible that a laboratory strain of BDV contaminated the brain material. Still, due to the extraordinary genome conservation of most BDV strains, the possibility that a human BDV pathogen exists that is identical to the strain that was isolated from a horse in the early 1980s in Germany cannot be ruled out.

Several other groups have reported the detection of BDV-specific nucleic acid from brain tissue. In a study using postmortem brain samples from 75 North American and European individuals with various brain disorders and healthy controls, BDV P transcripts were detected in 10 people with schizophrenia and in two samples from people who had suffered from bipolar disorder (M. Salvatore, S. Morzunov, M. Schwemmle, and W. I. Lipkin, Letter, Lancet 349:1813–1814, 1997). When samples from 13 of the 75 brains were sent for an independent analysis, only two of five positive samples could be confirmed and one sample from a patient with schizophrenia that was negative in the original investigation was now positive. Amplification products were sequenced and showed low sequence divergence from BDV strains He/80 and V, arguing that positive samples represented low-level laboratory strain contaminants. Yet the brain samples used for these independent analyses were obtained directly from the brain bank, making contamination unlikely. However, another group failed to demonstrate the presence of BDV RNA in some of these BDV-positive brain tissues, despite using a highly sensitive RT-nested PCR (Czygan et al., 1999).

In another investigation BDV-specific nucleic acid was found in brain tissue of healthy individuals (Haga et al., 1998). However, sequence analysis of the amplification products revealed identity to the laboratory strain, again questioning the origin of the BDV-specific nucleic acid.

A handicap in the investigation of BDV in humans is sample acquisition, i.e., that only blood from living individuals and postmortem brain material are available for testing. Therefore, it is almost impossible to compare data obtained from serological or RNA detection studies with blood to results obtained after investigations of brain tissue. Recently, Nakamura and colleagues were able to test brain tissue and blood from patients using RT-PCR to detect gene transcripts for nucleoprotein N and P. In one schizophrenic patient the cerebral cortex was positive for N and the hippocampus, pons, and cerebellum were positive for P. The P results were confirmed by in situ hybridization, and infectious virus was isolated from the tissue. After sequence analysis this isolate differed from the laboratory strain He/80 and V by 1.5 to 2.5%, suggesting that this virus might represent a true human isolate. However, it is difficult to exclude a contamination because the corresponding human isolate BDVHuP2br shows complete identity in the sequenced open reading frames to the laboratory strain BDV-MDCK commonly used in this laboratory (Staeheli et al., 2000). In addition, RT-PCR performed on whole blood from this patient failed to amplify BDV-specific gene transcripts.

In summary, since most of the RT-PCR products or virus isolates from brain tissue are identical in sequence to laboratory strains, one might be tempted to speculate that laboratory contaminations occurred in almost all cases of positive BDV results from human samples. However, due to the extraordinary high sequence conservation of BDV we cannot exclude that identical strains do exist in humans. Furthermore, the fact that positive samples were mostly found in either schizophrenic patients or in patients that suffered from hippocampus sclerosis supports the argument for the human origin of BDV in some of these samples.

Blood

In 1995 the first report that BDV-specific nucleic acid was found in three psychiatric patients appeared (Bode et al., 1995) (Table 4). Here, gene transcripts for N and P that differed from the two laboratory strains and among different patients were amplified. This finding that BDV-specific nucleic acid can be found in the blood of psychiatric patients was supported by two publications in 1995 by Kishi and coworkers, where some hundred blood samples were tested from patients in Japanese hospitals for the presence of BDV N gene transcripts (Kishi et al., 1995a; Kishi et al., 1995b). Sequence analyses of the amplified RT-PCR products showed divergences from He/80 and strain V of around 7%. Moreover, some of the transcripts showed either single point deletions or deletions of several nucleotides in the P gene, and so far, to our knowledge, nucleotide deletions

Table 4. Detection of BDV-specific nucleic acid in blood by RT-PCR

Reference	BDV gene(s)
Studies in which BDV-specific nucleic acid was detected	
Fukuda et al., 2001	P
Selten et al., 2000	P, N
Vahlenkamp et al., 2000	P, N
Tsuji et al., 2000	P, N
Nowotny et al., 2000	G, P, N
Chen et al., 1999	
Nakaya et al., 1999	P
Planz et al., 1999	P, N
Iwata et al., 1998	P
Iwahashi et al., letter	
Planz et al., letter	P, N
Iwahashi et al., 1997	
Takahashi et al., 1997	
Sauder et al., 1996	P, N
Nakaya et al., 1996	P
Kitani et al., 1996	
Kishi et al., 1995a	P
Kishi et al., 1995b	P
Kishi et al., 1996	P
Bode et al., 1995	P, N
Studies in which BDV-specific nucleic acid was not detected	
Evengard et al., 1999	
Kim et al., 1999	P[a]
Bachmann et al., 1999	N[a]
Lieb et al., letter	N[a]
Richt et al., 1997	
Sierra-Honigmann et al., 1995	

[a]Gene not detected.

in BDV transcripts or strains have never been reported. Besides the detection of BDV-specific nucleic acid in schizophrenic patients, BDV-RNA was found in the blood from patients that suffered from CFS, and BDV was isolated from PBMCs of an American patient with CFS (Bode et al., 1996; Kitani et al., 1996; Nakaya et al., 1996, 1999; N. Nowotny and J. Kolodziejek, Letter, *Lancet* 355:1462–1463, 2000). Nowotny and Kolodziejek were able to demonstrate BDV-specific nucleic acid for part of the N and G genes and the complete P and M genes of BDV for a total 1,398 bp. The sequences were unique and showed an overall nucleotide identity rate of 96 to 98% compared to other BDV sequences. Because of the large amount of sequenced nucleotides and the sequence divergences from other BDV sequences, these data suggested that, indeed, a clearly BDV-specific nucleic acid had been found in a human patient. However, based on the concerns that contamination with laboratory strains can occur and that other investigators were unable to find evidence for BDV infection in patients who suffered from CFS (Bode et al., 1992; Evengard et al., 1999; Yamaguchi et al., 1999), the results of Nowotny and Kolodziejek will be even more convincing after being confirmed in a BDV-free laboratory.

Several publications show the detection of BDV-specific nucleic acid in blood of psychiatric patients. Sauder et al. (1996) detected BDV RNA in PBMCs of psychiatric patients in Germany. When the gene products were sequenced, they revealed few differences from the laboratory strains He/80 and V. Out of 26 samples 11 were found to be positive for either P or N gene products and 6 samples tested positive for both P and N. Of these six samples, five were confirmed positive by RT-PCR by the laboratory in the United States. Because of the high frequency of positive samples, one might be tempted to speculate that contamination occurred, but since some BDV sequences differed from laboratory strains and the samples were tested in two independent laboratories, this seems to be unlikely. However, since the blood samples used for independent confirmation by the American group were obtained from the German BDV laboratory, accidental contamination with laboratory BDV strains cannot formally be excluded. Further, a detailed follow-up study of additional psychiatric patients from the same clinic revealed that no patients were positive for BDV RNA by RT-PCR (Lieb et al., letter).

Various publications concluded that BDV-RNA was present in PBMCs of schizophrenic patients (Iwahashi et al., 1997; K. Iwahashi, M. Watanabe, K. Nakamura, H. Suwaki, T. Nakaya, Y. Nakamura, H. Takahashi, and K. Ikuta, Letter, *Can. J. Psychiatry* **43**:197, 1998; Iwata et al., 1998; Chen et al., 1999; Vahlenkamp et al., 2000; Fukuda et al., 2001). In contrast, several groups failed to detect BDV RNA in PBMCs of schizophrenic patients or in PBMCs of patients that suffered from other psychiatric diseases (Sierra-Honigmann et al., 1995; Richt et al., 1997; Lieb et al., letter; Kim et al., 1999). In one report the prevalence of BDV RNA in psychiatric patients was not significantly different from that in healthy volunteers (Tsuji et al., 2000). Another report revealed that the frequencies of BDV RNA positivity in a group of healthy controls exceeded that in the group of patients (Selten et al., 2000).

The interpretation of these conflicting results is difficult. The inconsistent detection of BDV RNA in human blood samples can be due to differences in the initial amount of blood or sensitivity of the RT-PCR technique used. Clearly, the negative findings do not exclude the possibility that BDV can infect humans and could simply show that the detection of

BDV in human blood is far from being a trivial pursuit. Furthermore, these results may also reflect that both the percentage of BDV-positive patients and the amount of RNA in the blood is very low or that patient selection methods are not identifying the correct population for testing.

It remains unsolved whether BDV continuously persists in human blood as has been found in experimentally infected animals (Sierra-Honigmann et al., 1993; Furrer et al., 2001). In one study BDV was detected in a human when sampling occurred during an observation period of more than 8 months (O. Planz, C. Rentzsch, A. Batra, H. J. Rziha, and L. Stitz, Letter, *Lancet* **352**:623, 1998). Nevertheless, other studies showed that previously detected BDV can disappear from blood upon repeat testing (Bode et al., 1996).

It would be helpful to know the target cell population of the virus for the efficient detection of BDV in blood. Recently, it has been reported that human granulocytes were positive for BDV-RNA. This might explain why some groups failed to detect BDV in human blood, since granulocytes are lost after PBMC-Ficoll preparation of blood or after freezing of white blood cells (Planz et al., 1999). However, these findings have not been supported by other investigators, and given that several groups were able to amplify BDV-RNA from PBMCs, the data indicate that, in principle, BDV detection in PBMCs is possible.

In all but two publications the frequency of detection of BDV-RNA in blood of psychiatric patients always exceeded the frequency found in healthy controls. This supports the hypothesis that BDV can indeed be found in patients with psychiatric disorders; nevertheless, it does not support the opinion that BDV is the causative agent of these disorders. Sequence analyses performed with the amplified BDV-specific gene products showed either identity or slight differences compared to known laboratory strains, consistent with accidental contamination of samples with laboratory strains. Further, a comparison of all accessible sequences for the N gene of BDV demonstrated four distinct sequence clusters. In laboratories that use He/80 as their experimental strain, the sequence of the N gene obtained from human blood belonged to the He/80 cluster, whereas in laboratories that work with strain V the human sequences belonged to the strain V cluster. The only exception is the sequence published by Nowotny and Kolodziejek that fits in neither the He/80 nor the V clusters (Nowotny and Kolodziejek, letter). Therefore it is tempting to claim that indeed these investigators have a sequence that represents BDV from human origin. Nevertheless, the controversy over whether BDV is a pathogen in psychiatric patients ("pro") or whether all the positive RT-PCR results are due to laboratory contamination ("con") continues. Based on the currently available pro and con publications it is impossible to draw any firm conclusions. Since the contamination issue will always be raised in studies lacking independent confirmation, multicenter studies were recently initiated in Germany and Japan. There are no definite results yet, but with such studies there may be light at the end of the tunnel.

CLINICAL STUDIES OF HUMAN BDV INFECTION

Methodological concerns are substantial in human BDV studies, since increasing the sensitivity of methods is often accompanied by reduced specificity (Strongin, 1992), and blinded studies on BDV even suggested doubts about some standard techniques (C. M. Nübling, R. Kurth, and the Borna Virus Study Group, *Abstr. Borna Virus Meet. 1998*, 1998 [cited by Staeheli et al., 2000]). Therefore, concerns of serological methods needed to be considered when reviewing study results. Considering that the validity of studies with small sample size is apparently more affected by methodological or epidemiological variances than studies with large sample size, and recognizing an overall low prevalence of BDV infection in humans, only studies with a sample size of >500 using serological methods for documentation of BDV infection are discussed here; because of substantial concerns of contamination and false-positive results, all studies relying on PCR methods were excluded. Of a considerable number of studies done by serological methods studies were also excluded for small sample sizes; including samples from very different regions; or using newly introduced, unconfirmed serological methods. In addition to seroepidemiological survey studies, included are studies with BDV-seropositive results adding potentially important clinical disease information, using clinical diagnostics of central nervous system (CNS) infections in neurology and/or neuropsychiatry, e.g., brain imaging and CSF investigation.

There are two basically different models of BDV infection in animals: immunoincompetent or (early) perinatal BD and immunocompetent (or adult or adolescent) BD (Herzog et al., 1997), as discussed in chapter 5. Both perinatal BD and immunocompetent BD have been cited as possible models of human BDV infection. Infection of humans beyond the neonatal stage was suggested by seroepidemiological and clinical findings showing that BDV seroprevalence in surgical and neurological controls increased with age, a finding presumably indicating a lifelong risk of BDV infection in humans (Bechter et al., 1992a, 1992b, 1998). In addition, drug addicts were more frequently represented in the BDV-seropositive group than members of the control group in two studies (Bode et al., letter, 1988; Bechter et al., 1998), suggesting adult acquisition of BDV infection perhaps via intravenous blood contamination. Natural BD in animals is commonly an immunocompetent infection, though perinatal or subclinical BD may occur. Thus, both BD models are valid and may indeed serve as the human model: human BDV infection is possibly acquired anytime during prenatal, postnatal, or lifelong exposure to BDV.

Tolerant or nonpathogenic infections may lead into another type of pathogenesis, i.e., when quiescent virus is reactivated later and then, after reactivation, BD follows the immunocompetent model. BDV may also silently prime for and later trigger autoimmune disease by molecular mimicry (Theil et al., 2001). However, current investigations on BDV infection have not sufficiently well addressed these last two clinical presentations yet.

That BDV infection could induce human psychiatric disorders was initially hypothesized following analysis of results of an animal model of immunocompetent BD in tree shrews (Sprankel et al., 1978). Observed behavioral abnormalities during BDV encephalitis in those animals resembled specific psychiatric disorders, such as depression (Ludwig and Bode, 2000; Richt and Rott, 2001), with most important aspects of the BD model in tree shrews consistent with a spectrum of human psychiatric disorders (Bechter, 1998).

When just broadly considering possible clinical, epidemiological, and postmortem findings in human BD, we would expect the following:

1. In immunoincompetent human BD, symptoms would likely be detected early in infancy or childhood (e.g., autism) (see chapter 5). Within human postmortem brain one would find cellular abnormalities and possibly accompanying glia reactions, preferably in late-developing brain regions such as the cerebellum and dentate gyrus. Serum antibodies against BDV would be detected in infancy but must be differentiated in neonates from maternally transmitted antibodies. Perinatal BD could lead to smaller body size, as was found in BD in animals and in other pre- or perinatal human viral infections. Growth abnormalities would parallel neurodevelopmental abnormalities reflected, for example, in reduced skull and brain size. In a recent unique brain imaging study on monozygotic twins with schizophrenia, smaller whole cranial volumes appeared related to increased genetic risk, whereas smaller brain volumes with normal skull sizes appeared related to an exogenous factor presumably acquired later in life (Baaré et al., 2001).

2. Immunocompetent human BD could occur from days or weeks after birth until old age. Psychiatric symptoms and/or syndromes might be variable in presentation and might vary over time with phases and relapses, as seen in the BD model in tree shrews. BDV might also produce neurological symptoms or brain atrophy. Neurodevelopmental brain abnormalities would be absent or unrelated to BDV infection.

3. In both immunoincompetent and immunocompetent human BD, a subset of infected persons may never develop any psychiatric symptoms. In natural (immunocompetent) BD in horses, some seropositive animals never show any signs of disease (see chapter 4). Also, independent preexisting host factors might contribute to a variable range of psychiatric symptoms and syndromes in humans with immunoincompetent or immunocompetent BD.

It would be difficult to predict symptomatology and physical findings in human BDV infection to determine appropriate research approaches even if the methodological problems to assess human BDV infection did not exist. Current unknowns in human (and animal) BD include the following: age at infection, route of infection, dose of infectious virus, effects of genetic factors of the host, other independent preexisting factors in the individual, and the influence of general "brain reaction types" in known CNS infections, CNS inflammatory reaction, or any other secondary organic insult to the brain. Furthermore, diagnostic access to the brain and to brain function in humans is presently limited and the tests are somewhat insensitive.

Viral Hypothesis of Psychiatric Disorders

Although both immunoincompetent or immunocompetent human BD models may be linked to a range of psychiatric symptoms and syndromes, some major distinctive features should be identifiable, especially the early onset of symptoms (or lack of them) and specific postmortem brain findings. The use of valid and unambiguous laboratory methods is essential for BDV diagnosis, in a general setting of lack of knowledge about etiology and pathogenesis of psychiatric disorders. Following the discussion of the current evidence concerning whether human BDV infections exist or not, some general aspects regarding the present status of understanding the etiology and pathogenesis of psychiatric syndromes in known organic or secondary, especially infectious or inflammatory, brain disorders will be presented.

The hypothesis that viruses may cause psychiatric disorders, especially schizophrenia, has been voiced for nearly a century (O'Reilly, 1994) and is still hotly debated, reminiscent of the debates over the initial proposal of an infectious etiology of general paresis, later proved clearly to follow spirochete infection (Bechter, 1995). Regarding viruses, there were observations during and after the 1918–1919 influenza epidemic in which many adult-infected patients developed psychiatric syndromes identical to schizophrenia, depression, or other less well characterized psychiatric disorders (Menninger, 1925). The occasional occurrence of psychiatric disorders during or after various infectious or febrile diseases was subsequently increasingly recognized (Menninger, 1928). Since then, many infectious or inflammatory CNS disorders (and other organic brain diseases) presenting with exclusive or accompanying psychiatric symptoms have been described (Lishman, 1998). Nevertheless, over time the viral hypothesis decreased in psychiatric research, and the majority of present psychiatric textbooks do not even mention the term "encephalitis" or the viral hypothesis of psychiatric disorders or of schizophrenia outside a neurodevelopmental framework. However, recent research on the pathogenesis of viral infections suggests a freshly extended framework of interacting immunological and genetic factors (e.g., of inflammatory mediators such as a cytokine network) and other contributing factors (Pert et al., 1988; Eaves et al., 1988; Knight et al., 1992; Yolken and Torrey, 1995; Licinio and Wong, 1999; Pollmächer et al., 2000; Müller et al., 2000; Gonzalez-Dunia et al., 2000), making neuropsychiatric disturbances explainable in a general framework of still-hypothetical human viral infections (Yolken and Torrey, 2000). It seems that low acceptance of the hypothesis of viral etiologies in psychiatric research during recent decades stemmed from a long history of disappointments about this previously mainstream hypothesis, but convictions are changing. Although these findings await replication, recent detection of retroviral sequences in CSF of about 30% of acutely diseased schizophrenic patients greatly enhanced the viral hypothesis, suggesting endogenous retroviral reactivation or exogenous retroviral infection with secondary reactivation (Karlsson et al., 2001; D. A. Lewis, Commentary, *Proc. Natl. Acad. Sci. USA* **98**:4293–4294, 2001). In parallel, other research to improve diagnostic criteria and subclassification on a psychopathological level that hoped to eventually improve knowledge about etiologies of psychiatric disorders was disappointing (Goldberg and Weinberger, 1995; Hartmann, 1998; van Praag, 2000; Wittchen, 2000), and new ideas were needed. Indeed, this need may turn out to be, in certain respects, new reiterations of old ideas.

Validity and Specificity of Psychiatric Diagnostic Systems

Are certain clinical research problems unique to BD research, or are they general problems of clinical psychiatry? In fact, the validity of psychiatric diagnostic systems and nosology appears to be a general problem. During an ongoing process to improve psychiatric diagnostic systems over several decades, we now have the *Diagnostic and Statistical Manual of Mental Disorders,* 4th ed. (DSM-IV), and the *International Classification of Diseases,* 10th revision (ICD-10), as well as other research systems not in common use. There is broad agreement that DSM-IV and ICD-10 improve diagnostic reliability considerably, although further improvements are needed. However, the validity of DSM-IV and ICD-10 has been criticized and even challenged (Cooper, 1995, Goldberg and Weinberger, 1995; Hartmann, 1998; Wittchen, 2000; van Praag, 2000). Major criticisms of DSM-IV and ICD-10 are the confusing of valid clinical diagnosis (e.g., by not differentiating between etiology and pathogenesis), neglecting psychogenesis, and introducing new pseudoentities (van Praag, 2000).

Regarding the diagnostic crisis of present psychiatry one should recognize that known etiologies of psychiatric disorders are nonspecific (Buchsbaum and Rieder, 1979), e.g., that any known specific etiology can induce a range of psychiatric symptoms or syndromes, or given a level of symptoms or syndromes one is unable to differentiate their specific etiologies. It is often claimed that the old dichotomy between organic and functional disorders (or organic and endogenous [or, better, idiopathic] psychoses or disorders) and the previously established third category of psychogenic disorders appears outdated (Kaplan and Sadock, 1998). However, such claims are difficult to follow when trying to understand etiology and when facing the disappointing status of operationalization of clinical findings and respective evaluation.

To improve etiological research it was proposed, unsuccessfully in the case of DSM-IV and ICD-10, that specific biological markers be included the diagnostic categorization itself (Buchsbaum and Rieder, 1979; Wexler, 1992), and, thus, the lack of biological markers may represent a major shortcoming of these systems (van Praag, 2000). Since there is little advice to be found in DSM-IV or ICD-10 or in psychiatric textbooks about biological markers—e.g. findings in brain imaging, laboratory findings, and CSF findings—regarding a possible causal relationship to certain psychiatric disorders, or regarding differential diagnosis, such decisions are left to the clinician. There are many biological factors that are nevertheless recommended for investigation and careful evaluation by the clinician, who should first exclude an organic basis of primary psychiatric disorders. In other words, the construct validity of DSM-IV and ICD-10 is severely challenged (Newport and Nemeroff, 1999). In reality, evaluation of clinical findings is left to the clinician's training and skills, with understanding and interpretation open to great variance from experience and intuition and available or performed diagnostic means and tools.

Clearly, present psychiatry suffers from a lack of scientifically based expertise regarding evaluation of clinical findings and how to relate findings to causality of disorders. In clinical neurology one may find extended discussions and sophisticated studies addressing such questions as how findings are to be evaluated and how biological markers are to be related to neurological disease. However, in psychiatry evaluating clinical findings is much more difficult than evaluating the localizable and distinct symptoms and signs in clinical neurology. So, evaluation of etiologies of psychiatric disease is complicated, is not well understood, and often needs much clinical experience (Giedd, 2001). Thus, the clinical approach to causal inference in present psychiatry is not much beyond the status during the times of Kurt Schneider, who recommended that only meaningful findings ("belangvoller Befund") should be considered to be sufficient to explain certain psychiatric disorders. But what was meaningful was widely left open to the individual clinician, expertise, and subjective convictions. This is surprising, given that knowledge about the brain and diagnostic techniques and tools has greatly improved since that time.

Nosology and classifications remained a conundrum (Parshall and Priest, 1993). The old idea of Einheitspsychose (or unitary psychosis or continuum hypothesis) is again increasingly stressed (Kringlen, 1994; Nasrallah, 1994; Strömgren, 1994), meaning that there are no clear borders between disorders, or in other words, one can make differential typology, not differential diagnosis, of psychoses (Schneider, 1992). The overlap between schizophrenia and affective psychoses observed in the range of symptom patterns, in intraindividual disease courses, and in disease patterns within family trees might be explained by some common pathogenetic basis (Gross and Huber, 1993, Johnstone et al., 1996). So why has the promising idea to include specific biological markers (e.g., markers of BDV infection) in the diagnostic categorization itself continued to fail (Wexler, 1992; Buchsbaum and Rieder, 1979; van Praag, 2000)? It seems that problems such as nonspecificity of symptoms from specific etiologies, reflected in the clinician's view as overlap, and a general weakness of relationships between brain pathology and resulting symptoms are crucial factors which can probably be tackled in broad concerted research approaches only.

Thus, the situation in psychiatric research is generally difficult and complex. Although dealing with similar difficulties, the BDV research field has several advantages: at least one defined biological marker can be identified if BDV infection can be assessed by valid laboratory methods.

Furthermore, knowledge about natural BD in animals and well-studied experimental BD models provide a framework for research and analogy and, finally, conclusions. Furthermore, with research progress, new markers applicable in humans may also be developed.

Review of Selected Clinical Studies of Human BDV Infection

As outlined above, the studies presented are selected according to the following criteria: (i) studies done by serological methods, because the validity of serological methods appears acceptable, whereas the validity of PCR methods does not; (ii) studies with a sample size of >500, since smaller studies are difficult to evaluate because the overall prevalence of BDV may be low; and (iii) studies using clinical diagnostic methods such as brain imaging or CSF investigation in BDV-seropositive patients.

Seroepidemiology of BDV in humans

Rott et al. (1985) investigated BDV seropositivity by IFA in 979 patients, 694 hospitalized patients with various psychiatric diagnoses from Germany (mainly Würzburg), a group of patients from the United States (Philadelphia, Pa.) with major depression (Amsterdam et al., 1985), and controls ($n = 200$; 105 healthy controls; 95 nonpsychiatric patients). Anti-BDV serum antibodies were found in patients from Philadelphia with major depression (4.2%) and other psychiatric patients ($n = 694$) (1.6%) but were found in 0% of control subjects. The hypothesis was made of some relationship between exposure to BDV and development of an affective disorder.

Bechter et al. (1987) used IFA to screen psychiatric inpatients from the Günzburg clinics in Germany and found anti-BDV serum antibodies in 6.8% of patients ($n = 1.003$) with various psychiatric disorders. In a second screening study in the Günzburg clinics (Bechter et al., 1992a), a similar result was obtained: 5.9% of psychiatric inpatients ($n = 2,377$), 4.6% of neurological inpatients ($n = 1,791$), and 3.5% of surgical inpatients ($n = 569$) showed anti-BDV serum antibodies by IFA. A refined analysis of these data (Bechter et al., 1998; Bechter, 1998), showed that the (diagnostically not preselected) groups of psychiatric, neurological, and surgical inpatients from the Günzburg clinics were comparable with regard to age and sex distribution and that the BDV seroprevalence of 6% was statistically significantly increased in young psychiatric patients compared to <1% in surgical controls (ages between 17 and 30 years; odds ratio, 6.17). BDV seroprevalence increased with age in the surgical and neurological control patients from about 1 to 2% in 17 to 30 year olds to 5.5 to 6.5% in patients older than 70 years. Psychiatric diagnoses within the group of BDV-seropositive psychiatric patients were nearly identically distributed as in BDV-seronegative psychiatric patients, except that a significant, although slight, preference of drug addicts and an increased psychiatric comorbidity were seen in BDV-seropositive patients compared to pair-matched BDV-seronegative patients. Prevalences of BDV serum antibodies were similar for psychiatric inpatients on wards, chronic patients, and acute patients in clinic. BDV serum antibody titers were stable over years in some patients but declined in other patients (Bechter, 1998; Allmang et al., 2001). In BDV-seropositive neurological patients, meningoencephalitis was more frequently observed than in matched seronegative controls, suggesting occasional occurrence of BDV-related meningoencephalitis with neurological symptoms.

Bode et al. (letter, 1988) used IFA to identify BDV serum antibodies in 2% of patients with mental disorders, mainly depression, from the United States ($n = 642$), in 3.8% of drug abusers ($n = 106$), in 7.8% of HIV-infected people from West Germany ($n = 460$), and in 2% of controls from the United States and West Germany ($n = 540$). Age distribution of the populations was not reported. It was concluded that it remained open whether a correlation existed between BDV antibodies and psychiatric disorder. HIV infection was suggested to possibly activate the BD agent or induce cross-reactive autoantibodies.

Bode et al. (1992) further investigated sera of 2,876 adults from Europe, the United States, and Africa and of 220 children from Europe and Africa by IFA. Of healthy controls ($n = 483$) 2.35% were BDV seropositive; in the sample of the psychiatric patients with unipolar depression ($n = 363$) or bipolar depression ($n = 187$) 1.4 and 3.7% respectively, were BDV seropositive. In neurological patients BDV seroprevalences were as follows: in patients with MS, 13.2%; in HIV-infected patients, 13.9%; and in children with double infection from trypanosomiasis and malaria, 18.8%. The interpretation was that a latent BDV infection may have been reactivated by deteriorating health or immune status in such patients. The mean ages of patients with psychosis, patients with neurological disorders, patients with HIV infection, and healthy volunteers and blood donors were 45, 46, 35, and 33 years, respectively. The sex ratio (male to female) was 62:38 in psychiatric patients and 28:72 in healthy controls and blood donors.

Bode et al. (1993) further reported an intra-individual follow-up study on 70 psychiatric patients suffering from major depression, neurotic depression, or paranoid psychoses, taking three to four consecutive serum samples during one inpatient treatment. Using IFA, a total prevalence of anti-BDV antibody carriers of 20% was reported. However, while most patients were seronegative when admitted to the clinic, detectable antibody levels usually developed after 7 days of hospitalization. The mean period for seroconversion was 17.2 days. These results were interpreted as meaning that every third to every fourth patient with affective psychosis should be considered as latently infected with BDV expressing humoral response during acute disease episodes. However, these findings and the interpretation are difficult to understand considering that 60% of the patients suffered from chronic psychiatric disorders for at least 1 year before admission to the clinic and that many had previously experienced several disease episodes. Only 7% of the cohort studied were newly diagnosed.

Bode et al. (2001) recently published a dramatic finding that, if confirmed, reveals that "BDV-specific circulating immune complexes (CIC) and their interplay with free antibodies and plasma antigens (p40/p24) . . . indicate 10 times higher infection rates (up to 30% in controls, up to 100% in patients) than did previous serology" in patients with moderate or severe depression. Because of the "novel, easy-to-use diagnostic tools," confirmation of these findings should be a high priority. For the moment, these findings cannot be discussed from the clinician's point of view because of sparse clinical data in the report.

Sauder et al. (1996) found among 416 neuropsychiatric patients a BDV seroprevalence of 9.6% using a WBA, versus a 1.4% seroprevalence among 203 healthy controls. Psychiatric diagnoses included, among others, schizophrenia ($n = 114$), affective psychoses ($n = 52$), and neurological or personality disorders ($n = 54$). Most seropositive human sera recognized only one of the BDV protein antigens, N. Of 298 psychiatric patients whose diagnoses were known, fewer than 3% showed anti-BDV serum antibodies. Part of the patient group ($n = 202$) was matched by age and sex to surgery patient controls.

Using a WBA, Chen et al. (1999) found BDV serum antibodies in 12.1% of patients from Taiwan with chronic schizophrenia ($n = 314$) versus 2.9% of nonpsychotic controls, including blood donors and outpatients of a local community hospital ($n = 274$). These authors also reported anti-BDV serum antibodies in 12.1% of mental health workers ($n = 82$) and in 8.8% ($n = 132$) of family members of schizophrenic patients. The conclusion was that there exists a positive association with BDV or BDV-like virus infection and schizophrenia in the native population of Taiwan. Age and sex distributions between the psychiatric group and the controls were comparable.

Yamaguchi et al. (1999) investigated serum samples from 3,476 humans with various diseases using an ELISA-type assay. BDV seroprevalence was 3.08% in patients with schizophrenia ($n = 845$) and 3.59% in patients with mood disorders ($n = 251$). BDV seroprevalence was 0% in patients with other psychiatric diseases ($n = 323$), neurological diseases ($n = 114$), CFS ($n = 75$), HIV infection ($n = 85$), rheumatoid arthritis or systemic lupus erythematosus ($n = 50$), or leprosy ($n = 17$) (except for a single patient suffering from alcohol addiction plus AIDS plus dementia). BDV seropositivity was also reported in patients with various ocular diseases (1.36%; $n = 1,393$), blood donors (1.09%; $n = 917$), and patients who had received multiple transfusions (4.55%; $n = 66$). Seroprevalence in patients with schizophrenia was somewhat lower than that in patients with mood disorders; however, seroprevalence was still significantly increased in the schizophrenia group compared to blood donors (note the larger sample size of schizophrenic patients versus the mood disorder group). The patients were recruited from 11 hospitals in Japan. Mean ages were comparable between psychiatric patients and patients with ocular diseases but differed regarding other groups, e.g., blood donors. Sex ratios were comparable in psychiatric patients and patients with ocular diseases but differed in other subgroups, e.g., blood donors versus patients with neurological diseases, with alcohol addiction, with HIV infection, or with autoimmune diseases. The conclusion was that BDV infection seemed associated with psychiatric disorders.

Using the ECLIA method, Rybakowski et al. (2001) found anti-BDV serum antibodies in 2% of psychiatric patients ($n = 816$) recruited from seven regional mental hospitals from western Poland (anti-P and anti-N were tested). A recent-onset disease (ROD) group was arbitrarily defined by duration of symptoms of less than 1 year, in contrast to a long-duration group (LOD), defined by duration of illness of more than 1 year. In the ROD subgroup diagnoses included schizophrenia ($n = 21$) and various other syndromes such as affective and anxiety disorders. BDV seroprevalence in the ROD group was 10.2%, significantly increased compared to the 1.6% in the LOD group. The mean age of patients in the ROD group was 41 years, while that for the LOD group was 53 years. The conclusion was that BDV infection may initiate some psychiatric disorders.

Comment on seroepidemiological studies. The present status of knowledge about the epidemiology of BDV infection in human populations is at best preliminary. The various research groups used different serological methods, and results therefore cannot always be specifically compared. Validity was evaluated as generally acceptable, but some findings raised questions. When considering the major results in these studies with sample sizes of >500, it appears that most studies found an increased BDV seroprevalence in psychiatric patients and also in patients with other infectious disorders or intravenous drug addiction, as well as in contact persons of psychiatric patients. When summing up several studies in which IFA serology was done by one laboratory, a certain similarity of findings is recognized: in human populations from various regions, psychiatric patients rather consistently show an increased BDV seroprevalence (1.6 to 6.8%) compared to healthy or nonpsychiatric controls (0 to 3.5%) (Rott et al., 1985; Amsterdam et al., 1985; Bechter et al., 1987, 1992a). The laboratory doing IFA serology in these studies has accumulated extended experience in diagnostics of natural BD in animals, especially horses. In the horse system it was shown that IFA was highly sensitive and specific, as demonstrated by comparing findings in blood, CSF, and postmortem brains (Herzog et al., 1994). Although not firmly established BDV seroprevalence may increase with age in the healthy population (Bechter et al., 1992, 1998) and in recent-onset psychiatric disorder (Rybakowski et al., 2001), with the latter finding also suggesting that BDV may initiate psychiatric disorders. An increase in BDV seroprevalence in drug addicts (Bode et al., letter, 1988; Bechter et al., 1998) would correlate with a transmissible agent acquired during adolescence or adulthood presumably. However, we cannot exclude the possibility that human anti-BDV antibodies may be recognizing a cross-reacting BDV-related infectious agent (Allmang et al., 2001). Overall the present findings on possible BDV infection in humans are preliminary though intriguing and need further study.

Clinical studies of BDV-seropositive humans

Seroepidemiological studies suggesting that BDV infection may be more frequent in psychiatric patients than in controls and may possibly initiate psychiatric disorders supported the need to address the question of the etiologic, causal, or contributory role of BDV in seropositive patients. Established clinical methods to diagnose previous or active brain infections, brain inflammatory disorders, or neurodevelopmental disturbances include brain imaging and CSF investigation. A few such studies have been done with BDV-seropositive patients.

In two imaging studies, BDV-seropositive psychiatric patient groups were compared to matched seronegative controls. Lateral brain ventricles were larger and whole-brain volumes were smaller when estimated under blinded conditions in BDV-seropositive psychiatric patients with affective disorders or with personality disorders (Bechter et al., 1994). Larger putamen volumes and smaller amygdala-hippocampal complexes were also found in BDV-seropositive schizophrenic patients (Waltrip et al., 1995). These preliminary findings are consistent with an inflammatory-atrophic process initiated by BDV.

Three CSF investigation studies have been performed with BDV seropositive patients. Amsterdam et al. (1985) found no BDV antibodies in the CSF of five BDV-seropositive subjects by IFA. Bechter et al. (1995) detected BDV antibodies in the CSF of 12% (n = 38) of BDV-seropositive patients with acute schizophrenic or affective psychoses. When compared to BDV antibody level in the sera of these patients, the level of BDV-specific antibodies within CSF was considerably increased (CSF index > 10) beyond the level explained by passive transfer of BDV IgG antibodies through the blood-CSF barrier, (normal index value, 1 to 1.5). In samples from a CSF bank of psychiatric (n = 128) and neurological (n = 102) patients, BDV antibodies were found in two patients with major depression and in one patient with cerebrovascular disease (M. Deuschle, L. Bode, I. Heuser, J. Schmider, and H. Ludwig, Letter, *Lancet* **352**:1828–1829, 1998). However, the question as to whether these antibody levels were raised above the level passively transmitted through the blood-CSF barrier could not be addressed because simultaneous serum samples were not available from these subjects.

Mild BDV encephalitis: one possible view of human BD

Established clinical methods such as magnetic resonance imaging (MRI) and CSF investigation may be too insensitive to detect "mild encephalitis," a term proposed recently (Bechter, 1998, 2001a, 2001b). MRI is usually normal even in patients with meningoencephalitis with significant neurological symptoms (Osborn, 1994), and normal lumbar CSF values do not exclude encephalitis (Gerber et al., 1998). To diagnose mild BDV encephalitis by established clinical methods, therefore, may be a matter of chance or timing (e.g., may be possible only during certain disease stages). Thus, the rare cases presenting with CSF pathological findings may demonstrate only the tip of the iceberg.

It is possible that human BDV infection is preferably acquired during immunocompetence, be it during adolescence or adulthood, and that the time point of infection is in some way related to the onset of disease. It is also possible that later reactivation and relapses or even chronic disease can occur. Regardless of timing of infection, there are many that believe that mild BDV encephalitis may represent an underlying cause sufficient to explain one or more psychiatric disorders. Psychiatric disorders induced from mild BDV encephalitis may have a large range of psychiatric symptoms or syndromes, as illustrated by the variability of BD in animals and in diseases caused by other viral etiologies of human psychiatric disorders. In the individual case, the observed psychiatric symptomatology may depend upon contributing factors such as genetic, immunological, and other independent, preexisting factors.

In a recent study of patients with herpes simplex virus encephalitis, it was demonstrated that PCR was the method of choice in diagnostics of early stages of herpes simplex virus encephalitis; however, about 2 weeks later PCR was found to be insensitive, but specific IgG antibodies appeared to increase within CSF (Sauerbrei et al., 2000). In later stages of encephalitis the exclusive pathological finding may indeed be an increase of agent-specific immunoglobulin G beyond the level explained by passive transfer through the blood-brain barrier (Reiber, 1998). When considering the analogous findings in BDV-seropositive humans, mild BDV encephalitis was a plausible hypothesis and interpretation of the findings (Bechter et al., 1995, Bechter 2001a, 2001b). In 12% of acutely diseased BDV-seropositive patients with affective or schizophrenic psychoses, CSF BDV IgG antibodies were increased. BDV-specific IgG was found to be increased within the CSF of one patient during acute schizophrenic psychosis but was normal when investigated 5 years later when the patient was in remission (Bechter et al., 1996). In recent-onset schizophrenia, CSF proteins were increased about twofold above normal during the most acute phase of disease but by only 6 weeks later were normalized (Bechter et al., 1999).

QYNAD is a pentapeptide found to be increased in CSF from patients with various inflammatory neurological disorders including Guillain-Barré syndrome, an autoimmune inflammatory neurological disorder. QYNAD is newly classified as endocaine and may explain part of the disturbed CNS function during inflammatory neurological disorders (Brinkmeier et al., 2000), along with other humoral factors (Waxman, 2000). In four BDV-seropositive patients with therapy-resistant schizophrenic psychosis (one patient; DSM-IV 295.30, ICD-10.F20.09 diagnosis) or therapy-resistant affective disorders (three patients with major depression; DSM-IV 296.2x, ICD-10:F32.x diagnosis), QYNAD in CSF was increased about two- to four-fold above normal (Bechter et al., 2000, 2001a, 2001b). Analyses of the T-cell repertoire of CSF lymphocytes from three of these patients demonstrated oligoclonal expansion of the V-β-chain, to be interpreted as a specific immune activation within the CSF spaces (Oleszak et al., 2001), similar to findings in experimental models of virus-induced autoimmune encephalitis (Oleszak et al., 1995).

Experimental treatments for BDV-seropositive patients

Amantadine. An antiviral activity of amantadine in vitro and a therapeutic effect in vivo in a patient with bipolar depression have been reported (Bode et al., letter, 1997). Several open (nonblinded) clinical trials suggested an antidepressive effect of amantadine in patients assumed to be infected by BDV (Ferszt et al., 1999a, 1999b; Dietrich et al., 2000a, 2000b; Spannhuth et al., 2000). However, while many patients were relatively mildly depressed outpatients, the therapeutic effect was at best moderate, and most importantly, the therapeutic effect did not correlate with detection of BDV. Since an antidepressive effect of amantadine has been reported, presumably related to neuronal transmitter systems (Lieb et al., letter; Huber et al., 1999), the effects of amantadine, if any, on the clinical symptoms of these patients may not be related to effects of amantadine on BDV.

In a recent double-blind, randomized, crossover study, amantadine sulfate was tested against placebo in 10 patients, usually as an add-on medication to an existing antidepressant regimen. This study found that 200 mg of amantadine sulfate daily was significantly superior to placebo (Dietrich et al., 2000b). Again it remains an open question as to whether the improvement from the amantadine medication was related to BDV infection or simply to the known antidepressant effects of amantadine (Huber et al., 1999). In single case trials in standard-therapy-resistant, BDV-seropositive inpatients with severe major depression ($n = 8$; Hamilton depression scale, >28) 200 mg of amantadine daily showed no beneficial effect (K. Bechter, unpublished results).

CSFF. About 10 years ago cerebrospinal fluid filtration (CSFF) was introduced as an experimental treatment in severe Guillain-Barré syndrome resistant to plasmapheresis (Wollinsky et al., 1994). The therapeutic effect of CSFF in Guillain-Barré syndrome was recently shown in a randomized clinical trial (Wollinsky et al., 2001). Now CSFF was more broadly used as an adjuvant therapy in various severe or therapy-resistant CNS inflammatory neurological disorders, including viral or bacterial meningoencephalitis, therapy-resistant lupus erythematosus encephalitis, therapy-resistant MS, and others. It was suggested that filtration reduces the CSF concentrations of various endotoxins or inflammatory cytokines and other possibly damaging proteins or peptides (Rother et al., 1995).

Under the hypothesis that mild BDV encephalitis may underlie some affective or schizophrenic psychoses in BDV-seropositive psychiatric patients, we introduced CSFF in patients with therapy-resistant schizophrenia or major depression (Bechter et al., 1999, 2000, and unpublished). CSFF was performed via a catheter placed into the subarachnoid spaces at a lumbar site, and about 300 ml of CSF was filtered by an automatic syringe pump over a Pall-CSF1E filter daily for 5 consecutive days. During CSFF the previous psychopharmacological treatments remained unchanged. We observed a striking improvement of psychopathology and test performance in the patients experimentally treated thus far ($n = 4$). However, three patients relapsed 1 to 3 weeks after the first CSFF series, but therapeutic effect was again seen after a second CSFF series was initiated, and the therapeutic benefit proved to be of longer duration (catamnesis of 1 to 3 years). Within the CSFs of these patients QYNAD was mildly to moderately increased as compared to that in patients with Guillain-Barré syndrome (Bechter et al., 2000; Bechter, et al., 2001). During CSFF the concentration of QYNAD was reduced to normal levels (unpublished results). The therapeutic effect from CSFF included reduced psychopathology and cognitive disturbances. Cognitive disturbances were therapy resistant prior to CSFF, suggesting that improvement of cognitive disturbances during CSFF was related to removing QYNAD. However, CSFF treatment is in a very early experimental stage, and no conclusions of causal association can be made.

Psychiatry's Role in Identification of the Clinical Outcomes of Human BDV Infection

In this section, the issue of BDV-associated psychiatric disease is placed into the larger framework of psychiatric approaches and accepted wisdom. Clearly, some of the discord among scientists studying the issue of BDV infection of humans relates to the tangible problems within the basic science field, e.g., BDV assays for infection or within the clinical research field, e.g., clinical study design. However, there are also larger issues within the field of psychiatry regarding the assignment of an infectious etiology to a psychiatric disease or diseases.

Symptoms, syndromes, and diagnosis in "organic" psychiatric disorders

Consideration of various organic, infectious, or inflammatory CNS disorders known to underlie psychiatric symptoms and syndromes may help to evaluate possible associations between BDV infection and psychiatric disorders. In recognition of very contrary points of view in current psychiatry (e.g., the outdated terminology of organic brain syndromes according to the DSM-IV authors; Spitzer et al., 1992; Kaplan and Sadock, 1998), it seems appropriate to try to understand apparently similar problems involved in the BD research field.

AERT. According to Bonhoeffer (1917), acute exogenous reaction type (AERT) follows various organic insults to the brain and was characterized by disturbance of consciousness.

MTE. The mixed-type encephalopathies (MTE) are similar to Bonhoeffer's description of AERT and are frequently observed in neurology and intensive care medicine. Diagnosis of MTE is mainly or exclusively based on psychopathology since neurological deficits (e.g., MRI abnormalities) are often lacking, and only severe MTE regularly shows electroencephalogram abnormalities (Niedermeyer et al., 1999). MTE apparently represents an organic brain syndrome, but surprisingly, even with modern technologies, MTE remains difficult or impossible to objectify and, instead, is often diagnosed exclusively from psychopathological symptoms (Niedermeyer et al., 1999). Although the polyetiological origin of MTE is known, specific pathogenesis remains speculative, seemingly related to diffuse and mainly metabolic pathology within the brain (Niedermeyer et al., 1999). Indeed, less-severe brain pathology (compared to MTE) may underlie severe psychiatric disorders.

Chronic organic psychosyndrome or brain syndrome. The concept of a chronic organic psychosyndrome (or brain syndrome) was developed and, according to Kurt Schneider, graded into three levels (Huber, 1999); pseudoneurasthenia (mild), organic personality disorder (medium), and dementia (severe). A prerequisite to diagnose any organic psychosyndrome was that a certain well-described psychopathological syndrome was preceded or paralleled by a sufficient cause (*belangvoller Befund*) to be identified, for example, by electroencephalogram, carotid compression tomography, MRI, laboratory findings, and medical illness.

Symptomatic psychosis. Symptomatic psychosis appears related to identifiable brain pathology associated with psychosis and is another type of organic brain syndrome. This entity is typically an acute or subacute syndrome of schizophrenic or affective type, usually lacking the lead symptom of AERT, disturbed consciousness (Gross et al., 1989; Bechter, in press).

Understanding organic insults and psychiatric disease

Many researchers increasingly recognize the power of analogies evolving from psychiatric disorders termed secondary to medical illness for etiological research on the so-called primary psychiatric disorders (Newport and Nemeroff, 1999). The best-understood example is secondary mania, which is reliably diagnosed and presents with a long list of known but vastly differing etiologies, including even a list of infections (Strakowsky and Sax, 2000). The proximity between entry of an assumed cause and onset of symptoms is considered the most important identifier of a causal link, even when details of the pathogenesis may remain hidden. A full understanding of the pathogenetic chain would indeed be more convincing; however, this may be asking too much. In many human psychiatric disorders as well as infectious diseases, only some relevant or initiating factors are definitely known.

Zarin and Earls (1993) proposed that the formulation of a diagnostic system should be developed with respect to the intended goal; i.e., the clinician needs a diagnostic system that allows him or her to decide what to investigate further in the individual patient, how to evaluate certain findings from evidence with previous or similar cases, and what can be concluded or not from the findings. All available diagnostic systems of psychiatric disorders are based on plausibility, not final proof; therefore, the argument against the concept of organic psychosyndromes that they lack proof (Kaplan and Sadock, 1998) is not convincing. Indeed, researchers on the etiology of psychiatry disorders have accepted the proposed terminology of DSM-IV that any known organic etiologies are termed secondary instead of organic (compare Sax and Strakowsky, 1999).

Researchers are increasingly emphasizing the notion that etiological research may indeed be important to understanding better the so-called primary disorders (Strakowsky and Sax, 2000), which appear to be idiopathic, given that, in medicine, an understanding of etiology is thought to be important for therapy (Newport and Nemeroff, 1999). Primary mania or bipolar disorder, for example, may arise from abnormalities within the same brain regions found to be affected in secondary mania (Strakowsky and Sax, 2000). Going just one step further, the only difference between primary and secondary mania may be the understanding of the initiating step, not yet identified in so-called primary mania. It can be safely stated, at least in known etiologies, that psychiatric syndromes are nonspecific, be they mania, depression, or schizophrenia. Respective known etiologies are overshadowed by a long list of rare but possible etiologies. Over time, the contribution of viral infections has been assumed to be both low and high, and in any case, viruses still remain a hypothetical cause of psychiatric disease (Yolken and Torrey, 2000).

Organic psychiatric disease with known etiology but multiple disease manifestations: Huntington's disease. In contrast to the well-defined but poorly explained examples of organic psychosyndromes or psychiatric disorders, consider the etiology of Huntington's disease, now clearly defined by expanded triplet repeats in the genome. Clinical diagnosis can be easily made by the characteristic motor symptoms. However, a variety of psychiatric symptoms can be observed preceding the onset of motor symptoms or may even remain the only clinical manifestation of Huntington's disease. These psychiatric manifestations may range from nonspecific personality problems to minor symptoms such as apathy or sleep disorder, to alcohol abuse, to symptomatic schizophrenia, to symptomatic obsessive-compulsive disorder, or to so-called organic personality disorder. Surprisingly, a considerable number of people with triplet repeats remains free of symptoms (Shiwach, 1994; Wagle et al., 2000). Thus, despite having a defined genetic etiology, Huntington's disease is an impressive example of the nonspecificity of psychiatric symptoms, since the reason for these vast differences in disease manifestations remains unknown.

Psychiatric symptoms and syndromes related to known infectious or inflammatory CNS disorders. *Syphilis and GP.* There are many examples of psychiatric disorders from underlying brain infectious and/or inflammatory disorders (Lishman, 1998), including large epidemics or endemics with broad impact on clinical psychiatry. The most important example of an infectious brain disorder with a greater likelihood of psychiatric than neurological symptoms was GP, a form of chronic syphilis and the etiology behind about 20% of psychiatric disorders treated in European psychiatric clinics around 1900. Today, research history on GP often seems misunderstood (Bechter, 1995). An initial hypothesis that syphilis represented an underestimated risk factor of GP was formulated in 1857 by Esmarch and Jessen, but it took about 20 years until this hypothesis was confirmed in systematic epidemiological studies showing that syphilis frequently preceded GP (performed by Mendel around 1880). However, although these studies showed a high incidence of syphilis before the onset of GP, Mendel's conclusion was vigorously disputed and resulted in a more cautious reformulating of the hypothesis, suggesting that syphilis represented just one among many other risk factors. Subsequently, however, epidemiological studies replicated and extended Mendel's findings. Later, by using refined methods, the proportion of cases preceded by syphilis was recognized to be even higher and the hypothesis that syphilis was an important risk factor was generally accepted. Histopathologists had long argued against a causal model, because brain inflammation was prominent in acute syphilis whereas neuronal degeneration was characteristic of GP.

Newly introduced methods (e.g., serology according to the Wassermann reaction or CSF investigation by lumbar puncture according to the method of Quincke) and postmortem detection of spirochetes (in few brains) by Noguchi and Moore in 1913 completed the evidence that syphilis was the cause of GP. Nevertheless, the idea that syphilis might be the underlying cause of GP continued to be criticized until about 1900 or even until 1910. Finally around 1930, when many clinical studies had addressed such aspects as familiarity, transmission, and course of disease, sufficient evidence was accumulated to support the infectious causality hypothesis, arguing against the hereditary hypothesis or a type of vulnerability stress model. Furthermore, degenerative phenomena similar to findings in GP were demonstrated to occur similarly within the brains of dogs with experimental trypanosomiasis, and so recognizing degeneration as one specific type of pathogenesis in infectious brain disorders completed the pathogenetic puzzle. In retrospect, from a clinician's point of view, the most critical enigma for elucidation of causality of spirochetes for GP was that only about 4% of individuals suffering from syphilis eventually developed GP; in other words, the low pathogenicity risk confused and weak-ened causal conclusions. It is interesting that the hypothesis arose from the few cases in whom GP developed very rapidly soon after primary acute syphilis, critically observed and interpreted by gifted clinicians (Esmarch and Jessen, 1857), although not formulated specifically as a causality hy-pothesis. It is further interesting to note that the degenerative phenomena in GP or, similarly, in HIV infection, are still not well understood today.

HIV. The HIV epidemic is a large, current medical problem, and psy-chiatric syndromes are often related to HIV infection. Surprisingly, although a lot of postmortem brains have been investigated and several ex-perimental models exist, the pathogenesis of HIV-associated psychiatric syndromes is not sufficiently understood (for reviews, see Kaul [2001] and Rausch and Stover [2001]). HIV invasion into the brain probably occurs soon after infection, but only a proportion of infected patients develop AIDS dementia complex (ADC), often years after infection. ADC only poorly correlates with inflammatory cell numbers within the brain but rather seems related to poorly defined humoral factors, possibly produced by inflammatory cells. A variety of psychiatric syndromes are found to be increased in HIV-infected people, with ADC representing just a severe, late stage preceded by nonspecific symptoms or so-called organic brain syn-dromes, ranging from pseudoneurasthenia to organic personality disor-der. In some patients symptomatic psychoses are observed, although the frequency of such psychoses is not very high (Perkins et al., 1993, 1995, Maj et al., 1994; Huber, 1999; Rabkin et al., 1997; Baldassarre et al., 1998; Carson et al., 1998; Susser et al., 1997; Sax and Strakowsky, 1999). Symptomatic psychoses include manic-depressive or schizophrenic types and appear re-lated to an underlying organic brain pathology resulting from HIV infec-tion. A recently proposed model of the pathological interacting processes leading to CNS disease in a portion of HIV-infected patients (Garther and Liu, 2002) is very tempting and would fit in well with or demonstrate one case of the mild encephalitis hypothesis of psychiatric disorder.

Other examples. Other well-known but not well-understood examples of infectious or inflammatory CNS disorders present with a broad variety of psychiatric syndromes, apparently resulting from organic or brain pathological processes (Lishman, 1998; Strakowsky and Sax, 2000). For ex-ample, a disease often hypothesized to have an infectious etiology or trig-ger, MS, is sometimes preceded and frequently accompanied by depression or difficult-to-classify psychiatric disturbances or symptomatic psychoses (Skegg et al., 1988; Stenager and Jensen, 1988). Lyme disease may be ac-companied or preceded by various psychiatric syndromes such as para-noia, dementia, schizophrenia, bipolar disorder, panic attacks, major de-pression, anorexia, or other difficult-to-classify depressive states, although the majority of cases present with a characteristic neurological syndrome (Logigian et al., 1990; Fallon and Nields, 1994; Oschmann et al., 1998).

Prenatal or perinatal infections. Generally, symptoms in pre- or perinatal infection are early and rather severe compared to adult infections with the same agents. For example, symptoms and brain findings in transplacental or intrapartum HIV infection are more severe and disease course is more rapidly progressive than in adult infection (Rausch and Stover, 2001). Prenatal rubella syndrome is a comparably well-studied infection that often induces a neurodevelopmental disorder. In an original birth cohort prenatally exposed to the 1964 rubella pandemic in New York, there was an increased risk of autism, separation anxiety disorder, and impaired social relations (Chess et al., 1971). In part of this cohort a recent follow-up investigation analyzed participants who reached a mean age of 33.8 years (Brown et al., 2001). Of these individuals only 41.5% remained healthy (without any psychiatric diagnoses), 20% presented with schizophrenia spectrum disorders, 26% presented with affective disorders, and 12.5% presented with childhood disorders and atypical psychiatric or psychosocial problems. Within the schizophrenia spectrum disorder group, a subgroup developed schizophrenic-type psychosis preceded by a continuous decline of intelligence quotient (IQ) from childhood to adolescence. Overall risk of schizophrenia spectrum disorders was 10-fold increased in the rubella-exposed birth cohort, and this finding was considered to indicate a causal relationship, although definite pathogenesis of psychiatric disorders remained open. The authors suggested that rubella infection may have initiated a cascade of events in the developmental framework and that these data support the neurodevelopmental hypothesis of schizophrenia. On the other hand, the authors recognized another study, showing that active rubella infection persisted in some infants as late as 18 months following birth (South and Sever, 1985); thus, continuous viral effects on brain development during the postnatal period therefore cannot be excluded. Some active, mild inflammation may possibly continue for years until adolescence or adulthood, also explaining the continuous decline of IQ and development of schizophrenic psychosis only in a subgroup over time. Indeed, some indication of continuous inflammatory processes over the years appears to exist in prenatal rubella syndrome (Craighead, 2000).

Etiology, pathogenesis, causality, and organic brain syndrome: a critical reconsideration

Most human disorders have a multiconditional etiopathogenesis, especially medical disorders with unknown etiology and pathogenesis, when relevant factors are not yet identified. An example is gastric ulcer, explained over many years by an interactional psycho-acido-stress model. Now an infection with *Helicobacter pylori* is understood to be the most important etiological or causal factor (conditio sine qua non), although this pathogen is neither present in all gastric ulcers nor independent from other contributing factors. However, when *H. pylori* is successfully treated, other contributing factors seem no longer to be relevant. So is *H. pylori* causal then? In our usual understanding of causality, probably yes.

It seems that etiology and pathogenesis are often not exactly defined and not unambiguously understood. For example, we usually consider a bone fracture as causally related to a preceding crash or insult. However, other contributing factors may be even more important when considering the whole interactional framework, including factors leading eventually to the crash or insult. For the surgeon's view it is sufficient and important to consider whether a crash and related circumstances were sufficient to explain the fracture; if there are doubts, the surgeon should investigate whether predisposing factors such as osteoporosis, endocrine abnormalities, or hereditary bone disease may have contributed to the fracture. For the epidemiologist, it might be important to understand psychological factors or factors in the environment (e.g., car traffic or weather) contributing to the event, and from the epidemiologist's view it might be important to recommend educational programs or improve traffic regulation to prevent bone fractures in a general population. In fact, the approach of preventing bone fractures might be superior to research on surgical treatments.

The example of bone fracture is a simple one because the immediate pathogenetic chain is short. However, in psychiatric disorders the pathogenetic chain appears extended, and therefore the importance of single or initiating factors is more likely confused, hidden, or weakened. Broad scientific approaches are generally required to understand all contributing factors but may not be helpful when trying to understand relevant factors. One single initiating factor may make the difference. The above analogies illustrate the present problems of diagnostic categorization and understanding pathogenesis of psychiatric disorders.

In conclusion, many factors contribute to disease but may not necessarily exclude a specific, causal factor. For causal inferences there is no absolute need to understand any detail of pathogenesis, and it may be sufficient to recognize only a definite time relationship between the initiating event and the outcome. However, when regarding infectious or inflammatory brain disorders, a time relationship will be difficult to demonstrate if inflammation is mild, persistent, and insidious in onset and leads slowly to pathologic change of the CNS, as suggested for human BDV infections. In addition, the relationship between brain pathology and development of psychiatric symptoms is generally weak and therefore confusing for re-search approaches, because the importance of single factors is hard to determine. Furthermore, dysfunction of certain brain systems or of neurons does not always mean disease (Klein, 1999). Compensatory mechanisms may counteract and may differ in various individuals or at various time points, since the "fantastically complex brain" (Klein, 1999) is immanently difficult to understand even by complex research approaches and techni-cal tools.

Pathogenicity (the ratio of diseased to infected patients) is low in most viral and bacterial infections (Anderson and May, 1991; Mims et al., 1995). For example, only about 4 to 8% of individuals with syphilis eventually develop GP, or only about 2% of people infected by poliovirus develop paresis. This makes research on diseases in populations rather confusing in that seroprevalence rates in those with disease may be similar to those in the normal population.

Klein (1999) concluded that a causal relationship should have two components: "that something has really gone wrong involuntarily (dis-ease) and the results (illness) are sufficiently major to ratify the exempt sick role." This proposal is convincing although difficult to establish in clinical settings. Well-accepted diagnostic systems often cannot provide reliable criteria for how findings are to be evaluated and how causal relationships are to be identified. But apparently only a combination of clinical and epi-demiological findings, experience with many psychiatric disorders with identified etiologies and treatments, and analogies to experimental and natural infections will allow causal conclusions to be drawn. The impor-tance of a broad view was elegantly illustrated by van Praag (2000). He compared the problems of psychiatric diagnostics with a simple problem in internal medicine: the definition of pathological blood pressure, which was not determined by statistical abnormality within a population but came from understanding the harmful role of blood pressure when in-creased over some level, correlated with risk of reduced life expectancy.

The primary research goal in elucidating the possible association of BDV with human psychiatric disorders should be to identify the initiating event and relevant factors, closely guided by experience in research in other infectious or inflammatory neurological disorders and by develop-ing new sensitive diagnostic approaches.

REFERENCES

Allmang, U. M. Hofer, S. Herzog, K. Bechter, and P. Staeheli. 2001. Low avidity of human serum antibodies for Borna disease virus antigens questions their diagnostic value. *Mol. Psychiatry* 6:329–333.

Amsterdam, J. D., A. Winokur, W. Dyson, S. Herzog, F. Gonzalez, R. Rott, and H. Koprowski. 1985. Borna disease virus: a possible etiologic factor in human affective disorders? *Arch. Gen. Psychiatry* **42:**1093–1096.

Anderson, R. M., and R. M. May. 1991. *Infectious Diseases of Humans, Dynamics and Control.* Oxford University Press, Oxford, United Kingdom.

Auwanit, W., P. I. Ayuthaya, T. Nakaya S. Fujiwara, T. Kurata, K. Yamanishi, and K. Ikuta. 1996. Unusually high seroprevalence of Borna disease virus in clade E human immunodeficiency virus type 1-infected patients with sexually transmitted diseases in Thailand. *Clin. Diagn. Lab. Immunol.* **3:**590–593.

Baaré, W. F., C. J. van Oel, H. E. Hulshoff, H. G. Schnack, S. Durston, M. M. Sitskoorn, and R. S. Kahn. 2001. Volumes of brain structures in twins discordant for schizophrenia. *Arch. Gen. Psychiatry* **58:**33–40.

Bachmann, S., P. Caplazi, M. Fischer, F. Ehrensperger, and R. W. Cone. 1999. Lack of association between Borna disease virus infection and neurological disorders among HIV-infected individuals. *J. Neurovirol.* **5:**190–195.

Baldassarre, S. F., C. Blancolilli, F. M. Serpelloni, and L. Bartoli. 1998. Early neuropsychological impairment in HIV-seropositive intravenous drug users: evidence from the Italian multicentre neuropsychological HIV study. *Acta Psychiatr. Scand* **97:**132–138.

Bechter, K. 1995. Research strategies in 'slow' infections in psychiatry. *Hist. Psychiatry* **6:**503–511.

Bechter, K. 1998. Borna Disease Virus. Mögliche Ursache neurologischer und psychiatrischer Störungen des Menschen, vol. 89. *In* H. Hippius, W. Janzarik, and C. Müller (ed.), *Monographien aus dem Gesamtgebiete der Psychiatrie.* Steinkopff, Darmstadt, Germany.

Bechter, K. 2001a. Mild encephalitis underlying psychiatric disorder—a reconsideration and hypothesis exemplified on Borna disease. *Neurol. Psychiatry Brain Res.* **9:**55–70.

Bechter, K. 2001b. New findings suggesting that mild Borna disease virus encephalitis underlies some affective or schizophrenic disorders and experimental treatments. *Adv. Biol. Psychiatr.* **20:**53–60.

Bechter, K. Basic symptoms in symptomatic schizophrenia. *Neurol. Psychiatry Brain Res.,* in press.

Bechter, K., M. Bauer, H. C. Estler, S. Herzog, R. Schüttler, and R. Rott. 1994. MRI findings in Borna disease virus seropositive psychiatric patients and controls an extended study. *Nervenarzt* **65:**169–174.

Bechter, K., S. Herzog, P. Aulkemeyer, F. Weber, and H. Brinkmeier. 2001. Detecting the endocaine QYNAD within cerebrospinal fluids of patients with Borna virus-related psychosis. *World J. Biol. Psychiatry* **2:**59S.

Bechter, K., S. Herzog, W. Behr, and R. Schüttler. 1995. Investigations of cerebrospinal fluid in Borna disease virus seropositive psychiatric patients. *Eur. Psychiatry* **10:**250–258.

Bechter, K., S. Herzog, H. C. Estler, and R. Schüttler. 1998. Increased psychiatric comorbidity in Borna disease virus seropositive psychiatric patients. *Acta Psychiatr. Belg.* **98:**190–204.

Bechter, K., S. Herzog, B. Fleischer, R. Schüttler, and R. Rott. 1987. Magnetic resonance imaging in psychiatric patients with and without serum antibodies against Borna disease. *Nervenarzt* **58:**617–624.

Bechter, K., S. Herzog, V. Schreiner, H. Brinkmeier, P. Aulkemeyer, F. Weber, and R. Schüttler. 2000. Borna disease virus related therapy resistant depression improved after cerebrospinal fluid filtration. *J. Psychiatr. Res.* **34:**393–396.

Bechter, K., S. Herzog, V. Schreiner, K. W. Wollinsky, and R. Schüttler. 1999. Cerebrospinal fluid filtration in a case of schizophrenia related to 'subclinical' Borna disease virus encephalitis, p. 19–35. *In* N. Müller (ed.), *Psychiatry Psychoneuroimmunology, and Viruses. Key Top Brain Research.* Springer, Vienna, Austria.

Bechter, K., S. Herzog, and R. Schüttler. 1992a. Possible significance of Borna disease for humans. *Neurol. Psychiatry Brain Res.* **1**:23–29.

Bechter, K., S. Herzog, and R. Schüttler. 1992b. Borna disease virus. Possible causal agent in psychiatric and neurological disorders in two families. *Psychiatry Res.* **42**:291–294.

Bechter, K., S. Herzog, and R. Schüttler. 1992c. Case of neurological and behavioral abnormalities: due to Borna disease virus encephalitis? *Psychiatry Res.* **42**:193–196.

Bechter, K., S. Herzog, and R. Schüttler. 1996. Borna disease virus: possible cause of human neuropsychiatric disorders. *Neurol. Psychiatry Brain Res.* **4**:45–52.

Bode, L., R. Durrwald, F. A. Rantam, R. Ferszt, and H. Ludwig. 1996. First isolates of infectious human Borna disease virus from patients with mood disorders. *Mol. Psychiatry* **1**:200–212.

Bode, L., R. Ferszt, and G. Czech. 1993. Borna disease virus infection and affective disorders in man. *Arch. Virol.* **7**(Suppl.):159–167.

Bode, L., P. Reckwald, W. E. Severus, R. Stoyloff, R. Ferszt, D. E. Dietrich, and H. Ludwig. 2001. Borna disease virus-specific circulating immune complexes, antigenemia, and free antibodies—the key marker triplet determining infection and prevailing in severe mood disorders. *Mol. Psychiatry* **6**:481–491.

Bode, L., S. Riegel, W. Lange, and H. Ludwig. 1992. Human infections with Borna disease virus: seroprevalence in patients with chronic diseases and healthy individuals. *J. Med. Virol.* **36**:309–315.

Bode, L., W. Zimmermann, R. Ferszt, F. Steinbach, and H. Ludwig. 1995. Borna disease virus genome transcribed and expressed in psychiatric patients. *Nat. Med.* **1**:232–236.

Bonhoeffer, K. 1917. Die exogenen Reaktionstypen. *Arch. Psychiatr. Nervenkr.* **58**:58–70.

Briese, T., J. C. de la Torre, A. Lewis, H. Ludwig, and W. I. Lipkin. 1992. Borna disease virus, a negative-strand RNA virus, transcribes in the nucleus of infected cells. *Proc. Natl. Acad. Sci. USA* **89**:11486–11489.

Briese, T., M. Hornig, and W. I. Lipkin. 1999. Bornavirus immunopathogenesis in rodents: models for human neurological diseases. *J. Neurovirol.* **5**:604–612.

Briese, T., A. Schneemann, A. Lewis, A. J. Park, S. Kim, H. Ludwig, and W. I. Lipkin. 1994. Genomic organization of Borna disease virus. *Proc. Natl. Acad. Sci. USA* **91**:4362–4366.

Brinkmejer, H., P. Aulkemeyer, K. H. Wollinsky, and R. Rudel. 2000. An endogenous pentapeptide acting as a sodium channel blocker in inflammatory autoimmune disorders of the central nervous system. *Nat. Med.* **6**:808–811.

Brown, A. S., P. Cohen, J. Harkavy-Friedman, V. Babulas, D. Malaspina, J. M. Gorman, and E. S. Susser. 2001. Prenatal rubella, premorbid abnormalities, and adult schizophrenia. *Biol. Psychiatry* **49**:473–486.

Buchsbaum, M. S., and R. O. Rieder. 1979. Biologic heterogeneity and psychiatric research. *Arch. Gen. Psychiatry* **36**:1163–1169.

Carbone, K. M., T. R. Moench, and W. I. Lipkin. 1991. Borna disease virus replicates in astrocytes, Schwann cells and ependymal cells in persistently infected rats: location of viral genomic and messenger RNAs by in situ hybridization. *J. Neuropathol. Exp. Neurol.* **50**:205–214.

Carson, A. J., R. Sandler, F. N. Owino, F. O. G. Matete, and E. C. Johnstone. 1998. Psychological morbidity and HIV in Kenya. *Acta Psychiatr. Scand.* **97**:267–271.

Chen, C. H., Y. L. Chiu, F. C. Wei, F. J. Koong, H. C. Liu, C. K. Shaw, H. G. Hwu, and K. J. Hsiao. 1999. High seroprevalence of Borna virus infection in schizophrenic patients, family members and mental health workers in Taiwan. *Mol. Psychiatry* **4**:33–38.

Chess, S., S. Korn, and P. Fernandez. 1971. Psychiatric disorders of children with congenital rubella. Brunner/Mazel, New York, N. Y.

Cooper, J. E. 1995. On the publication of the Diagnostic and Statistical Manual of Mental Disorders: Fourth Edition (DSM-IV). *Br. J. Psychiatry* **166**:4–8.

Craighead, J. E. 2000. *Pathology and Pathogenesis of Human Viral Disease.* Academic Press, San Diego, Calif.

Cubitt, B., and J. C. de la Torre. 1997. Amantadine does not have antiviral activity against Borna disease virus. *Arch. Virol.* **142:**2035–2042.

Cubitt, B., C. Oldstone, and J. C. de la Torre. 1994. Sequence and genome organization of Borna disease virus. *J. Virol.* **68:**1382–1396.

Czygan, M., W. Hallensleben, M. Hofer, S. Pollak, C. Sauder, T. Bilzer, I. Blumcke, P. Riederer, B. Bogerts, P. Falkai, M. J. Schwarz, E. Masliah, P. Staeheli, F. T. Hufert, and K. Lieb. 1999. Borna disease virus in human brains with a rare form of hippocampal degeneration but not in brains of patients with common neuropsychiatric disorders. *J. Infect. Dis.* **180:**1695–1699.

Davies, J. R., Grunert, R. R., and C. E. Hoffmann. 1965. Influenza virus growth and antibody response in amantadine-treated mice. *J. Immunol.* **95:**1090–1094.

de la Torre, J. C., L. Bode, R. Durrwald, B. Cubitt, and H. Ludwig. 1996. Sequence characterization of human Borna disease virus. *Virus Res.* **44:**33–44.

Dietrich, D. E., L. Bode, C. W. Spannhuth, T. Lau, T. J. Huber, B. Brodhun, H. Ludwig, and H. M. Emrich. 2000a. Amantadine in depressive patients with Borna disease virus (BDV) infection an open trial. *Bipol. Disord.* **2:**65–70.

Dietrich, D. E., A. Kleinschmidt, U. Hauser, U. Schneider, C. W. Spannhuth, K. Kipp, T. J. Huber, B. M. Wieringa, H. M. Emrich, and S. Johannes. 2000b. Word recognition memory before and after successful treatment of depression. *Pharmacopsychiatry* **33:**221–228.

Eaves, L. 1988. Genetics, immunology, and virology. *Schizophr. Bull.* **14:**365–382.

Esmarch, F., and W. Jessen. 1857. Syphilis und Geistesstörung. *Allg. Z. Psychiatr.* **14:**20–36.

Evengard, B., T. Briese, G. Lindh, S. Lee, and W. I. Lipkin. 1999. Absence of evidence of Borna disease virus infection in Swedish patients with chronic fatigue syndrome. *J. Neurovirol.* **5:**495–499.

Fallon, B. A., and J. A. Nields. 1994. Lyme disease: a neuropsychiatric illness. *Am. J. Psychiatry* **151:**1571–1583.

Ferszt, R., K. P. Kühl, L. Bode, E. W. Severus, B. Winzer, A. Berghofer, G. Beelitz, B. Brodhun, B. Müller-Oerlinghausen, and H. Ludwig. 1999a. Amantadine revisited: an open trial of amantadinesulfate treatment in chronically depressed patients with Borna disease virus infection. *Pharmacopsychiatry* **32:**142–147.

Ferszt, R., E. Severus, L. Bode, M. Brehm, K. P. Kühl, H. Berzewski, and H. Ludwig. 1999b. Activated Borna disease virus in affective disorders. *Pharmacopsychiatry* **32:**93–98.

Formella, S., C. Jehle, C. Sauder, P. Staeheli, and M. Schwemmle. 2000. Sequence variability of Borna disease virus: resistance to superinfection may contribute to high genome stability in persistently infected cells. *J. Virol.* **74:**7878–7883.

Fu, Z. F., J. D. Amsterdam, M. Kao, V. Shankar, H. Koprowski, and B. Dietzschold. 1993. Detection of Borna disease virus-reactive antibodies from patients with affective disorders by western immunoblot technique. *J. Affect. Disord.* **27:**61–68.

Fukuda, K., K. Takahashi, Y. Iwata, N. Mori, K. Gonda, T. Ogawa, K. Osonoe, M. Sato, S. Ogata, T. Horimoto, T. Sawada, M. Tashiro, K. Yamaguchi, S. Niwa, and S. Shigeta. 2001. Immunological and PCR analyses for Borna disease virus in psychiatric patients and blood donors in Japan. *J. Clin. Microbiol.* **39:**419–429.

Furrer, E., T. Bilzer, L. Stitz, and O. Planz. 2001. Neutralizing antibodies in persistent Borna disease virus infection: prophylactic effect of gp94-specific monoclonal antibodies in preventing encephalitis. *J. Virol.* **75:**943–951.

Ganguli, R., B. S. Rabin, and J. S. Brar. 1992. Antinuclear and gastric parietal cell autoantibodies in schizophrenic patients. *Biol. Psychiatry* **32:**735–738.

Gartner, S., and Y. Lin. 2002. Insights into the role of immune activation in HIV neuropathogenesis. *J. Neurovirol.* **8:**69–75.

Gerber, J., H. Tumani, H. Kolenda, and R. Nau. 1998. Lumbar and ventricular CSF protein, leukocytes, and lactate in suspected bacterial CNS infections. *Neurology* 51:1710–1714.

Giedd, J. N. 2001. Neuroimaging of pediatric neuropsychiatric disorders. Is a picture really worth a thousand words? *Arch. Gen. Psychiatry* 58:443–444.

Goldberg, T. E., and D. R. Weinberger. 1995. A case against subtyping in schizophrenia. *Schizophr. Res.* 17:147–152.

Gonzalez-Dunia, D., B. Cubitt, F. A. Grasser, and J. C. de la Torre. 1997. Characterization of Borna disease virus p56 protein, a surface glycoprotein involved in virus entry. *J. Virol.* 71:3208–3218.

Gonzalez-Dunia, D., M. Watanabe, S. Syan, M. Mallory, E. Masliah, and J. C. de la Torre. 2000. Synaptic pathology in Borna disease virus persistent infection. *J. Virol.* 74:3441–3448.

Gross, G., and G. Huber. 1993. Premorbid personality in schizophrenia: the contribution of European long-term studies. *Neurol. Psychiatry Brain Res.* 2:14–20.

Gross, G., G. Huber, and M. Linz. 1989. The problem of 'symptomatic schizophrenia' and 'symptomatic cyclothymia'. *Zentbl. Neurol. Psychiatr.* 251:323–332.

Gutierrez, J., and C. Maroto. 1996. Are IgG antibody avidity assays useful in the diagnosis of infectious diseases? A review. *Microbios* 87:113–121.

Haga, S., M. Yoshimura, Y. Motoi, K. Arima, T. Aizawa, K. Ikuta, M. Tashiro, and K. Ikeda. 1997. Detection of Borna disease virus genome in normal human brain tissue. *Brain Res.* 770:307–309.

Hallensleben, W., M. Zocher, and P. Staehell. 1997. Borna disease virus is not sensitive to amantadine. *Arch. Virol.* 142:2043–2048.

Hartmann, L. 1998. Child and adolescent psychiatry research remains a challenge. *Am. J. Psychiatry* 155:453–454.

Herzog, S., K. Frese, J. A. Richt, and R. Rott. 1994. Ein Beitrag zur Epizootiologie der Bornaschen Krankheit beim Pferd. *Wien. Tierarztl. Monschr.* 81:374–379.

Herzog, S., I. Pfeuffer, K. Haberzetti, H. Feldmann, K. Frese, K. Bechter, and J. A. Richt. 1997. Molecular characterization of Borna disease virus from naturally infected animals and possible links to human disorders. *Arch. Virol.* 131(Suppl.):183–190.

Horimoto, T., H. Takahashi, M. Sakaguchi, K. Horikoshi, S. Iritani, H. Kazamatsuri, K. Ikeda, and M. Tashiro. 1997. A reverse-type sandwich enzyme-linked immunosorbent assay for detecting antibodies to Borna disease virus. *J. Clin. Microbiol.* 35:1661–1666.

Huber, G. 1999. *Psychiatrie. Lehrbuch für Studierende und Ärzte*, 6th ed. Schattauer, Stuttgart, Germany.

Huber, T. J., D. E. Dietrich, and H. M. Emrich. 1999. Possible use of amantadine in depression. *Pharmacopsychiatry* 32:47–55.

Iwahashi, K., M. Watanabe, K. Nakamura, H. Suwaki, T. Nakaya, Y. Nakamura, H. Takahashi, and K. Ikuta. 1997. Clinical investigation of the relationship between Borna disease virus (BDV) infection and schizophrenia in 67 patients in Japan. *Acta Psychiatr. Scand.* 96:412–415.

Iwata, Y., K. Takahashi, X. Peng, K. Fukuda, K. Ohno, T. Ogawa, K. Gonda, N. Mori, S. Niwa, and S. Shigeta. 1998. Detection and sequence analysis of Borna disease virus p24 RNA from peripheral blood mononuclear cells of patients with mood disorders or schizophrenia and of blood donors. *J. Virol.* 72:10044–10049.

Johnstone, E. C., J. Connelly, C. D. Frith, M. T. Lambert, and D. G. C. Owens. 1996. The nature of 'transient' and 'partial' psychoses: findings from the Northwick Park 'functional' psychosis study. *Psychol. Med.* 26:361–369.

Kaplan, H. I., and B. J. Sadock. 1998. *Kaplan and Sadock's Synopsis of Psychiatry Behavioral Sciences/Clinical Psychiatry*, 8th ed. Williams & Wilkins, Baltimore, Md.

Karlsson, H., S. Bachmann, J. Schröder, J. McArthur, E. F. Torrey, and R. H. Yolken. 2001. Retroviral RNA identified in the cerebrospinal fluids and brains of individuals with schizophrenia. *Proc. Natl. Acad. Sci. USA* **98:**4634–4639.

Kaul, M., G. A. Garden, and S. A. Lipton. 2001. Pathways to neuronal injury and apoptosis in HIV-associated dementia. *Nature* **410:**988–994.

Kim, Y. K., S. H. Kim, S. H. Choi, Y. H. Ko, L. Kim, M. S. Lee, K. Y. Suh, D. I. Kwak, K. J. Song, Y. J. Lee, R. Yanagihara, and J. W. Song. 1999. Failure to demonstrate Borna disease virus genome in peripheral blood mononuclear cells from psychiatric patients in Korea. *J. Neurovirol.* **5:**196–199.

Kishi, M., Y. Arimura, K. Ikuta, Y. Shoya, P. K. Lai, and M. Kakinuma. 1996. Sequence variability of Borna disease virus open reading frame II found in human peripheral blood mononuclear cells. *J. Virol.* **70:**635–640.

Kishi, M., T. Nakaya, Y. Nakamura, M. Kakinuma, T. A. Takahashi, S. Sekiguchi, M. Uchikawa, K. Tadokoro, K. Ikeda, and K. Ikuta. 1995a. Prevalence of Borna disease virus RNA in peripheral blood mononuclear cells from blood donors. *Med. Microbiol. Immunol.* **184:**135–138.

Kishi, M., T. Nakaya, Y. Nakamura, Q. Zhong, K. Ikeda, M. Senjo, M. Kakinuma, S. Kato, and K. Ikuta. 1995b. Demonstration of human Borna disease virus RNA in human peripheral blood mononuclear cells. *FEBS Lett.* **364:**293–297.

Kitani, T., H. Kuratsune, I. Fuke, Y. Nakamura, T. Nakaya, S. Asahi, M. Tobiume, K. Yamaguti, T. Machii, R. Inagi, K. Yamanishi, and K. Ikuta. 1996. Possible correlation between Borna disease virus infection and Japanese patients with chronic fatigue syndrome. *Microbiol. Immunol.* **40:**459–462.

Klein, D. F. 1999. Harmful dysfunction, disorder, disease, illness and evolution. *J. Abnorm. Psychol.* **108:**421–429.

Knight, J., A. Knight and G. Ungvari. 1992. Can autoimmune mechanisms account for the genetic predisposition to schizophrenia? *Br. J. Psychiatry* **160:**533–540.

Kringlen, E. 1994. Is the concept of schizophrenia useful from an aetiological point of view? A selective review of findings and paradoxes. *Acta Psychiatr. Scand.* **90**(Suppl. 384)**:**17–25.

Kubo, K., T. Fujiyoshi, M. M. Yokoyama, K. Kamei, J. A. Richt, B. Kitze, S. Herzog, M. Takigawa, and S. Sonoda. 1997. Lack of association of Borna disease virus and human T-cell leukemia virus type 1 infections with psychiatric disorders among Japanese patients. *Clin. Diagn. Lab. Immunol.* **4:**189–194.

Lange, W., and G. Jaeschke. 1987. Influenza epidemic in horses in West Berlin 1983–1985. 2. Virological and serological findings. *Dtsch. Tierarztl. Wochenschr.* **94:**157–160. (In German.)

Legros, S., J. Mendlewicz, and J. Wybran. 1985. Immunoglobulins, autoantibodies and other serum protein fractions in psychiatric disorders. *Eur. Arch. Psychiatry Neurol. Sci.* **235:**9–11.

Lehtonen, O. P., and O. H. Maurman. 1986. Avidity of IgG antibodies against mumps, parainfluenza 2 and Newcastle disease viruses after mumps infection. *J. Virol. Methods* **14:**1–7.

Licinio, J., and M. L. Wong. 1999. The role of inflammatory mediators in the biology of major depression: central nervous system cytokines modulate the biological substrate of depressive symptoms, regulate stress-responsive systems, and contribute to neurotoxicity and neuroprotection. *Mol. Psychiatry* **4:**317–327.

Lishman, W. A. 1998. *Organic Psychiatry. The Psychological Consequences of Cerebral Disorder,* 3rd ed. Blackwell Science, Oxford, United Kingdom.

Logigian, E. L., R. F. Kaplan, and A. C. Steere. 1990. Chronic neurologic manifestations of Lyme disease. *N. Engl. J. Med.* **323:**1438–1444.

Ludwig, H., and L. Bode. 2000. Borna disease virus: new aspects on infection, disease, diagnosis and epidemiology. *Rev. Sci. Tech.* **19:**259–288.

Maj, M., R. Jannsen, F. Starace, M. Zaudig, P. Satz, B. Sughondhabirom, M. A. Luabeya, R. Riedel, D. Ndetei, and H. M. Calil. 1994. WHO neuropsychiatric AIDS study, cross-sectional phase I. *Arch. Gen. Psychiatry* **51:**39–49.

Menninger, K. A. 1928. The schizophrenic syndrome as a product of acute infectious disease. *Arch. Neurol. Psychiatry* **20:**464–481.

Menninger, K. A. 1994. Influenza and schizophrenia. *Am. J. Psychiatry* **151:**183–187.

Mims, C. A., N. J. Dimmock, A. Nash, and J. Stephen. 1995. *Mims' Pathogenesis of Infectious Disease,* 4th ed. Academic Press, London, United Kingdom.

Moryl, E., W. Danysz, and G. Quack. 1993. Potential antidepressive properties of amantadine, memantine and bifemelane. *Pharmacol. Toxicol.* **72:**394–397.

Müller, N., M. Riedel, M. Ackenheil, and M. J. Schwarz. 2000. Cellular and humoral immune system in schizophrenia: a conceptual re-evaluation. *World J. Biol. Psychiatry* **1:**173–179.

Nakaya, T., H. Takahashi, Y. Nakamura, S. Asahi, M. Toblume, H. Kuratsune, T. Kitani, K. Yamanishi, and K. Ikuta. 1996. Demonstration of Borna disease virus RNA in peripheral blood mononuclear cells derived from Japanese patients with chronic fatigue syndrome. *FEBS Lett.* **378:**145–149.

Nakaya, T., H. Takahashi, Y. Nakamura, H. Kuratsune, T. Kitani, T. Machii, K. Yamanishi, and K. Ikuta. 1999. Borna disease virus infection in two family clusters of patients with chronic fatigue syndrome. *Microbiol. Immunol.* **43:**679–689.

Nasrallah, H. A. 1994. The continuum of psychoses between schizophrenia and bipolar disorder: the neuroanatomic evidence. *Neurol. Psychiatry Brain Res.* **2:**206–209.

Newport, D. J., and C. B. Nemeroff. 1999. Depression in the medically ill, p. 57–104. *In* M. Tohen (ed.), *Comorbidity in Affective Disorders.* Marcel Dekker, New York, N.Y.

Niedermeyer, E., M. Ribeiro, and S. Hertz. 1999. Mixed-type encephalopathies: preliminary considerations. *Clin. Electroencephalogr.* **30:**12–15.

Nowotny, N., J. Kolodzlejek, C. O. Jehle, A. Suchy, P. Staeheli, and M. Schwemmle. 2000. Isolation and characterization of a new subtype of Borna disease virus. *J. Virol* **74:**5655–5658.

Oleszak, E. L., J. Kuzmak, B. Hogue, R. Parr, E. W. Collisson, L. S. Rodkey, and J. L. Leibowitz. 1995. Molecular mimicry between Fc receptor and S peplomer protein of mouse hepatitis virus, bovine corona virus, and transmissible gastroenteritis virus. *Hybridoma* **14:**1–8.

Oleszak, E. L., W. L. Lin, J. R. Chang, S. Herzog, and K. Bechter. 2001. Clonally expanded T cells are present in the CSF of patients with major depression. *World J. Biol. Psychiatry* **2:**60S.

O'Reilly, R. L. 1994. Viruses and schizophrenia. *Aust. N. Z. J. Psychiatry* **28:**222–228.

Osborn, A. G. 1994. *Diagnostic Neuroradiology.* Mosby, St. Louis, Mo.

Oschmann, P., W. Dorndorf, C. Hornig, C. Schafer, H. J. Wellensiek, and K. W. Pflughaupt. 1998. Stages and syndromes of neuroborreliosis. *J. Neurol.* **245:**262–272.

Parshall, A. M., and R. G. Priest. 1993. Nosology, taxonomy and the classification conundrum of the functional psychoses. *Br. J. Psychiatry* **162:**227–236.

Perkins, D. O., E. J. Davidson, J. Leserman, D. Liao, and D. L. Evans. 1993. Personality disorder in patients infected with HIV: a controlled study with implications for clinical care. *Am. J. Psychiatry* **150:**309–315.

Perkins, D. O., J. Leserman, R. A. Stern, S. F. Baum, D. Liao, R. N. Golden, and D. L. Evans. 1995. Somatic symptoms and HIV infection: relationship to depressive symptoms and indicators of HIV disease. *Am. J. Psychiatry* **152:**1776–1781.

Pert, C. B., J. G. Knight, P. Laing, and M. A. K. Markwell. 1988. Scenarios for a viral etiology of schizophrenia. *Schizophr. Bull.* **2:**243–247.

Planz, O., C. Rentzsch, A. Batra, T. Winkler, M. Buttner, H. J. Rziha, and L. Stitz. 1999. Pathogenesis of Borna disease virus: granulocyte fractions of psychiatric patients harbor infectious virus in the absence of antiviral antibodies. *J. Virol.* **73:**6251–6256.

Pollmacher, T., M. Haack, A. Schuld, T. Kraus, and D. Hinze-Selch. 2000. Effects of antipsychotic drugs on cytokine networks. *J. Psychiatr. Res.* **34:**369–382.

Rabkin, J. G., R. R. Goetz, R. H. Remien, J. B. W. Williams, G. Todak, and J. M. Gorman. 1997. Stability of mood despite HIV illness progression in a group of homosexual men. *Am. J. Psychiatry* **154:**231–238.

Rausch, D. M., and E. S. Stover. 2001. Neuroscience research in AIDS. *Prog. Neuro-Psychopharmacol. Biol. Psychiatry* **25:**231–257.

Reiber, H. 1998. Cerebrospinal fluid: physiology, analysis and interpretation of protein patterns for diagnosis of neurological diseases. *Mult. Scler.* **4:**99–107.

Richt, J. A., R. C. Alexander, S. Herzog, D. C. Hooper, R. Kean, S. Spitsin, K. Bechter, R. Schuttler, H. Feldmann, A. Heiske, Z. F. Fu, B. Dietzschold, R. Rott, and H. Koprowski. 1997. Failure to detect Borna disease virus infection in peripheral blood leukocytes from humans with psychiatric disorders. *J. Neurovirol.* **3:**174–178.

Richt, J. A., and R. Rott. 2001. Borna disease virus: a mystery as an emerging zoonotic pathogen. *Vet. J.* **161:**24–40.

Rother, S., K. D. Knoblauch, and M. Kirschfink. 1995. Filtration of liquor cerebrospinalis (CSF-filtration): technical concept and filter performance under in vitro conditions. *Neuropsychiatrie* **9:**82–85.

Rott, R., S. Herzog, K. Bechter, and K. Frese. 1991. Borna disease, a possible hazard for man? *Arch. Virol.* **118:**143–149.

Rott, R., S. Herzog, B. Fleischer, A. Winokur, J. Amsterdam, W. Dyson, and H. Koprowski. 1985. Detection of serum-antibodies to Borna disease virus in patients with psychiatric disorders. *Science* **228:**755–756.

Rybakowski, F., T. Sawada, and K. Yamaguchi. 2001. Borna disease virus-reactive antibodies and recent-onset psychiatric disorders. *Eur. Psychiatry* **16:**191–192.

Sauder, C., and J. C. de la Torre. 1998. Sensitivity and reproducibility of RT-PCR to detect Borna disease virus (BDV) RNA in blood: implications for BDV epidemiology. *J. Virol. Methods* **71:**229–245.

Sauder, C., A. Müller, B. Cubitt, J. Mayer, J. Steinmetz, W. Trabert, B. Ziegler, K. Wanke, N. Mueller-Lantzsch, J. C. de la Torre, and F. A. Grässer. 1996. Detection of Borna disease virus (BDV) antibodies and BDV. RNA in psychiatric patients: evidence for high sequence conservation of human blood-derived BDV RNA. *J. Virol.* **70:**7713–7724.

Sauerbrei, A., U. Eichhorn, G. Hottenrott, and P. Wutzler. 2000. Virological diagnosis of herpes simplex encephalitis. *J. Clin. Virol.* **17:**31–36.

Sax, K. W., and S. M. Strakowsky. 1999. The co-occurrence of bipolar disorder with medical illness, p. 213–228. *In* M. Tohen (ed.), *Comorbidity in Affective Disorders.* Marcel Dekker, New York, N.Y.

Schneider, K. 1992. *Clinical Psychopathology,* 14th ed. Thieme, Stuttgart, Germany.

Schupbach, J., A. Baumgartner, and Z. Tomasik. 1988. HTLV-1 in Switzerland: low prevalence of specific antibodies in HIV risk groups, high prevalence of cross-reactive antibodies in normal blood donors. *Int. J. Cancer* **42:**857–862.

Schwemmle, M. 1999. Progress and controversy in Bornavirus research: a meeting report. *Arch. Virol.* **80:**97–100.

Selten, J. P., K. van Vliet, W. Pleyte, S. Herzog, H. W. Hoek, and A. M. van Loon. 2000. Borna disease virus and schizophrenia in Surinamese immigrants to the Netherlands. *Med. Microbiol. Immunol.* (Berlin) **189:**55–57.

Shankar, V., M. Kao, A. N. Hamir, H. Sheng, H. Koprowski, and B. Dietzschold. 1992. Kinetics of virus spread and changes in levels of several cytokine mRNAs in the brain after intranasal infection of rats with Borna disease virus. *J. Virol.* **66:**992–998.

Shiwach, R. 1994. Psychopathology in Huntington's disease patients. *Acta Psychiatr. Scand.* **90:**241–246.

Sierra-Honigmann, A. M., K. M. Carbone, and R. H. Yolken. 1995. Polymerase chain reaction (PCR) search for viral nucleic acid sequences in schizophrenia. *Br. J. Psychiatry* **166**:55–60.

Sierra-Honigmann, A. M., S. A. Rubin, M. G. Estafanous, R. H. Yolken, and K. M. Carbone. 1993. Borna disease virus in peripheral blood mononuclear and bone marrow cells of neonatally and chronically infected rats. *J. Neuroimmunol.* **45**:31–36.

Sirota, P., M. A. Firer, K. Schild, A. Tanay, A. Elizur, D. Meytes, and H. Slor. 1993. Autoantibodies to DNA in multicase families with schizophrenia. *Biol. Psychiatry* **33**:450–454.

Skegg, K., P. A. Corwin, and D. C. G. Skegg. 1988. How often is multiple sclerosis mistaken for a psychiatric disorder? *Psychol. Med.* **18**:733–736.

South, M., and J. Sever. 1985. Teratogen update: the congenital rubella syndrome. *Teratology* **31**:297–307.

Spannhuth, C. W., D. E. Dietrich, L. Bode, T. Lau, T. J. Huber, H. Ludwig, and H. M. Emrich. 2000. Mögliche prädiktive Faktoren zur Amantadinbehandlung bei BDV-infizierten depressiven Patienten. *Nervenarzt* **71**(Suppl 1):S150.

Spitzer, R. L., M. B. First, J. B. Williams, K. Kendler, H. A. Pincus, and G. Tucker. 1992. Now is the time to retire the term 'organic mental disorders.' *Am. J. Psychiatry* **149**:240–244.

Sprankel, H., K. Richarz, H. Ludwig, and R. Rott. 1978. Behavior alterations in tree shrews (*Tupala glis*, Diard 1820) induced by Borna disease virus. *Med. Microbiol. Immunol.* **165**:1–18.

Staeheli, P., C. Sauder, J. Hausmann, F. Ehrensperger, and M. Schwemmle. 2000. Epidemiology of Borna disease virus. *J. Gen. Virol.* **81**:2123–2135.

Stenager, E., and K. Jensen. 1988. Multiple sclerosis: correlation of psychiatric admissions to onset of initial symptoms. *Acta Neurol. Scand.* **77**:414–417.

Stitz, L., O. Planz, and T. Bilzer. 1998. Lack of antiviral effect of amantadine in Borna disease virus infection. *Med. Microbiol. Immunol.* (Berlin) **186**:195–200.

Strakowsky, S. M., and K. W. Sax. 2000. Secondary mania. A model of the pathophysiology of bipolar disorder?, p. 13–29. *In* J. C. Soares and S. Gershon (ed.), *Bipolar Disorders. Basic Mechanisms and Therapeutic Implications.* Marcel Dekker, New York, N.Y.

Strömgren, E. 1994. The unitary psychosis (Einheitspsychose) concept: past and present. *Neurol. Psychiatry Brain Res.* **2**:201–205.

Strongin, W. 1992. Sensitivity, specificity, and predictive value of diagnostic tests: definitions and clinical applications, p. 211–222. *In* E. H. Lennette (ed.), *Laboratory Diagnosis of Viral Infections,* 2nd ed. Marcel Dekker, New York, N.Y.

Susser, E., P. Colson, L. Jandorf, A. Berkman, J. Lavelle, S. Fennig, C. Waniek, and E. Bromet. 1997. HIV infection among young adults with psychotic disorders. *Am. J. Psychiatry* **154**:864–866.

Takahashi, H., T. Nakaya, Y. Nakamura, S. Asahi, Y. Onishi, K. Ikebuchi, T. A. Takahashi, T. Katoh, S. Sekiguchi, M. Takazawa, H. Tanaka, and K. Ikuta. 1997. Higher prevalence of Borna disease virus infection in blood donors living near thoroughbred horse farms. *J. Med. Virol.* **52**:330–335.

Theil, J. D., I. Tsunoda, F. Rodriguez, J. L. Whitton, and R. S. Fujinami. 2001. Viruses can silently prime for and trigger central nervous system autoimmune disease. *J. Neurovirol.* **7**:220–227.

Tsuji, K., K. Toyomasu, Y. Imamura, H. Maeda, and T. Toyoda. 2000. No association of borna disease virus with psychiatric disorders among patients in northern Kyushu, Japan. *J. Med. Virol.* **61**:336–340.

Vahlenkamp, T. W., H. K. Enbergs, and H. Muller. 2000. Experimental and natural borna disease virus infections: presence of viral RNA in cells of the peripheral blood. *Vet. Microbiol.* **76**:229–244.

van Praag, H. M. 2000. Nosologomania: a disorder of psychiatry. *World J. Biol. Psychiatry* **1**:151–158.

Wagle, A. C., S. A. Wagle, I. S. Marková, and G. E. Berrios. 2000. Psychiatric morbidity in Huntington's disease: the current view. *Neurol. Psychiatry Brain Res.* **8:**5–16.

Waltrip, R. W., II, R. W. Buchanan, A. Summerfelt, A. Breier, W. T. Carpenter, Jr., L. N. Bryant, S. A. Rubin, and K. M. Carbone. 1995. Borna disease virus and schizophrenia. *Psychiatry Res.* **56:**33–44.

Waxman, S. G. 2000. Do 'demyelinating' diseases involve more than myelin? *Nat. Med.* **6:**738–73.

Wexler, B. E. 1992. Beyond the Kraepelinean dichotomy. *Biol. Psychiatry* **31:**539–541.

Wittchen, H. U. 2000. Epidemiological research in mental disorders: lessons for the next decade of research—the NAPE Lecture 1999. *Acta Psychiatr. Scand.* **101:**2–10.

Wollinsky, K. H., P. J. Hülser, H. Brinkmeier, P. Aulkemeyer, W. Bössenecker, K. H. Huber-Hartmann, P. Rohrbach, H. Schreiber, F. Weber, M. Kron, G. Büchele, H. H. Mehrkens, A. C. Ludolph, and R. Rüdel. 2001. CSF filtration is an effective treatment of Guillain-Barré syndrome: a randomized clinical trial. *Neurology* **57:**774–780.

Wollinsky, K. H., P. J. Hülser, H. Brinkmeier, H. H. Mehrkens, H. H. Kornhuber, and R. Rüdel. 1994. Filtration of cerebrospinal fluid in acute inflammatory demyelinating polyneuropathy (Guillain-Barre syndrome). *Ann. Med. Intern.* **145:**451–458.

Yamaguchi, K., T. Sawada, T. Naraki, R. Igata, Yi, H. Shiraki, Y. Horii, T. Ishii, K. Ikeda, N. Asou, H. Okabe, M. Mochizuki, K. Takahashi, S. Yamada, K. Kubo, S. Yashiki, R. W. Waltrip, and K. M. Carbone. 1999. Detection of Borna disease virus-reactive antibodies from patients with psychiatric disorders and from horses by electrochemiluminescence immunoassay. *Clin. Diagn. Lab. Immunol.* **6:**696–700.

Yolken, R. H., and E. F. Torrey. 1995. Viruses, schizophrenia and bipolar disorders. *Clin. Microbiol. Rev.* **8:**131–145.

Yolken, R. H., and E. F. Torrey. 2000. Hypothesis of a viral etiology in bipolar disorder, p. 305–315. *In* J. C. Soares and S. Gershon (ed.), *Bipolar Disorders. Basic Mechanisms and Therapeutic Implications.* Marcel Dekker, New York, N.Y.

Zarin, D. A., and F. Earls. 1993. Diagnostic decision making in psychiatry. *Am. J. Psychiatry* **150:**197–206.

Index